A Dimensional Approach to Schizotypy

Simone Cheli • Paul H. Lysaker
Editors

A Dimensional Approach to Schizotypy

Conceptualization and Treatment

Springer

Editors
Simone Cheli
Department of Psychology
St. John's University
Rome, Italy

Center for Psychology and Health
Tages Charity
Florence, Italy

Paul H. Lysaker
Richard L Roudebush VA Medical Center
Department of Psychiatry
Indianapolis, IN, USA

Indiana University School of Medicine
Department of Psychiatry
Indianapolis, IN, USA

ISBN 978-3-031-41787-0 ISBN 978-3-031-41788-7 (eBook)
https://doi.org/10.1007/978-3-031-41788-7

This Springer imprint is published by the registered company Springer Nature Switzerland AG
The registered company address is: Gewerbestrasse 11, 6330 Cham, Switzerland

Paper in this product is recyclable.

Schizotypy generally represents a set of personality traits observable in the general population, as well as in patients prior to their first psychotic episode, and their nonschizophrenic relatives. Based on its ability to travel up and down the typical-to-atypical continuum, schizotypy has earned provisional status as an endophenotype on the path to schizophrenia, as well as being a useful model for understanding the dimensional reconceptualization of the personality-psychopathology continuum. In this thoughtful edited volume, Cheli and Lysaker build on these foundations by bringing together leaders in the field of schizotypy, personality and schizophrenia with the goal of translating complex research findings into practical, useful and clinically relevant information. They succeed in this goal with masterful integration of the research and clinical literature highlighting transdiagnostic processes central to the human experience such as metacognition, mentalizing, attachment, self- and interpersonal criticism that can be targeted in treatment. The result is a ground-breaking volume that articulates a set of theoretically grounded and evidence-based clinical guidelines sensitive to the human experience beyond signs and symptoms. This book is a must-read for anyone working at the complex intersection of personality, psychopathology and psychosis. It conveys a compassionate yet empirically rich message of hope – not only that recovery is possible, but that clinicians can play a critical role in realizing it.

—Carla Sharp, *Department of Psychology, University of Houston, Houston, Texas, USA*

A Dimensional Approach to Schizotypy includes contributions from a number of researchers at the forefront of psychopathology and psychiatric nosology. The editors provide us with a 30,000-foot view of current-day schizotypy, accompanied by fascinating clinical theory and an updated discussion of transdiagnostic clinical implications. These chapters also include important new information on unique cultural perspectives, encouraging better representation of global populations, critical for the generalizability and public health impact of our research. Overall, these chapters will provide academic researchers and postgraduate students with a strong grasp of schizotypy within the framework of new and expanded nosologies. It will also appeal to clinicians considering the symptoms of schizotypy across the lifespan and across evidence-based therapy modalities. Beautifully presented and very informative, this book will be an important resource for early career trainees and established faculty alike.

—Anna Docherty, *Department of Psychiatry, Huntsman Mental Health Institute, University of Utah School of Medicine, Salt Lake City, UT, USA*

Foreword

Historically, schizotypy has been primarily the focus of research scientists who sought to delineate a diagnosis that might presage schizophrenia or appear in the close relatives of patients with schizophrenia diagnoses. This is a noble and important tradition. By clearly defining relevant features and criteria, early identification of a schizotypy diagnosis could lead to substantial reduction of the risk for a subsequent transition to a fully justified schizophrenia diagnosis.

Nevertheless, this approach, focused on identifying putatively categorical diagnostic entities and "hyper-splitting" psychotic phenomena into numerous supposedly distinguishable categories, is waning. The categorical diagnostic paradigm in authoritative nosologies such as the DSM and ICD is at odds with a substantial empirical literature. The contemporary literature is replete with evidence that psychopathological signs and symptoms do not delineate categories in nature. Rather, signs and symptoms are organized into dimensional spectrums of human variation, without bright dividing lines to distinguish "normality" from "abnormality."

In this way, the current volume could not be timelier. This remarkable book brings together many influential scholars under the general rubric of dimensional approaches to schizotypy and can thereby serve as a real boon to both scientists and practitioners. Coverage of the current literature is extensive, and goes well beyond schizotypy research per se. Indeed, focal research on schizotypy as a psychopathological phenomenon is covered thoroughly yet is only one aspect of a much more comprehensive volume. In this way, schizotypy is now brought directly into contemporary paradigms for understanding psychopathology, such as the Hierarchical Taxonomy of Psychopathology (HiTOP; Chap. 3). In addition, transdiagnostic perspectives are closely tethered to a variety of useful and clinically near perspectives on effective intervention, such as mentalization approaches (Chap. 17) and clinical staging (which nicely merges the need for early intervention with a focus on reducing progression to later stages of illness; Chap. 20).

We live in exciting and interesting times in terms of effective empirical reconceptualization of psychopathology. This volume points the way toward how dimensional reconceptualization can go well beyond the pages of scholarly journals and benefit the lives of persons whose hopes and dreams are stymied because their schizotypal experiences diminish their efforts to pursue their goals.

University of Minnesota
Minneapolis, MN, USA

Robert F. Krueger, PhD

Preface: Schizotypy from a Clinical Point of View

The very idea of editing this book is based on an observation shared by the two of us: the vast and sophisticated literature on schizotypy has often been far from clinical practice. Great minds and theories have emerged and then been transferred to fascinating books, but the ambition of finding solid mechanisms of onset has seemingly diverted attention from practical work with patients. And the more the models become abstract, the more clinicians may distance themselves from them. Although nearly a century has passed since the first attempts to develop psychotherapy for people diagnosed with schizophrenia, many mental health professionals overtly or covertly think that recovery is not possible. Pioneers such as Harry Stack Sullivan, Frieda Fromm-Reichman, William R.D. Fairbairn and Donald D. Jackson seemingly appear too distant in time to be of daily inspiration.

All the authors of this book instead share the idea that recovery is possible and the construct of schizotypy is extremely helpful in pursuing it. Indeed, schizotypy refers to a wide continuum of experiences, ranging from subclinical or even healthy manifestations to severe forms of disorders such as schizophrenia. After the first systematic formulation by Paul E. Meehl (1962) in the early sixties, the construct of schizotypy attracted research which has corroborated the evidence that schizotypy may refer to a feature of personality and psychopathology not simply overlapping with schizophrenia-like phenomena. From this broad and fully dimensional perspective, schizotypy becomes a useful and unifying construct that can foster clinical research and practice (Kwapil & Barrantes-Vidal, 2015).

Recent advances, such as the Alternative Model of Personality Disorders (AMPD) and the Hierarchical Taxonomy of Psychopathology (HiTOP), have pursued this vision, looking for a rapprochement between clinical and research practice and overcoming the limits of categorical diagnosis (Hopwood, 2018; Kotov et al., 2020; Krueger & Markon, 2011). Although diagnostic categories seem to give us immediate reassurance in understanding the problem presented, they may also result in limited predictivity for the clinician and stigmatization of the patient. Beyond the known problems in comorbidity, categories make clinical work significantly more complicated than dimensions. First, we lose the complexity and uniqueness of one's life, focusing instead on symptoms and criteria. Consequently, subjective and intersubjective experience is not the core of conceptualization as it is in most models of psychotherapy. Finally, with this approach a person is understood through a single moment of crisis, rather than along an individual trajectory made up of memories, emotions and traits referable to temperament and personality.

Over a century of studies on what characteristics are premorbid to a diagnosis of schizophrenia or occurring among relatives of those diagnosed with schizophrenia have made schizotypy an extremely fertile and challenging field. This book is aimed at extending previous knowledge by bringing attention to clinically relevant mechanisms and psychotherapeutic interventions targeting these mechanisms. The chapters are organized into three sections: (I) schizotypy as a feature of personality and psychopathology; (II) transdiagnostic mechanisms in schizotypy; and (III) finally, integrated interventions for those struggling with schizotypy.

In Part I, we establish a common ground by defining schizotypy as a feature of personality and psychopathology from a dimensional and unifying point of view. Diverse perspectives are shown so as to clarify how broad and articulated the field is. Despite the complexity and lack of clinical guidelines, schizotypy is one of the dimensions of psychopathology that has collected a vast amount of biopsychosocial and evolutionary evidence. The rise of schizotypy and its clinical manifestation is linked with the rise of, at phylogenetic and ontogenetic level, the most distinctive feature of humanity: that is our complex and tricky social brain. In Chap. 1, Snyder and colleagues summarize the vast literature on neurodevelopmental aspects of schizotypy. They clearly highlight the complexity of the field, and how little is known so far. Clinically speaking and consistent with the broad and multifaceted dimension of schizotypy, it is difficult to identify specific targets or biomarkers. In Chap. 2, Cheli and Brüne discuss the proximate and evolutionary factors involved in schizotypy. By following Tinbergen's famous four ethological questions, they explore the many models that have been proposed. Again, a unifying theory cannot be presented, just the importance of considering schizotypy through a multidimensional framework. Then, Minor and colleagues (Chap. 4) try to answer a fascinating question: Which mechanisms may explain the schizotypal impairment in social functioning? They summarize four main potential explanations related to social, cognitive, anticipated pleasure and emotion regulation deficits. In Chap. 5, Skodlar and Henriksen explore the vast phenomenological literature about schizophrenia and psychosis and offer a nuanced look at schizotypy. The leading thread of a disordered self may be considered the core of their reflections. In Chap. 6, Barrantes-Vidal and Kwapil summarize the history of the complex construct of schizotypy and how it has been assessed over time through diverse measures. They help us understand how decade after decade there has been a convergence on specific features, namely positive, negative and disorganized features. Finally, Chap. 7 proposes a transcultural perspective to schizotypy. Deeley widely considers how cultural and religious contexts and backgrounds may shape our suffering and the expression of it.

In Part II, we take a step toward clinical practice. Five transdiagnostic mechanisms are defined and discussed from a clinical point of view. A common framework emerges that posits how human suffering is always located on the fringe between one's own and others' experiences. Thus, constructs referring to metacognition and mentalizing are presented together with the ones of attachment, interpersonal criticism and self-criticism. We speculate how these modern constructs may parallel and extend beyond the early intuitions of aforementioned pioneers (i.e., Sullivan, Fromm-Reichman, etc.). Psychopathology is possibly a failure in the capacity to interconnect our lives with the ones of the surrounding others. This then results in a loss of the sense of ourselves, our purposes and meaning. Lysaker and Wiesepape (Chap. 8) introduce the construct of metacognition as a complex and nuanced understanding of one's own and others' mental states. They summarize how this can be considered an architecture of the self that when impaired may result in the emergence of severe manifestations of schizotypy ranging from at high-risk states to personality disorders and psychosis. Then, Salaminios and Debanné (Chap. 9) summarize existing knowledge about the pivotal role of mentalizing in human development and in the onset of psychopathology. They focus on a growing body of evidence about the intertwined path of attachment, trauma and mentalizing along the schizotypy continuum. Consistent with this, Berry and colleagues (Chap. 10) review scientific literature about attachment and how this early pattern shapes and predicts the onset of severe psychopathology, such as psychosis, and informs a deep understanding of the therapeutic relationship with those struggling with schizotypy. The last two chapters of Part II explore the role of self-criticism and interpersonal criticism, respectively. Gilbert (Chap. 11) presents an evolutionary model of self-criticism that is consistent with an extensive literature about its transdiagnostic role in psychopathology. When people struggle with emotional suffering, those with heightened self-criticism are at higher risk for severe manifestations such as those of schizotypy. Finally, Asan and colleagues (Chap. 12) introduce a broad interpersonal look at schizotypy that is consistent with an emerging conceptualization of personality disorders as interpersonal disorders. They clearly underline how threatening and distorted beliefs about others and one's relational life stand at the core of clinical manifestations of schizotypy.

Finally, in Part III, a collection of integrated interventions is presented. All these therapeutic approaches share a framework similar or even identical with one presented in previous chapters. The invited authors consider schizotypy as a continuum of different and interconnected clinical manifestations and their work as aimed at recovering the fracture between the subjective and intersubjective worlds. In spite of different backgrounds, these same authors frequently conceptualize and treat presenting problems in schizotypy in ways that share a commonality. They think that recovery is possible and that the patient's relationship with the therapist and significant others is possibly the main focus of intervention. Moreover, they look at uncommon experiences such as oddity and delusion as the person's attempt to maintain a sense of themselves, even if fragmented. The therapeutic stance is shaped by a compassionate curiosity in exploring these attempts. In Chap. 13, Turkington and Cioroboiu try to extend the application of cognitive behavioral therapy for psychosis (CBTp) to schizotypal traits. Relying upon solid evidence for CBTp, they present the case of a patient diagnosed with schizotypal personality disorder (SPD). Then, Murphy and Heriot-Maitland (Chap. 14) review the growing body of evidence supporting the effectiveness of compassion-focused therapy (CFT) for hearing voices and suggest possible application along the continuum of schizotypy. In Chaps. 15 and 16, two metacognitively oriented psychotherapies (MOPs) are presented. Wiesepape, Morris and Hasson-Ohayon (Chap. 15) suggest that metacognitive reflection and insight therapy (MERIT) can be effective in treating severe manifestations of schizotypy such as psychosis and schizophrenia. They also explore the feasibility of MERIT in those with schizotypal traits summarizing existing evidence and presenting a single case. In Chap. 16, Dimaggio and colleagues describe the procedure and techniques used in metacognitive interpersonal therapy (MIT) to target metacognitive impairment in those with personality disorders. They detail how MIT has been tailored to address schizotypal manifestations such as SPD, psychosis and other severe disorders. Subsequently, Cheli (Chap. 17) introduces a newly developed treatment to specifically target schizotypal traits, namely evolutionary systems therapy for schizotypy (ESTS). The structure of the intervention and supporting evidence are discussed, and particular attention is paid to the integrative model consisting of an evolutionary conceptualization of schizotypy, narrative and experiential techniques derived from MOP and CFT, respectively. In the following chapters, two psychodynamic oriented perspectives are discussed. First, Ridenour, Knauss and Pozzi (Chap. 18) show the application of mentalization-based treatment (MBT) to schizotypal traits and, specifically, SPD. They present a possible line of interventions distinguishing between inpatients and outpatients, highlighting the feasibility of MBT modes in conceptualizing psychopathology. Second, Pec and Probstova (Chap. 19) summarize the vast literature about psychoanalytic treatments for those with schizophrenia, psychosis and schizotypal traits. The intervention is presented in terms of promoting integration of the patient's internal experience. Then, Gundersen and colleagues (Chap. 20) review existing literature on treatments for schizotypy, suggesting on one hand the usefulness of CBT and MOP, and on the other hand a possible integrated approach that is consistent with the staging model of psychiatry. They also highlight the need for further evidence and research to define a clinical staging approach to schizotypy. Finally, in Chap. 21, Hayakawa and Kato suggest how the Japanese construct of hikikomori may foster the understanding of severe pathological withdrawal along the continuum of schizotypy. They present their integrated model of interventions and discuss similarities between hikikomori and negative symptoms.

In short, we have tried to put together different perspectives with a unique aim to foster our clinical understanding of effective conceptualizations and interventions. The multifaceted background detailed in Part I hopefully supports the understanding of the presented transdiagnostic processes (i.e., metacognition, mentalizing, attachment, self-criticism, interpersonal criticism) that in turn inform the clinical practices covered in the final part. Despite there being limited guidelines to rely upon, the authors have reported several inspiring suggestions and described promising treatments.

Our wish is that readers from the diverse fields of mental health may find in these chapters solid and fertile support for their professional challenges. The assumption that recovery is possible is reliable to the extent to which it is a daily practice. We thank the many authors from diverse backgrounds and heritages for their generous contribution to this mission. Although much needs to be done and our collection is certainly incomplete, this can be reputed as the first book entirely devoted to considering schizotypy as a personality dimension from a clinical point of view. And this means – from our point of view – looking at patients as active agents in their process of recovery and at therapists as co-experimenters in restoring the fracture between the subjective and intersubjective worlds of those struggling with schizotypy.

Rome, Italy Simone Cheli
Indianapolis, IN, USA Paul H. Lysaker

References

Hopwood, C. J. (2018). A framework for treating DSM-5 alternative model for personality disorder features. *Personality and Mental Health, 12*(2), 107–125. https://doi.org/10.1002/pmh.1414

Kotov, R., Jonas, K. G., Carpenter, W. T., Dretsch, M. N., Eaton, N. R., Forbes, M. K., Forbush, K. T., Hobbs, K., Reininghaus, U., Slade, T., South, S. C., Sunderland, M., Waszczuk, M. A., Widiger, T. A., Wright, A., Zald, D. H., Krueger, R. F., Watson, D., & HiTOP Utility Workgroup. (2020). Validity and utility of Hierarchical Taxonomy of Psychopathology (HiTOP): I. Psychosis superspectrum. *World Psychiatry, 19*(2), 151–172. https://doi.org/10.1002/wps.20730

Krueger, R. F., & Markon, K. E. (2011). A dimensional-spectrum model of psychopathology: Progress and opportunities. *Archives of General Psychiatry, 68*(1), 10–11. https://doi.org/10.1001/archgenpsychiatry.2010.188

Kwapil, T. R., & Barrantes-Vidal, N. (2015). Schizotypy: Looking back and moving forward. *Schizophrenia Bulletin, 41 Suppl 2*(Suppl 2), S366–S373. https://doi.org/10.1093/schbul/sbu186

Meehl, P. E. (1962). Schizotaxia, schizotypy, schizophrenia. *American Psychologist, 17*(12), 827–838. https://doi.org/10.1037/h0041029

Contents

Part I
Schizotypy as a Feature of Personality and Psychopathology

Chapter 1
The Neurodevelopmental Considerations of Schizotypy

Madeline E. Snyder, Jennifer M. Blank, Miranda A. Bridgwater, Maksim Giljen, Emily Petti, Jason Schiffman, and Elizabeth A. Martin

Introduction

Schizotypy is a multidimensional continuum of traits, symptoms, and impairment, which can range from subclinical to clinical levels of schizophrenia-spectrum psychopathology (Kwapil et al., 2018). Research has found that elevated schizotypy is associated with atypical neurodevelopmental trajectories throughout critical developmental periods (Kwapil & Barrantes-Vidal, 2012). More specifically, evidence suggests that schizotypy is related to neurodevelopmental divergences in neuroanatomy and physiology (e.g., Tonini et al., 2021), fluctuating asymmetry (FA) and minor physical anomalies (MPAs) (e.g., Compton & Walker, 2009), and neurological soft signs (e.g., Hirjak et al., 2018). Therefore, the neurodevelopmental correlates of schizotypy have emerged as an important area of research when investigating the onset and development of schizophrenia-spectrum psychopathology throughout the lifespan.

Schizotypy is often conceptualized as a dimensional construct comprised of three dimensions—positive, negative, and disorganized, though assessments can range from continuous trait measures to categorical, clinical diagnoses made through structured interviews.[1] Dimensional schizotypy levels are often measured

[1] Measurement impacts interpretation of outcomes in all research. Although beyond the scope of this chapter, future work should consider how differences in the measurement of schizotypy could impact our ability to compare outcomes across studies.

M. E. Snyder · J. M. Blank · M. A. Bridgwater · M. Giljen · E. Petti · J. Schiffman ·
E. A. Martin (✉)
Department of Psychological Science, University of California, Irvine, CA, USA
e-mail: snyderme@uci.edu; jmblank@uci.edu; mbridgwa@uci.edu; mgiljen@uci.edu; epetti@uci.edu; jason.schiffman@uci.edu; emartin8@uci.edu

S. Cheli, P. H. Lysaker (eds.), *A Dimensional Approach to Schizotypy*,
https://doi.org/10.1007/978-3-031-41788-7_1

using self-report assessments such as the Wisconsin Schizotypy Scales (Chapman et al., 1978; Eckblad & Chapman, 1983; Eckblad et al., 1982), Schizotypal Personality Questionnaire (Raine, 1991), and the Multidimensional Schizotypy Scale (Kwapil et al., 2018). Across scales, positive schizotypy is defined by psychotic-like experiences such as perceptual aberrations, magical thinking, and pathological levels of paranoia. Negative schizotypy is defined by characteristics such as restricted affectivity, social withdrawal, motivational deficits, and anhedonia. Disorganized schizotypy is defined by disruptions in typical cognitive, speech, and behavioral patterns (Kwapil et al., 2018). As a result, research exploring a neurodevelopmental model of schizotypy provides insight on how divergences in neuromaturation may relate to the expression of characteristics associated with these distinct dimensions.

Using the aforementioned assessments, researchers can measure individuals' levels of seemingly heritable, trait-like characteristics of schizotypy that have been linked to neurodevelopmental irregularities and schizophrenia-spectrum disorder liability (Kwapil & Barrantes-Vidal, 2012). Although present in the general population, schizotypy-related features are observed more frequently in individuals who meet diagnostic criteria for schizophrenia-spectrum disorders and their first-degree relatives (Debbané et al., 2015). Research suggests that schizotypy levels have genetic underpinnings (e.g., twin studies; see Kwapil & Barrantes-Vidal, 2012 for a review), and are especially predictive of vulnerability for psychosis in individuals with a genetic high-risk (Debbané et al., 2015). Environmental factors such as childhood maltreatment (Kwapil & Barrantes-Vidal, 2012), maternal stress during pregnancy, and chronic stress throughout the lifespan (Walker & Diforio, 1997) also appear to have an important role in the manifestation of heightened schizotypy. It is likely that in the etiology of schizotypy and related characteristics, genetic and environmental components interact as early as fetal development to alter neurodevelopmental trajectories and promote the emergence of characteristics associated with a greater vulnerability for psychosis (Kwapil & Barrantes-Vidal, 2012).

In addition to etiological risk factors for heightened schizotypy, it is prudent to consider biological and behavioral correlates of schizotypy when investigating the neurodevelopment of schizophrenia-spectrum psychopathology across the lifespan. These biomarkers and associated behavioral risk factors may combine additively or interact to increase individual risk of transitioning to high-risk states or acute psychosis throughout different stages of development (Kwapil & Barrantes-Vidal, 2012). Select biomarkers associated with schizotypy, such as cortisol exposure (Walker et al., 2008), can potentially be measured as early as fetal development. However, due to the barriers of studying the early stages of fetal development (e.g., time, money, invasive procedures), researchers frequently opt for other methods. Such methods include studying biomarkers and related behavioral risk factors during postnatal developmental periods (e.g., early childhood; Chan et al., 2011). These biological and behavioral risk factors provide valuable information about the phenotypic expression of schizotypy.

Despite potential caveats (e.g., few replications of some findings, some studies with small samples), there is substantial evidence to suggest that overall schizotypy, or a unidimensional conceptualization of schizotypy that includes characteristics from multiple dimensions, as well as distinct dimensions of schizotypy, have links to atypical neurodevelopment. This evidence comes from a diverse range of studies that use varying assessments of schizotypy, different sampling procedures, and samples differing in size and average schizotypy severity. Thus, this chapter provides a broad overview and summary of the available research on links between overall and multidimensional schizotypy severity and important neurodevelopmental outcomes across the lifespan.

Neuroanatomy and Physiology

There is robust evidence for various neuroanatomical correlates of overall schizotypy and its dimensions (see Tonini et al., 2021 for a review). Neuroimaging research in schizotypy has spanned the developmental stages of late childhood and adolescence (e.g., Derome et al., 2020) to adulthood (e.g., Pfarr & Nenadic, 2020). As a result, the study of brain development using neuroimaging techniques has been a promising avenue for distinguishing biomarkers for psychosis risk and determining how these biomarkers may relate to overall and dimensional schizotypy levels across the lifespan.

Neuroanatomical Abnormalities and Schizotypy

Given that neuroanatomy, or the structure of the central nervous system, forms during fetal development and develops throughout the lifespan, research exploring the prevalence of structural anomalies in schizotypy provides evidence for a neurodevelopmental model of schizotypy. A systematic review by Tonini et al. (2021) summarizes a large body of neuroimaging research of predominantly adult samples (though select studies included adolescents), which suggests neuroanatomical variations associated with schizotypy can be observed across a range of schizophrenia-spectrum psychopathology severity. Preliminary evidence supporting possible links between neuroanatomical anomalies and dimensions of schizotypy comes from various studies. For example, Pfarr and Nanadic (2020) studied a sample of healthy adults ($N = 104$; $M_{age} = 24.9$; $SD_{age} = 4.7$) while Derome et al. (2020) tracked a cohort of community adolescents across a five-year period ($N = 110$; $M_{age} = 15.98$; $SD_{age} = 1.83$; range 12–20). In addition, Koo et al. (2006) studied a subsample of women with schizotypal personality disorder ($n = 32$; $M_{age} = 30$; $SD_{age} = 9.2$), and Asami et al. (2013) studied a subsample of men with schizotypal personality disorder ($n = 54$) in comparison to adult controls ($N = 108$; $M_{age} = 37.9$; $SD_{age} = 10.4$). Across studies, and across levels of schizophrenia-spectrum psychopathology severity, the specificity of the associations between neuroanatomical anomalies and individual dimensions of schizotypy appears to fluctuate depending on the brain region or structure being measured (Tonini et al., 2021).

The inconstant specificity of neuroanatomical correlates can be observed across the different dimensions of schizotypy, particularly disorganized schizotypy. There is some evidence that disorganized schizotypy is associated with lower gray matter volume (GMV) in the bilateral superior frontal gyrus and anterior cingulate cortex in healthy adults (Pfarr & Nanadic, 2020). In addition, in a five-year longitudinal study of adolescents, only the subsample of adolescents with elevated disorganized schizotypy levels had significant left lateral ventricle enlargement, which suggests that enlargement of the lateral ventricle may begin earlier in the neurodevelopmental process than the first-episode of psychosis, as has been previously hypothesized (Derome et al., 2020). In the same adolescent sample, only the elevated disorganized schizotypy subsample had GMV reductions in the bilateral hippocampi, a structural abnormality that is frequently observed in schizophrenia (Derome et al., 2020). Taken together, these findings suggest that some neuroanatomical abnormalities may be dimension-specific when studying the correlates of schizotypy.

Like disorganized schizotypy, negative schizotypy is associated with volumetric reductions in the superior frontal gyrus and anterior cingulate cortex in healthy adults. Unlike disorganized schizotypy, however, the relation between negative schizotypy and these structural variants appears to be specific to the left hemisphere (Pfarr & Nanadic, 2020). Thus, disorganized and negative schizotypy may have shared and unique associations with these cortical regions when assessed across both hemispheres. At the same time, in samples with schizotypal personality disorder, negative and positive schizotypy scores were associated with reduced GMV in the caudate nucleus (Koo et al., 2006) while only negative schizotypy was associated with reduced GMV in temporal regions (Asami et al., 2013). Altogether, while these studies are limited in sample size and replication, extant research seems to provide some support for the multidimensionality of schizotypy in relation to neuroanatomical features across a range of ages and schizotypy severity.

Neurophysiological Abnormalities and Schizotypy

Neurophysiology is the study of the functions of the nervous system, and there is an extensive and diverse body of research on the neurophysiological underpinnings of schizotypy. The following section will review various neurophysiological correlates of schizotypy during the neurodevelopmental process: the neuroendocrine system, regional activation, functional connectivity, and electrophysiological activity. This section provides an overview of select neurophysiological biomarkers associated with heightened schizotypy/schizotypy dimensions and describes how these biomarkers may relate to the neurodevelopmental mechanisms of schizophrenia-spectrum psychopathology.

The Neuroendocrine System and Schizotypy

Hypothalamic–Pituitary–Adrenal (HPA) Axis The HPA axis is a neuroendocrine system that is responsible for cortisol secretion in response to stressors, as well as modulation of cortisol levels via negative feedback to the hypothalamus. Consequently, the HPA axis is thought to play an important role in the diathesis–stress model of psychosis. Work by Walker and colleagues has been critical in illuminating the association between HPA axis irregularities and psychosis risk (e.g., Walker & Diforio, 1997; Walker et al., 2008). Walker and Diforio (1997) assert that dysregulation of the HPA axis may be the result of developmental irregularities at different stages of neurodevelopment, including during fetal development and post-birth. This dysregulation may result in hypersensitivity to stress and may increase vulnerability for psychosis. While cortisol secretion changes throughout typical neurodevelopment, the steady increase throughout childhood and more notable rise in adolescence may help explain why attenuated symptoms of psychosis often emerge during this period (Walker & Diforio, 1997). In studies of people with schizophrenia-spectrum disorders, baseline cortisol secretion is greater on average than cortisol secretion in typically developing people, indicating dysregulation in this system in individuals with schizophrenia-spectrum psychopathology. Cortisol secretion has been found to be associated with both negative and positive symptoms—although more strongly to negative symptoms—in schizophrenia-spectrum disorders, and appears to increase prior to psychotic relapse (Walker & Diforio, 1997). In sum, anomalous cortisol secretion rates in the HPA axes of individuals with and at-risk for psychosis are a pertinent consideration when investigating potential neurodevelopmental mechanisms of elevated schizotypy.

Neural Activation, Connectivity, and Schizotypy

Regional Activation Extant literature finds that schizotypy is related to heterogeneous levels of blood-oxygen-level dependent (BOLD) activation across brain regions (see Tonini et al., 2021 for a review). BOLD signals are metabolic markers that provide an estimate of neuronal activity and metabolic efficiency in a given brain region (Deco et al., 2011). Research using BOLD activation has built evidence for potential neurophysiological mechanisms, such as abnormal regional activation, for preeminent risk factors of schizophrenia (e.g., motor dysfunction, minor neurological deficits; Hirjak et al., 2018). For example, in a sample ($N = 32$) of individuals with schizophrenia-spectrum disorders ($M_{age} = 40.2$; $SD_{age} = 9.1$) and controls ($M_{age} = 37.4$; $SD_{age} = 7.0$), preliminary evidence suggests that negative schizotypy is positively related to BOLD signals in the inferior frontal gyrus during a social cognition task involving imitating another individual's hand movements. These findings suggest that greater effort is used during basic imitation tasks among individuals with schizophrenia-spectrum disorders (Thakkar et al., 2014). Therefore, given its role in action goal processing and communication via imitative movements, anomalous activation in the inferior frontal gyrus may be linked to negative schizotypy and may provide preliminary evidence for the involvement of social cognition in motor control (Ettinger et al., 2015).

Beyond potential biomarkers for atypical motor control, many empirical studies involving social cognition in clinical and nonclinical samples (k = 16) in adolescence and adulthood (M_{age} = 15.9–38.8) suggest that schizotypy is related to anomalous activation across multiple brain regions (see Tonini et al., 2021 for a review). This pattern of activation has been found when individuals are processing self-other information, or stimuli/information related to oneself as well as stimuli/information related to other people or external sources. Multiple studies have found that overall schizotypy is related to greater BOLD signaling in the posterior cingulate cortex and insular regions in adolescents and adults when processing self-related information (e.g., when attributing an adjective to oneself; Tonini et al., 2021). Furthermore, there is some evidence to suggest that negative and disorganized schizotypy are associated with greater BOLD signaling across regions when processing other-related information, while positive schizotypy is associated with greater BOLD signaling across regions when processing self-related information (Di Plinio et al., 2020). Conversely, overall schizotypy is associated with lower BOLD signaling in the frontal, anterior cingulate, and striatal cortices when processing self-related information in adolescent and adult samples (Tonini et al., 2021). Altogether, the literature suggests that overall and dimensional schizotypy levels may be related to atypical neurophysiological mechanisms during activities involving social cognitive processing across adolescence and adulthood. Thus, in attempting to conceptualize a neurodevelopmental pathway toward schizophrenia-spectrum psychopathology later in life, aberrations in regional activation may be valuable biomarkers of psychosis risk.

Functional Connectivity Functional connectivity, which can often be reliably predicted by structural connectivity in the brain, is a measure of fluctuations in BOLD signals over time and characterizes dynamic (or "functional") connections across neural networks (Deco et al., 2011). Adolescence is a critical window of development when the maturation of neural networks (e.g., auditory, attention) occurs. This maturation process results in complex, large-scale networks that integrate disconnected local networks such that the adolescent brain can more efficiently process complex stimuli from the environment (Lagioia et al., 2010). Researchers have proposed that disturbances in this integration process could result in aberrant neural connectivity and maturation, potentially representing a biomarker of vulnerability for schizotypy and related psychopathology (Lagioia et al., 2010).

The dimensions of schizotypy have both shared and disparate associations with functional connectivity in large-scale, interhemispheric brain networks. For example, during resting-state fMRI scans in a sample of help-seeking and community adolescents (N = 39; age 12–20), Lagioia and colleagues (2010) found that all three schizotypy dimensions were positively related to intrinsic functional connectivity in the visual network, while only disorganized schizotypy was negatively related to intrinsic functional connectivity in the auditory network. There is also some evidence that adults with schizophrenia-spectrum disorders show similar patterns of anomalous neurophysiological activity in these same neural networks (e.g., Spencer, 2008). Thus, the similar results in adult samples with schizophrenia-spectrum disorders and in the help-seeking and community adolescent sample suggest that childhood and adolescence may be key periods for disruptions in typical functional connectivity maturation in individuals with elevated schizotypy (Lagioia et al., 2010).

Neural Activity and Schizotypy

Electrophysiology Altered electrophysiological events or activity, or atypical brain waves, related to the processing of different kinds of information (e.g., visual, auditory, language) are associated with higher levels of schizotypy (Ettinger et al., 2015). In their qualitative review, Ettinger et al. (2015) describe how schizotypy is related to visual abnormalities, such as difficulties with depth perception and backward masking, or the presentation of a target stimulus followed by a second "masking" stimulus, making it difficult to perceive the target. Schizotypy is also positively associated with aberrant P100 event-related potentials, or brain waves occurring 80–120 ms following a stimulus (Ettinger et al. 2015). Relatedly, deficits in early visual processing and related desynchronization in oscillatory activity across visual networks are not only associated with overall levels of schizotypy but also may be associated with levels of positive and disorganized schizotypy individually (Cappe et al., 2012; Richardson & Gruzelier, 1994). At the same time, there is evidence of abnormalities related to processing emotion-evoking visual stimuli across schizotypy dimensions. More specifically, although individuals with positive schizotypy and individuals with negative schizotypy (specifically social anhedonia) both show greater late positive potential (LLP) amplitudes when passively viewing unpleasant images (Martin et al., 2017), they show divergent responses to pleasant images. Whereas individuals with positive schizotypy show greater increases in LLP amplitudes when passively viewing positive images (Martin et al., 2017) and when viewing pleasant images with increasing motivational salience (Martin et al., 2020), individuals with negative schizotypy do not. Thus, across studies and stimuli types, aberrant electrophysiological activity related to visual processing appears to be an important neurological correlate of overall schizotypy and its dimensions.

Anomalies in neurophysiology related to visual processing may be a biological pathway between early life and later schizophrenia-spectrum psychopathology levels in individuals with heightened schizotypy. Scientists theorize that abnormalities in the temporally sensitive and spatially insensitive magnocellular pathway of the visual cortex are one of the underlying mechanisms for atypical visual processing in individuals with greater levels of schizotypy (Richardson & Gruzelier, 1994). The magnocellular pathway is continuously developing throughout the lifespan, beginning during the first trimester of fetal development (Porges & Furman, 2011), and processing speed deficits involving visual stimuli in individuals at-risk for psychosis can be measured as early as childhood (age 8–12; Niarchou et al., 2013). Thus, it is possible that neural mechanisms associated with risk for schizophrenia-spectrum psychopathology—such as those related to P100 discoordination—may begin to develop years or even decades before psychosis symptom onset (Porges & Furman, 2011).

Overall, neuroanatomical and neurophysiological abnormalities—two biomarkers of risk for psychosis—can manifest during fetal and postnatal development (Kwapil & Barrantes-Vidal, 2012). Studies have explored the full spectrum of schizophrenia-spectrum psychopathology from samples with no psychiatric history (e.g., Di Plinio et al., 2020) to clinical samples (e.g., Thakkar et al., 2014), and there is evidence for both similar and disparate neurological correlates of schizotypy and schizophrenia-spectrum disorders (Ettinger et al., 2015). Furthermore, existing literature not only supports the notion that overall schizotypy levels are positively associated with anomalies in brain development but also suggests that some neural abnormalities may be uniquely associated with specific dimensions of schizotypy (see Tonini et al., 2021 for a review). Thus, neuroanatomy and neurophysiology are essential to consider when investigating neurodevelopmental outcomes in relation to overall and multidimensional schizotypy.

Fluctuating Asymmetry and Minor Physical Anomalies

Two physical biomarkers that are relatively easy to measure postnatally and reflect underlying disruptions in neurodevelopment include fluctuating asymmetry and minor physical anomalies. Fluctuating asymmetry (FA) refers to variations in traits that are normally symmetrical in the population (e.g., ear width, space between fingers; Yeo et al., 2007). One area of FA that has been widely studied in schizophrenia-spectrum disorders is dermatoglyphic asymmetry, which refers to the asymmetry of ridges on the hands and feet of the left and right side of the body (see Golembo-Smith et al., 2012 for a review). Minor physical anomalies (MPAs) are subtle irregularities appearing in the head, face, and limbs that typically have minimal impact on physical appearance and functioning (Compton & Walker, 2009). While both FA and MPAs are physical abnormalities that impact similar regions of the body, they are considered to be different constructs due to divergences in their theorized developmental mechanisms and the measures used to assess them (Compton & Walker, 2009; Yeo et al., 2007). However, the similarities between FA and MPAs suggest that both emerge during the first or second trimester of pregnancy (Compton & Walker, 2009). This period in fetal development is associated with the formation of the ectoderm, which is responsible for the development of both internal and external structures, including the skin, hair, eyes, teeth, and mouth (traits often impacted by FA and MPAs; Ansari & Pillarisetty, 2021). The ectoderm also gives rise to the neuroectoderm, which is responsible for the development of the central and peripheral nervous systems (Ansari & Pillarisetty, 2021). Relatedly, MPAs in particular have been found to be associated with increased levels of cortisol, suggestive of dysregulation in the HPA axis (Mittal et al., 2007). For this reason, the emergence of both FA and MPAs is believed to reflect disruptions in neurodevelopment that may also lead to irregularities in brain development.

FA, MPAs, and Schizotypy

Robust evidence suggests that individuals with schizophrenia as well as individuals with heightened levels of schizotypy tend to have greater incidences of both FA and MPAs (for reviews see Chan et al., 2011 and Compton & Walker, 2009). Research exploring the relation between FA and specific dimensions of schizophrenia-spectrum disorders, on the other hand, has produced extremely varied results. Some studies focusing specifically on dermatoglyphics have found FA to be associated with specific dimensions of schizotypy (e.g., Stephan-Otto et al., 2020), while others have found no relation between FA and specific schizotypy dimensions (Kwapil & Barrantes-Vidal, 2012). Similarly, reports of associations between MPAs and dimensions of schizophrenia-spectrum disorders have been mixed. Some studies have found MPAs to be associated with negative schizotypy, particularly when additional deficits were present along with genetic risk for schizophrenia (Blanchard et al., 2010; Hans et al., 2009). Furthermore, one study of first-degree relatives of individuals with schizophrenia (n = 25) and controls (n = 38) found MPAs to be related to distinct dimensions of schizotypy (Bollini et al., 2007). Specifically, Bollini et al. (2007) found that in controls, assessor-measured MPAs of the hands had moderate to strong associations with interviewer-rated disorganized schizotypy levels ($r_s = 0.45$, $p < 0.003$), while MPAs of the feet had moderate to strong associations with interviewer-rated positive schizotypy levels ($r_s = 0.46$, $p < 0.003$). No relation, however, was found between interviewer-rated MPAs and overall schizotypy levels in first-degree relatives of individuals with schizophrenia (Bollini et al., 2007). Contrary to these findings, other studies have reported no relation between MPAs and schizotypy levels (see Compton & Walker, 2009 for a review). Although in need of replication, the variable findings across studies seem to suggest that FA and MPAs have stronger associations with general risk for schizophrenia-spectrum psychopathology in comparison to specific dimensions of schizophrenia-spectrum psychopathology.

Neurological Soft Signs

Neurological soft signs, or subtle neurological deficits related to anomalous sensory and motor coordination, may indicate an underlying biological vulnerability for developing a schizophrenia-spectrum disorder (Ettinger et al., 2015). Schizotypy is positively associated with neurological soft signs and related cognitive deficits in both community and at-risk samples (Kwapil & Barrantes-Vidal, 2012). Studies have found that across different stages of development, individuals with heightened schizotypy demonstrate measurable differences in neurological soft signs when compared to their same-aged peers with low schizotypy (e.g., Siddi et al., 2017; Steffens et al., 2018). Furthermore, like schizotypy levels, neurological soft signs appear to be positively associated with MPAs (see Kwapil & Barrantes-Vidal, 2012 for a review). Thus, these non-specific and subtle neurological impairments, which are associated with minor cognitive deficits and can be measured behaviorally, are thought to be important behavioral risk factors for schizophrenia-spectrum psychopathology development.

Motor Control and Schizotypy

Heightened schizotypy is associated with motor control impairments, or individual differences in the ability to control movements such as gait abnormalities, imprecise movements, and oculomotor impairments (Ettinger et al., 2015). Neurological soft signs, including motor control, persist throughout the lifespan and impact developmental trajectories. They also potentially share some etiological mechanisms with other neurodevelopmental correlates of schizotypy (e.g., MPAs; Kwapil & Barrantes-Vidal, 2012). For example, in a sample of adolescents oversampled for schizotypal personality disorder ($N = 114$; age 12–18), greater dyskinesias, or involuntary movements, were associated with more MPAs (Mittal et al., 2007). This preliminary evidence suggests that underlying neural mechanisms of motor impairments may emerge around the same time as MPAs—during early fetal development. Consequently, individuals with heightened schizotypy may possess some risk factors for psychosis throughout their lifespan.

Oculomotor impairments, similar to peripheral motor impairments, have been measured in relation to schizotypy to identify connections with motor control capabilities. In their qualitative review, Ettinger et al. (2015) described how multiple studies of community samples have found that schizotypy is related to greater difficulties with oculomotor smooth pursuit (i.e., visually tracking a moving target) and antisaccade performance (i.e., suppressing the reflex to look at a non-target stimulus and voluntarily look at a target stimulus). As a result, healthy adults with heightened schizotypy demonstrate more subtle, but very similar, oculomotor impairments in comparison to individuals with schizophrenia-spectrum disorders (Ettinger et al., 2015). Research with nonclinical samples has also shown preliminary evidence that positive and negative schizotypy are associated with greater smooth pursuit deficits and direction errors during antisaccade tasks (e.g., Holahan & O'Driscoll, 2005). Overall, these behavioral risk factors provide some evidence for the theory that specific dimensions of schizotypy are related to disparate levels of risk for schizophrenia-spectrum psychopathology.

Cognitive Functioning and Schizotypy

Brain development, which begins in utero, is related to cognitive development and consequently, cognitive functioning. While there are numerous cognitive deficits associated with schizotypy, these deficits are often more subtle than the deficits observed in individuals with schizophrenia-spectrum disorders (Siddi et al., 2017). As a result, research on neurological soft signs frequently examines associations between schizotypy and many cognitive outcomes (e.g., Siddi et al., 2017; Steffens et al., 2018). While studies have investigated a range of cognitive outcomes in relation to schizotypy, cognitive control and working memory are areas of research that stand out as being particularly important. This importance stems from a crucial developmental shift in executive functioning that occurs during adolescence and is related to changes in neurophysiology (Bathelt et al., 2018; Crone & Steinbeis, 2017).

Cognitive control, which is defined as individuals' ability to control their thoughts and behaviors to achieve their goals, is believed to be related to the maturation of the dorsolateral and ventromedial prefrontal cortex during adolescence (Crone & Steinbeis, 2017). Steffens et al. (2018) investigated the relationship between overall and individual dimensions of schizotypy and components of cognitive control. Their meta-analysis, which included community and college samples, found that positive schizotypy ($k = 18$; $n = 1692$) and negative schizotypy ($k = 19$; $n = 1846$) had small significant associations with shifting, or the ability to flexibly shift attention across tasks or stimuli ($gs = 0.18$). Negative schizotypy ($k = 12$; $n = 1772$) had a very small but significant association with updating, or the ability to process and maintain accurate mental representations in working memory ($g = 0.11$). Neither overall nor dimensional schizotypy were significantly associated with inhibition ($ps > 0.05$) (Steffens et al., 2018). Altogether, these findings suggest that measuring schizotypy as a unidimensional construct may overlook the nuances of the schizotypy spectrum and unique relations between dimensions of schizotypy and cognitive control abilities. This concept is important when investigating the roles of schizotypy and cognitive risk factors in the development of schizophrenia-spectrum psychopathology across the lifespan.

Like cognitive control, working memory (WM), or the ability to consciously hold and process information in the mind, is a key component of cognitive functioning (Bathelt et al., 2018). WM impairments are considered a fundamental symptom of schizophrenia-spectrum disorders. Consequently, greater WM impairments may be a cognitive risk factor related to one's likelihood of experiencing full-threshold psychosis in the future in individuals with high schizotypy (Siddi et al., 2017). Research with youth aged 6–16 suggests that during earlier neurodevelopment in younger children, interhemispheric connectivity plays a significant role in WM abilities. Conversely, evidence also suggests that WM abilities have a stronger link to cortical thickness in the left occipitotemporal cortex in older children. Thus, in the typically maturing brain, there appear to be adjustments in the primary neural mechanisms for WM as a result of shifts from relying on a large-scale distributed network to relying on localized neural connections (Bathelt et al., 2018). Adolescents with schizophrenia-spectrum disorders (age 12–24), however, have significantly thinner left occipitotemporal cortical thickness, as well as delayed maturation in this region (Zalesky et al., 2015). Thus, it is possible that neural mechanisms for WM impairments may become more apparent following the shift to reliance on localized circuits in later childhood. In sum, this research provides initial evidence for the development of risk factors for psychosis throughout later childhood development, suggesting that some biomarkers and behavioral risk factors for schizophrenia-spectrum psychopathology may be linked to aberrant neuromaturational processes in later childhood and adolescence.

Conclusion

Schizotypy is associated with a range of aberrant neurodevelopmental outcomes across the domains of neuroanatomy and physiology, FA and MPAs, and neurological soft signs, with some providing links to specific dimensions (e.g., bilateral hippocampal GMV reductions and disorganized schizotypy; Derome et al., 2020). Conversely, some abnormalities (e.g., FA, MPAs) may not be related to specific dimensions of schizotypy but instead may be related to a general risk for schizophrenia-spectrum psychopathology (Compton & Walker, 2009). Like schizophrenia-spectrum disorders, elevated schizotypy is heterogeneous in (sub) clinical presentation, resulting in variable levels of positive, negative, and disorganized characteristics across individuals (Kwapil et al., 2018). Therefore, the measurement of dimensional levels of schizotypy may be valuable in informing the selection of optimal therapeutic interventions for individuals with elevated schizotypy.

Anomalous neuromaturational trajectories may act as the building blocks of the developmental pathway to schizophrenia-spectrum psychopathology (Kwapil & Barrantes-Vidal, 2012). It is important to note, however, that research has found that heightened schizotypy is also associated with other psychopathological outcomes (e.g., mood and substance use disorders; Kwapil et al., 2013). Given that these psychopathologies often manifest at greater rates in people with schizophrenia-spectrum disorders and sometimes share biomarkers of risk (e.g., MPAs in autism-spectrum disorder and schizophrenia-spectrum disorders; Compton & Walker, 2009), it seems that schizotypy may have predictive value for clinical outcomes beyond psychosis risk. Future research can improve the specificity of clinical predictions by using multidimensional schizotypy measures given evidence that individual dimensions (e.g., positive and negative) are uniquely predictive of long-term risk for different schizophrenia-spectrum disorders (Kwapil et al., 2013).

In addition to current limitations in the specificity of clinical predictions based on schizotypy levels, research on the neurodevelopmental correlates of multidimensional schizotypy is still sparse in samples of younger children and older adults. Longitudinal studies measuring facets of neurodevelopment across different developmental stages are needed to address gaps in the literature. For example, it is unclear if different neural abnormalities are present since birth or manifest later in the lifespan. Thus, similar to the 5-year study of adolescents by Derome et al. (2020), researchers could investigate neuroanatomical and physiological outcomes in younger children with heightened schizotypy over time. Overall, further research is needed on the neurodevelopmental correlates of multidimensional schizotypy. This area of study appears to be a fruitful topic for future scientific investigations as we continue to analyze how specific neurodevelopmental aberrancies relate to schizotypy and its dimensions.

References

Ansari, A., & Pillarisetty, L. S. (2021). Embryology, ectoderm. In *StatPearls [Internet]*. StatPearls Publishing.

Asami, T., Whitford, T. J., Bouix, S., Dickey, C. C., Niznikiewicz, M., Shenton, M. E., et al. (2013). Globally and locally reduced MRI gray matter volumes in neuroleptic-naive men with schizotypal personality disorder: Association with negative symptoms. *JAMA Psychiatry, 70*(4), 361–372. https://doi.org/10.1001/jamapsychiatry.2013.665

Bathelt, J., Gathercole, S. E., Johnson, A., & Astle, D. E. (2018). Differences in brain morphology and working memory capacity across childhood. *Developmental Science, 21*(3), e12579. https://doi.org/10.1111/desc.12579

Blanchard, J. J., Aghevli, M., Wilson, A., & Sargeant, M. (2010). Developmental instability in social anhedonia: An examination of minor physical anomalies and clinical characteristics. *Schizophrenia Research, 118*(1–3), 162–167. https://doi.org/10.1016/j.schres.2009.10.028

Bollini, A. M., Compton, M. T., Esterberg, M. L., Rutland, J., Chien, V. H., & Walker, E. F. (2007). Associations between schizotypal features and indicators of neurological and morphological abnormalities. *Schizophrenia Research, 92*(1–3), 32–40. https://doi.org/10.1016/j.schres.2007.01.018

Cappe, C., Herzog, M. H., Herzig, D. A., Brand, A., & Mohr, C. (2012). Cognitive disorganisation in schizotypy is associated with deterioration in visual backward masking. *Psychiatry Research, 200*, 652–659. https://doi.org/10.1016/j.psychres.2012.07.001

Chan, R. C., Stone, W. S., & Hsi, X. (2011). Neurological and neuropsychological endophenotypes in schizophrenia spectrum disorders. In *Handbook of Schizophrenia Spectrum Disorders* (Vol. II, pp. 325–349). Springer. https://doi.org/10.1007/978-94-007-0831-0_13

Chapman, L. J., Chapman, J. P., Raulin, M. L., & Edell, W. S. (1978). Schizotypy and thought disorder as a high risk approach to schizophrenia. In G. Serban (Ed.), *Cognitive Defects in the Development of Mental Illness* (pp. 351–360). Brunner/Mazel.

Compton, M. T., & Walker, E. F. (2009). Physical manifestations of neurodevelopmental disruption: Are minor physical anomalies part of the syndrome of schizophrenia? *Schizophrenia Bulletin, 35*(2), 425–436. https://doi.org/10.1093/schbul/sbn151

Crone, E. A., & Steinbeis, N. (2017). Neural perspectives on cognitive control development during childhood and adolescence. *Trends in Cognitive Sciences, 21*(3), 205–215. https://doi.org/10.1016/j.tics.2017.01.003

Debbané, M., Eliez, S., Badoud, D., Conus, P., Flückiger, R., & Schultze-Lutter, F. (2015). Developing psychosis and its risk states through the lens of schizotypy. *Schizophrenia Bulletin, 41*(suppl_2), S396–S407. https://doi.org/10.1093/schbul/sbu176

Deco, G., Jirsa, V. K., & McIntosh, A. R. (2011). Emerging concepts for the dynamical organization of resting-state activity in the brain. *Nature Reviews Neuroscience, 12*(1), 43–56. https://doi.org/10.1038/nrn2961

Derome, M., Zöller, D., Modinos, G., Schaer, M., Eliez, S., & Debbané, M. (2020). Developmental trajectories of subcortical structures in relation to dimensional schizotypy expression along adolescence. *Schizophrenia Research, 218*, 76–84. https://doi.org/10.1016/j.schres.2020.02.005

Di Plinio, S., Perrucci, M. G., Aleman, A., & Ebisch, S. J. (2020). I am me: Brain systems integrate and segregate to establish a multidimensional sense of self. *NeuroImage, 205*, 116284. https://doi.org/10.1016/j.neuroimage.2019.116284

Eckblad, M. L., & Chapman, J. (1983). Magical ideation as an indicator of schizotypy. *Journal of Consulting and Clinical Psychology, 51*, 215–225. https://doi.org/10.1037/0022-006X.51.2.215

Eckblad, M. L., Chapman, L. J., Chapman, J. P., & Mishlove, M. (1982). *The revised social anhedonia scale*. University of Wisconsin. Unpublished test.

Ettinger, U., Mohr, C., Gooding, D. C., Cohen, A. S., Rapp, A., Haenschel, C., & Park, S. (2015). Cognition and brain function in schizotypy: A selective review. *Schizophrenia Bulletin, 41*(suppl_2), S417–S426. https://doi.org/10.1093/schbul/sbu190

Golembo-Smith, S., Walder, D. J., Daly, M. P., Mittal, V. A., Kline, E., Reeves, G., & Schiffman, J. (2012). The presentation of dermatoglyphic abnormalities in schizophrenia: A meta-analytic review. *Schizophrenia Research, 142*(1–3), 1–11. https://doi.org/10.1016/j.schres.2012.10.002

Hans, S. L., Auerbach, J. G., Nuechterlein, K. H., Asarnow, R. F., Asarnow, J., Styr, B., & Marcus, J. (2009). Neurodevelopmental factors associated with schizotypal symptoms among adolescents at risk for schizophrenia. *Development and Psychopathology, 21*(4), 1195–1210. https://doi.org/10.1017/S0954579409990113

Hirjak, D., Meyer-Lindenberg, A., Kubera, K. M., Thomann, P. A., & Wolf, R. C. (2018). Motor dysfunction as research domain in the period preceding manifest schizophrenia: A systematic review. *Neuroscience & Biobehavioral Reviews, 87*, 87–105. https://doi.org/10.1016/j.neubiorev.2018.01.011

Holahan, A. L. V., & O'Driscoll, G. A. (2005). Antisaccade and smooth pursuit performance in positive-and negative-symptom schizotypy. *Schizophrenia Research, 76*(1), 43–54. https://doi.org/10.1016/j.schres.2004.10.005

Koo, M. S., Levitt, J. J., McCarley, R. W., Seidman, L. J., Dickey, C. C., Niznikiewicz, M. A., et al. (2006). Reduction of caudate nucleus volumes in neuroleptic-naive female subjects with schizotypal personality disorder. *Biological Psychiatry, 60*(1), 40–48. https://doi.org/10.1016/j.biopsych.2005.09.028

Kwapil, T. R., & Barrantes-Vidal, N. (2012). Schizotypal personality disorder: An integrative review. In *The Oxford Handbook of Personality Disorders*. https://doi.org/10.1093/oxfordhb/9780199735013.013.0021

Kwapil, T. R., Gross, G. M., Silvia, P. J., & Barrantes-Vidal, N. (2013). Prediction of psychopathology and functional impairment by positive and negative schizotypy in the Chapmans' ten-year longitudinal study. *Journal of Abnormal Psychology, 122*(3), 807–815. https://doi.org/10.1037/a0033759

Kwapil, T. R., Gross, G. M., Silvia, P. J., Raulin, M. L., & Barrantes-Vidal, N. (2018). Development and psychometric properties of the multidimensional Schizotypy scale: A new measure for assessing positive, negative, and disorganized schizotypy. *Schizophrenia Research, 193*, 209–217. https://doi.org/10.1016/j.schres.2017.07.001

Lagioia, A., Van De Ville, D., Debbané, M., Lazeyras, F., & Eliez, S. (2010). Adolescent resting state networks and their associations with schizotypal trait expression. *Frontiers in Systems Neuroscience, 4*, 35. https://doi.org/10.3389/fnsys.2010.00035

Martin, E. A., Karcher, N. R., Bartholow, B. D., Siegle, G. J., & Kerns, J. G. (2017). An electrophysiological investigation of emotional abnormalities in groups at risk for schizophrenia-spectrum personality disorders. *Biological Psychology, 124*, 119–132. https://doi.org/10.1016/j.biopsycho.2017.02.001

Martin, E. A., Li, L. Y., & Castro, M. K. (2020). Electrophysiological responses to images ranging in motivational salience: Attentional abnormalities associated with schizophrenia-spectrum disorder risk. *Scientific Reports, 10*(1), 1–13. https://doi.org/10.1038/s41598-020-61504-2

Mittal, V. A., Dhruv, S., Tessner, K. D., Walder, D. J., & Walker, E. F. (2007). The relations among putative biorisk markers in schizotypal adolescents: Minor physical anomalies, movement abnormalities, and salivary cortisol. *Biological Psychiatry, 61*(10), 1179–1186. https://doi.org/10.1016/j.biopsych.2006.08.043

Niarchou, M., Zammit, S., Walters, J., Lewis, G., Owen, M. J., & van den Bree, M. B. (2013). Defective processing speed and nonclinical psychotic experiences in children: Longitudinal analyses in a large birth cohort. *American Journal of Psychiatry, 170*(5), 550–557. https://doi.org/10.1176/appi.ajp.2012.12060792

Pfarr, J. K., & Nenadić, I. (2020). A multimodal imaging study of brain structural correlates of schizotypy dimensions using the MSS. *Psychiatry Research: Neuroimaging, 302*, 111104. https://doi.org/10.1016/j.pscychresns.2020.111104

Porges, S. W., & Furman, S. A. (2011). The early development of the autonomic nervous system provides a neural platform for social behaviour: A polyvagal perspective. *Infant and Child Development, 20*(1), 106–118. https://doi.org/10.1002/icd.688

Raine, A. (1991). The SPQ: A scale for the assessment of schizotypal personality based on DSM-III-R criteria. *Schizophrenia Bulletin, 17*(4), 555–564. https://doi.org/10.1093/schbul/17.4.555

Richardson, A. J., & Gruzelier, J. (1994). Visual processing, lateralization and syndromes of schizotypy. *International Journal of Psychophysiology, 18*(3), 227–239. https://doi.org/10.1016/0167-8760(94)90009-4

Siddi, S., Petretto, D. R., & Preti, A. (2017). Neuropsychological correlates of schizotypy: A systematic review and meta-analysis of cross-sectional studies. *Cognitive Neuropsychiatry, 22*(3), 186–212. https://doi.org/10.1080/13546805.2017.1299702

Spencer, K. M. (2008). Visual gamma oscillations in schizophrenia: Implications for understanding neural circuitry abnormalities. *Clinical EEG and Neuroscience, 39*(2), 65–68. https://doi.org/10.1177/155005940803900208

Steffens, M., Meyhöfer, I., Fassbender, K., Ettinger, U., & Kambeitz, J. (2018). Association of schizotypy with dimensions of cognitive control: A meta-analysis. *Schizophrenia Bulletin, 44*(suppl_2), S512–S524. https://doi.org/10.1093/schbul/sby030

Stephan-Otto, C., Lombardini, F., Núñez, C., Senior, C., Ochoa, S., Usall, J., & Brébion, G. (2020). Fluctuating asymmetry in patients with schizophrenia is related to hallucinations and thought disorganisation. *Psychiatry Research, 285*, 112816. https://doi.org/10.1016/j.psychres.2020.112816

Thakkar, K. N., Peterman, J. S., & Park, S. (2014). Altered brain activation during action imitation and observation in schizophrenia: A translational approach to investigating social dysfunction in schizophrenia. *American Journal of Psychiatry, 171*(5), 539–548. https://doi.org/10.1176/appi.ajp.2013.13040498

Tonini, E., Quidé, Y., Kaur, M., Whitford, T. J., & Green, M. J. (2021). Structural and functional neural correlates of schizotypy: A systematic review. *Psychological Bulletin, 147*(8), 828. https://doi.org/10.1037/bul0000260

Walker, E. F., & Diforio, D. (1997). Schizophrenia: A neural diathesis-stress model. *Psychological Review, 104*(4), 667. https://doi.org/10.1037/0033-295X.104.4.667

Walker, E., Mittal, V., & Tessner, K. (2008). Stress and the hypothalamic pituitary adrenal axis in the developmental course of schizophrenia. *Annual Review of Clinical Psychology, 4*, 189–216. https://doi.org/10.1146/annurev.clinpsy.4.022007.141248

Yeo, R. A., Gangestad, S. W., & Thoma, R. J. (2007). Developmental instability and individual variation in brain development: Implications for the origin of neurodevelopmental disorders. *Current Directions in Psychological Science, 16*(5), 245–249. https://doi.org/10.1111/j.1467-8721.2007.00513

Zalesky, A., Pantelis, C., Cropley, V., Fornito, A., Cocchi, L., McAdams, H., et al. (2015). Delayed development of brain connectivity in adolescents with schizophrenia and their unaffected siblings. *JAMA Psychiatry, 72*(9), 900–908. https://doi.org/10.1001/jamapsychiatry.2015.0226

Chapter 2
Evolutionary Aspects of Schizotypy

Simone Cheli and Martin Brüne

Introduction

The study of schizotypy can be traced back to more than a century ago, when clinical authorities such as the Swiss psychiatrist Eugen Bleuler noticed recurring traits such as eccentricity among healthy relatives of individuals diagnosed with schizophrenia. Moreover, such traits have also been associated with premorbid or "prodromal" states of psychosis. Both terms, schizophrenia and schizotypy, share a common etymological origin and are derived from the Greek root *schizo* (literally meaning to split) (Bleuler, 1911).

Since the 1960s, a growing body of research, pioneered by Paul Meehl (1962) and others, sought to identify genetic and environmental risk factors for schizophrenia, suggesting that some unknown dominant "schizogene" associated with unfavorable rearing environments could lead to a phenotypic expression referred to as "schizotypy" (Meehl, 1962). In fact, Meehl believed that the "schizogene" was common in human populations, but that the transition to manifest schizophrenia was comparably rare. Indeed, more recent studies report that schizotypy—as a continuum of experiences ranging from subclinical or even psychologically healthy states to severe manifestations such as schizophrenia—would be present in almost

S. Cheli
Department of Psychology, St. John's University, Rome, Italy

Center for Psychology and Health, Tages Charity, Florence, Italy
e-mail: chelis@stjohns.edu

M. Brüne (✉)
Department of Psychiatry, Psychotherapy and Preventive Medicine, Research Division of Social Neuropsychiatry and Evolutionary Medicine, LWL University Hospital, Bochum, Germany

Ruhr University, Bochum, Germany
e-mail: martin.brune@ruhr-uni-bochum.de

S. Cheli, P. H. Lysaker (eds.), *A Dimensional Approach to Schizotypy*,
https://doi.org/10.1007/978-3-031-41788-7_2

10% of the general population (Kwapil & Barrantes-Vidal, 2015). These reports seem to be largely consistent with prevalence rates of schizotypal personality disorder (SPD) ranging between 0.6% and 4.6% in community samples (American Psychiatric Association, 2013), and more transitory clinical states such as psychotic experiences with an estimated rate ranging between 5.8% and 7.2% in the general population (Linscott & van Os, 2013; McGrath et al., 2015).

The construct of schizotypy as a taxon or continuum of seemingly anomalous experiences has somehow anticipated recent advances in psychopathology and an increasing interest in dimensional and transdiagnostic approaches to mental health. Personality models such as the five-factor model applied to schizotypy (FFM; Edmunson & Kwapil, 2013), the Alternative Model of Personality Disorder (AMPD; APA, 2013), and the Hierarchical Taxonomy of Psychopathology (HiTOP; Kotov et al., 2020) posit a continuum of experiences ranging from adaptive to maladaptive states throughout a few main dimensions. Accordingly, schizotypy would be better understood in terms of high scores of openness to experience introversion and neuroticism (FFM) that would parallel high scores of psychoticism and detachment (AMPD). Therefore, the focus of research interests in schizotypy has progressively shifted toward a functional understanding, which seems to be more consistent with an evolutionary approach to mental health (Millon, 2011). Indeed, Anthony Stevens and John Price (1996) were the first to suggest that schizotypal personality traits may be prominent and adaptive features of charismatic leadership, which fosters human groups to split up in subgroups and compete with one another (for resources and mating opportunities). This view has recently been seconded in Joseph Polimeni's (2012) analysis of shamanism in an evolutionary perspective.

These fresh and inspiring interpretations of schizotypy as an evolved phenotypic expression of certain personality traits may also shed a slightly different light on schizophrenia as a "disease entity." While we are not advocating the view that schizophrenia is adaptive, we believe that some of the clinical manifestations commonly diagnosed as "schizophrenia" may represent extremes of variations of traits that could be adaptive in specific environmental contexts.

Accordingly, the aim of this chapter is to review existing studies taking an evolutionary look at schizotypy, which includes work on evolutionary explanations of schizophrenia. Thus, we integrate studies on schizophrenia with those on schizotypy, since collective evidence on brain structure and genetics suggests that schizotypy overlaps with schizophrenia across multiple behavioral and neurobiological domains (Ettinger et al., 2014). The chapter starts with an overview of (some) proximate and evolutionary explanations of schizophrenia, following the framework proposed by the Dutch biologist Nikolaas Tinbergen (1963). Tinbergen defined four levels of analysis of behavior that refer to either proximate or evolutionary explanations. While the former entail the understanding of ontogeny (i.e., developmental history) and underlying mechanisms (i.e., causation) involved in a specific pattern of behaviors or physiological traits, the evolutionary explanations seek to explore the phylogeny (i.e., evolution) and adaptive value of these behaviors or traits. We then introduce evolutionary theories of personality, including the ones focusing on schizotypy and dimensional approaches to psychopathology, and finally discuss trends and future research in schizotypy.

Evolutionary Explanations of Schizophrenia

Schizophrenia has always represented a puzzling paradox in evolutionary studies (Brüne, 2004, 2022). Central to this enigma is the question of how genes predisposing individuals to schizophrenia could prevail in populations despite the huge evolutionary costs in terms of survival and reproduction associated with psychosis. In fact, one of the basic principles of evolutionary theory is that, if a trait persists over evolutionary time, it should offer a direct advantage in terms of survival and/or reproductive success. Another explanation could be that the effect is indirect, for example, there are other advantageous traits connected to the trait (i.e., there is an evolutionary trade-off). However, the heterogeneity of traits associated with schizophrenia (and schizotypy) makes the existence of a single evolutionary hypothesis highly unlikely, which is consistent with the polygenic nature of schizophrenia and the failure of attempts to identify single genes or neurophysiological aberrations capable of predicting the onset of psychotic symptoms (Smeland et al., 2020). Here, we briefly review some of the most important evolution-based explanations of schizophrenia. More exhaustive reviews can be found in Brüne (2022) or Allen (in press).

Ontogenetic Aspects

Evolutionary ontogenetic hypotheses have explored developmental instability models positing that schizophrenia may result from a failure in buffering the negative effects of multifaceted pathogens, toxins, and genetic or epigenetic mutations (Brüne, 2022). For example, Yeo et al. (1999) have focused on factors that may favor (or not favor) an organism in expressing their development in the face of perturbations. Those later diagnosed with schizophrenia would present an inability to soften the effects of deleterious mutations and environmental agents. For example, such impairments could be related to an asymmetry of bilateral traits that are symmetrical at the population level (i.e., fluctuation asymmetry). These traits include minor physical abnormalities (e.g., hypertelorism), delay in brain maturation causing abnormal brain lateralization (e.g., reduced dendritic branching, dysfunctional intra-/inter-hemispheric connectivity, etc.), or several other minimal physical anomalies (Crow, 1999; Davies, 2007; Mittal et al., 2007; Yeo et al., 1999).

Genetic Aspects

An advantage of the developmental instability models is that they have formulated and tested specific hypotheses related to a broad developmental pattern. However, such models partly disregard the complexity of clinical phenotypes and the role of genes. Indeed, there is robust evidence suggesting that schizophrenia is highly hereditable (Owen et al., 2007; Tienari et al., 2004). A recent genome-wide association study identified 120 genes putatively conveying genetic risk for schizophrenia (Trubetskoy et al., 2022). While no single locus associated with at least moderate effect size has been identified, the existing genetic studies of schizophrenia are consistent with the view that the clinical phenotype reflects an accumulation of alleles each of which is infrequent in the population but collectively very common. Keller and Miller (2006) proposed three evolutionary factors that favor the overcoming of a simplistic view of the link between genetics and psychopathology. First, alleles associated with a possible vulnerability were not necessarily harmful in ancestral environments (ancestral neutrality). Second, some "susceptibility" alleles may have increased human fitness in the evolutionary past (balancing selection). Third, severe mental disorders such as schizophrenia reflect the mutational load on thousands of genes underlying human behavior (polygenic mutation-selection balance). This latter explanation would be highly consistent with the complexity of schizophrenia, its prevalence, and fitness costs.

Social Aspects

While a large amount of variance in the expression of the schizophrenia phenotype is explained by genetic factors, a substantial part is not. For example, clinical observations and correlational studies support the idea that changes in social environments associated with or directly caused by social isolation, migration, changes in social status, or break-up of romantic relationships are associated with an increased risk for schizophrenia (Cantor-Grae & Selten, 2005; Michalska da Rocha et al., 2018; Ku et al., 2021). In addition, schizophrenia seems to be more prevalent in urban than in rural contexts (Pedersen et al., 2022) and can be associated with cultural transition periods (Torrey et al., 1974). Together, social stressors seem to contribute to the risk of schizophrenia, which is entirely consistent with evolutionary perspectives.

Our ancestors lived in small communities characterized by limited contacts with external conspecifics and tight interactions with members of one's own community. Accordingly, it has been suggested that schizophrenia could reflect an extreme variation of out-group intolerance, that is, individuals with higher genetic vulnerability, once exposed to novel or even distressful social conditions caused by migration, urbanicity, etc., may be at risk of developing schizophrenia (Abed & Abbas, 2011). This hypothesis is consistent with studies showing social hypervigilance in those diagnosed with psychosis (Garwood et al., 2015), and higher distress and more recurrently aggressive contents in those hearing voices in Western than in non-Western cultures (Luhrman et al., 2015). Despite the limited specificity of these social stress models, they offer a viable framework for the understanding of evolution-based proximate factors involved in schizophrenia.

Immunological Aspects

The recent SARS-CoV-2 pandemic has bolstered long-standing research exploring the association between intrauterine exposure to infectious agents and the risk for schizophrenia (Zimmer et al., 2021). Indeed, several authors have suggested that aberrant neurodevelopment secondary to viral transmission may be related to the later development of schizophrenia spectrum disorders. Bayer and colleagues (1999) proposed a two-hit hypothesis positing a first hit as a prenatal insult (e.g., intrauterine infection) and a second hit as affecting a developmentally vulnerable brain.

Another interesting infectious model of schizophrenia has been proposed with respect to a latent infection of *Toxoplasma gondii* (Delgado Garcia & Garcia Landa, 1979). *T. gondii* is a protozoic agent that infects warm-blooded animals, and it is estimated that about 3 billion humans worldwide are infected by it. Even though the majority of cases are clinically silent, the control of infection is regulated by several specific immunological responses, one of which is regulated by a major histocompatibility complex that is thought to play a role in the onset of schizophrenia (Blanchard et al., 2015; Flint & Munafò, 2014). Indeed, several studies suggest an association between *T. gondii* and schizophrenia. For example, individuals showing *T. gondii* antibodies have a 2.7-fold elevated risk for schizophrenia compared to the general population (Torrey et al., 2007). From an evolutionary point of view, it is interesting to note how rodents infected by *T. gondii* show potentially self-harmful and careless "suicidal" behavior. They lose their innate and adaptive avoidance of the odor of cat urine and instead are seemingly triggered to approach locations containing cat urine odor, that is, they dramatically increase their risk of being predated by enacting a nearly suicidal behavior (Flegr, 2007). Similar effects have been shown in chimpanzees losing their fear of leopards (Poirotte et al., 2016). Brüne (2019) has suggested that some behaviors associated with schizophrenia could be interpreted as a consequence of parasitic behavior manipulation, akin to what has been observed in nonhuman animals; however, this has not yet been systematically explored.

Phylogenetic Aspects

The paradox of schizophrenia has attracted evolutionary scientists to generate a couple of intriguing hypotheses about the phylogenetic origin of schizophrenia spectrum disorders and—more broadly—schizotypy. These studies are more strictly linked to Tinbergen's question about the potentially adaptive function of schizotypal or schizophrenia-like traits.

There is no convincing evidence to suggest that psychosis exists in nonhuman animals. Even though captive great apes often display behavioral abnormalities such as self-mutilation or inappropriate aggression, these behaviors resemble symptoms associated with depression, anxiety, and post-traumatic stress disorder but not schizophrenia spectrum disorders (Brüne et al., 2006). Second, recently evolved genomic regions in humans such as methylated regions (enriched in anatomically modern humans, or AMHs) are involved in the genetic risk for schizophrenia, suggesting that schizophrenia and related disorders seemingly appeared in *Homo sapiens* (Banerjee et al., 2018). Third, AMHs diagnosed with schizophrenia have less Neanderthal-derived genetic variation than controls, and having more Neanderthal admixture seemingly predicts less severe symptoms once diagnosed with schizophrenia (Gregory et al., 2021). Fourth, the evolution of neocortex in human lineage is seemingly associated with an evolutionary trade-off across different regions (amygdala, cingulate cortex) between greater information efficiency (efficient coding) and reduced robustness (synchronized neural activity) exposing AMHs to an increased risk for psychopathology (Pryluk et al., 2019). Finally, schizotypal traits would be related to genomic regions (e.g., prefrontal cortex) associated with distinctive higher cognitive functions of AMHs (e.g., mentalizing) and phylogenetically exposed to a strong selective pressure and, again, to a higher risk for severe mental disorders (Xu et al., 2015).

These studies do not precisely confirm any of the existing evolutionary hypotheses but strongly support a background assumption of them; schizophrenia spectrum disorders and schizotypal traits are specific to AMHs and possibly associated with the increasing complexity of the human brain.

This trade-off perspective considers schizotypal traits as a by-product of other adaptive traits. None of the theories considering schizotypy or psychosis as a trade-off of human brain evolution have prevailed, however. Crow was among the first to propose that schizophrenia emerged from a failure to establish hemispheric dominance for language (Crow, 1990, 1999). The resulting failure in the lateralization of these brain functions would have exposed humans to an impaired ability in distinguishing internal and external voices and so an increased risk for psychosis. Crow's model is consistent with reduced brain asymmetry observed in individuals with schizophrenia; however, Crow's hypothesis that this is related to a "speciation event" by a mutation in a single locus has been proven incorrect. Burns (2007) proposed a social brain theory of schizophrenia that is consistent with the social brain hypothesis (Dunbar, 2009). Accordingly, the rise of AMHs was associated with the evolution of increasingly complex brains due to greater complexity of the social environment, which, in turn, came at the cost of heightened risk of dysfunction. However, Burns' model lacks explanations as to why this vulnerability would specifically predispose one to psychosis (and not other mental disorders).

Evolutionary Insights About Variation in Personality

Considering how schizotypy emerged as a feature or organization of personality, with schizophrenia being the extreme expression of traits associated with schizotypy, we believe it can be extremely helpful to look at the evolution of personality in a more general evolutionary perspective.

From a scientific point of view, there has been a century-old debate as to what "personality" actually is. One difficulty, for instance, resides in the fact that conceptual frameworks of biologically-based individual differences in personality often overlap with more clearly behavior-regulating traits summarized under the term "temperament." While traits associated with "temperament" commonly entail endurance, impulsivity, stress reactivity, and so forth that can be linked to the function of neurochemical systems, "personality" is more strongly embedded in socio-cultural contexts (Trofimova et al., 2018). The lack of differentiating between "temperament" and "personality" is even reflected in widely acknowledged models of personality traits such as the FFM. Specifically, the dimensions "neuroticism" and "extraversion" are presumed to have a clearer biological basis (i.e., emotional stability, which is considered to be a temperamental factor) compared to the dimensions "agreeableness" and "conscientiousness," which are more deeply rooted in socio-cultural issues, including perspectives on morality (Trofimova et al., 2018). However, as Poortinga and van Hemert (2001) argue, there is nevertheless solid evidence for cross-cultural similarities in personality traits, even though there is room for expanding the "classic" five-factor model by considering additional factors. For example, in Chinese populations, the factor "interpersonal relatedness" has been demonstrated as highly relevant and may be underrepresented in "Western" approaches to describe personality dimensions (Poortinga & van Hemert, 2001).

In any event, in accordance with an evolutionary perspective, it is important to highlight that neither "temperament" nor "personality" are features unique to human beings. In fact, research suggests that differences in "temperament" even exist between colonies of social insects, such as ants, in terms of risk taking, food retrieval, and interaction with conspecifics, whereby "boldness" comes at the cost of higher mortality among worker ants (Blight et al., 2016). In less distantly related species to AMH, the evidence for individual differences in personality traits is even more clear. A plethora of research has shown differences in personality among a broad spectrum of vertebrates, most notably mammals (Gosling & John, 1999). In nonhuman primates, studies have demonstrated individual differences in timidity, assertiveness, sociability, impulsivity, and curiosity (Capitanio, 2004). In our closest extant relatives, the great apes, King et al. (2005) have shown that, in addition to the five factors known from human research, a sixth factor exists in chimpanzees, termed "dominance" (King et al., 2005; see also Uher & Asendorpf, 2008). Another line of research has reported that psychopathic traits can also reliably be measured in chimpanzees (Lilienfeld et al., 1999).

Together, the evidence of differences in temperament and personality between individuals of a broad range of animal species is overwhelming. A critical question is why such differences evolved. Wolf et al. (2007) suggested, from an adaptationist point of view, that life-history theory predicts individual differences in risk-taking behavior, boldness, and explorative behavior. Specifically, individuals of any species are predicted to be risk-averse (i.e., pursuing a "slow" life-history strategy) if future expectations are good with regard to the availability of crucial resources such as food, mates, etc. In contrast, individuals are expected to be more risk-prone in unpredictable environments ("fast" life-history strategy). This evolutionary principle is also applicable to personality traits and explains why some traits frequently co-occur (e.g., boldness, explorative behavior, and aggressiveness). The logic behind this is that reproductive activity is accelerated in environmentally poor conditions (at the cost of somatic maintenance), whereas delayed reproduction often paysoff in stable environments (Wolf et al., 2007).

While life-history theory explains differences between species in this regard (e.g., between elephants and mice), there is also mounting evidence to propose within-species differences in temperament and personality, depending on the *actual* or (as far as our own species is concerned) *perceived* resource availability. Figueredo et al. (2005) as well as Del Giudice (2015) have convincingly argued that individual differences in expectations with regard to future resource availability impact the development of personality dimensions in quite predictable ways. Accordingly, similar to what has been found in animals, risk-taking, sensation-seeking, impulsivity, and discounting of future rewards are much more likely to occur in individuals who actually live or perceive their environments as dangerous, unpredictable, or unstable. In contrast, conscientiousness and agreeableness (empathic concern) are underdeveloped in such circumstances. For reasons of space, these highly relevant aspects concerning human (personality) development cannot be described in every detail. Importantly, however, there is ample evidence supporting the view that early developmental contingencies (i.e., during early childhood and adolescence) are crucial with regard to the question of how exactly expectations about future resource availability are shaped by early environments, foremost by the behavior of caregivers, including their emotional availability and rearing styles (reviewed in Del Giudice, 2015). In fact, the quality of infant–caregiver interaction decisively impacts the development of the infant's "inner working model" and attachment style (Ellis et al., 2011).

Personality disorders can be seen as the extremes of variation of life-history strategies, whereby the term "strategy" does not involve conscious reflection or decision-making. In a nutshell, Cluster B personality disorders (according to DSM-5) largely reflect "fast" strategies associated with the goal of immediate resource extraction, whereas Cluster C personality disorders reside more in the "slow" lane. Detailed analyses for psychopathy (Mealey, 1995; Glenn et al., 2011), antisocial personality disorder (Troisi, 2005), and borderline personality disorder

(Brüne, 2016) illustrate how early environmental contingencies can shape (unconsciously pursued) behavioral strategies in terms of interpersonal functioning and mating.

Life-history theory would also posit differences between male and female individuals of the same species (as defined biologically), with males usually pursuing "faster" strategies than females, partly depending on their differential parental investment in offspring (which is usually higher in females than males). Consistent with this assumption, Del Giudice et al. (2012) reported differences in personality between men and women across a broad range of traits. For example, "boldness" was considerably more prevalent in men compared to women, whereas "warmth" was rated higher in women than men (Del Giudice et al., 2012). How can all this inform the study of schizotypy?

Evolutionary Aspects of Schizotypy

Several scholars have proposed selective advantages of schizotypal traits, and thus indirectly, of psychosis. According to the hypotheses of Price and Stevens (1998)—probably the first evolutionary account specific to schizotypy—schizotypal traits would have played a role in promoting divergent thinking associated with two main advantages: a proneness to religious leadership and so to the generation of new ideas and perspectives, plus a dispersal of human communities around the world due to the tendency of group splitting. The original formulation of the model by Price and Stevens (1998) was highly speculative and very much relied on group selection, which is hotly debated among evolutionary scientists, though the model is consistent with more recent evolutionary accounts of the evolution of religion (Dunbar, 2022).

In contrast, Nettle (2001) and Del Giudice (2010) have argued in favor of sexual selection being involved in the emergence of schizotypal traits. While natural selection implies that a trait is adaptive if it directly increases the chances of survival and reproduction, sexual selection suggests that a few traits that are seemingly associated with a handicap—such as the peacock's tail—promote mate attraction, but not necessarily survival. Accordingly, schizotypy could be linked to a short-term, promiscuous, and possibly polygamous mating strategy (Del Giudice, 2010). This interpretation, however, is incompatible with the sexual selection hypotheses of schizophrenia. Shaner et al. (2004), for example, considered signs and symptoms associated with schizophrenia as "low fitness" variants of sexually selected traits.

The role of sexual selection in understanding schizotypy and its association with putatively adaptive traits gives rise to a more integrated look that is consistent with modern dimensional approaches to psychopathology. Indeed, several studies have postulated an evolutionary relationship between schizotypal traits and creativity, yet others do not support this connection (Kozbelt et al., 2014).

Moreover, Cheli (2023) has proposed a hypothesis integrating evolutionary and dimensional models of schizotypy. Consistent with existing knowledge on FFM,

AMPD, and HiTOP (Cicero et al., 2019), Cheli identified two personality traits—openness to experience and introversion—that may clinically manifest in the form of psychoticism and detachment, respectively, if excessively present. In fact, high scores of openness have been related to creativity and superior intellect, at the risk of being disadvantageous through an increased susceptibility for psychosis. In contrast, high levels of introversion can be useful (and adaptive) as a risk-minimizing strategy, especially with respect to social threats, but fraught with a heightened risk for pathological social withdrawal (Moorman & Samuel, 2018; Verbeke & De Clercq, 2014; Keyes et al., 2013; Zimmermann et al., 2022). If these two traits (i.e., openness to experience and introversion) co-exist—due to differential vulnerabilities to environmental contingencies—individuals may fail in "socializing" their creativity, which may eventually lead to distorted cognitions, emotions, and behaviors. In such circumstances, the putative advantages of creativity in terms of superior reproductive success would cause rigid uniqueness-maximizing (i.e., high degrees of psychoticism) and risk-minimizing (i.e., high detachment) strategies resulting in severe disorders such as SPD and psychosis. Accordingly, a person would perceive any negative judgment about their own bizarre beliefs as a threatening experience, frequently fueled by self-critical doubts about her own wishes and choices. This could create a vicious cycle, where the more threatening the beliefs are, the higher is the psychosocial distress. Conversely, high levels of psychosocial distress may activate rigid defense strategies, which may entail even stronger attempts to stabilize a fragile self by increasing one's self-perception as unique, and by avoiding risks of failure in the social domain. This is consistent with correlational studies showing how developmental stressors (e.g., childhood maltreatment), self-criticism, social rank, and shame are associated with a higher risk for schizotypal manifestations (Cheli et al., 2021; Varese et al., 2012; Wood & Irons, 2016). These factors could either be related to evolutionary trade-offs, such as the costly evolution of the social brain, or to reproductive advantages in terms of sexual selection, such as the proactive role of creativity (Burns, 2007; Del Giudice, 2018; Zwir et al., 2022). Moreover, this interpretation is also compatible with growing evidence suggesting that the activation of the threat-response system may have a vagally mediated dampening effect on prefrontal cortex activity, which, in turn, may further impair mentalizing (Luyten & Fonagy, 2015; Petrocchi & Cheli, 2019). In sum, openness to experience and introversion may represent the basic personality dimensions, which, in the context of unfavorable gene-environment interactions, may lead to pathological manifestations in terms of psychoticism and detachment (AMPD).

Conclusions

Schizotypy, as a personality organization possibly leading to severe mental disorders such as schizophrenia, is an evolutionary enigma. Despite numerous efforts, there is as yet no conclusive answer to the question whether schizotypy represents an evolutionary trade-off or a sexually selected phenotype.

Del Giudice (2018) has argued that studies showing a reduced fecundity of people with schizophrenia (and their relatives) are inconclusive and not suitable to refute an explanation involving sexual selection. More specifically, in his view, an effective comparison would not be between individuals diagnosed with schizophrenia and their siblings, but instead, between individuals with schizophrenia and people expressing high levels of schizotypal traits without significant impairments. This perspective seems to be consistent with a dimensional approach to psychopathology such as the one proposed by FFM, AMPD, and HiTOP, even though the latter has been criticized for its possible theoretical limitations (Haeffel et al., 2022). Indeed, the focus of Del Giudice's model (life-history theory) is an integrated framework in accounting how individual differences in development, physiology, and behavior arise from trade-offs in survival (natural selection) and reproduction (sexual selection). Therefore, dimensions of psychopathology may support an effective comparison between persons with the same traits but different manifestations (e.g., clinical, subclinical, healthy).

From a phylogenetic point of view, it would seem that the evolution of schizotypal traits is strongly connected with the history of our species. Indeed, our closest extant relatives, the great apes may display signs of distress resembling (or being homologous to) psychiatric disorders, however, with the exception of schizophrenia. Similarly, humans with larger Neanderthal genetic admixture have a reduced risk for schizophrenia, and less severe symptoms when diagnosed with a psychotic disorder (Gregory et al., 2021). The majority of existing evolutionary explanations links these and other findings to the emergence of our costly social brain and the complexity of human traits. However, we now know that individual differences in temperament and personality are not unique to AMH (Capitanio, 2004; Uher & Asendorpf, 2008). Individual differences in openness to experience and introversion surely exist in other species, too, yet the peculiar association of these traits as a potential "risk combination" of personality dimensions has not been studied in non-human animals. From this perspective, schizotypy, comprising both creativity and social avoidance, is difficult to assign to a "fast" or "slow" life-history strategy. While Del Giudice (2018) promotes the view that creativity could increase mating success (thus arguing in favor of a "fast" strategy), introversion (conceptualized as the opposite of extraversion) clearly resides on the "slow" end of life-history strategies (in favor of long-term mating). Existing studies on schizotypy suggest a complexity that would be consistent with neither a unidimensional look at schizotypal traits nor, consequently, a unique reproduction strategy (Brüne, 2022; Cicero et al., 2019). This broader perspective, as recently suggested by Cheli (2023), entails that individuals with high levels of openness to experience and introversion are more vulnerable to adverse rearing conditions including childhood maltreatment. Accordingly, these personality traits, in the presence of schizotypal traits, may reduce one's capacity to utilize one's creative potential in socially beneficial ways, and instead, promote a risk-minimizing (i.e., detachment) and uniqueness-maximizing (i.e., psychoticism) strategy. Thus, the potential reproduction advantage of creativity would disappear and may even be disadvantageous (both socially and reproductively).

To sum up, we believe that future research should explore the intersection of different proximate and evolutionary explanations, rather than searching for a single one factor. The evolved psychosocial mechanisms related to schizotypy—as any other human feature—can be better understood by considering how advantages and disadvantages are interconnected, consistent with Tinbergen's framework.

References

Abed, R. T., & Abbas, M. J. (2011). A reformulation of the social brain theory for schizophrenia: The case for out-group intolerance. *Perspectives in Biology and Medicine, 54*(2), 132–151. https://doi.org/10.1353/pbm.2011.0020

Allen, J. S. (in press). Schizophrenia – Embracing the spectrum. In N. Diederich, C. Goetz, M. Brüne, & K. Amunts (Eds.), *The evolutionary roots of human brain disease*. Oxford University Press.

American Psychiatric Association. (2013). *The diagnostic and statistical manual of mental disorders – Fifth edition (DSM-5)*. American Psychiatric Association Publishing.

Banerjee, N., Polushina, T., Bettella, F., Giddaluru, S., Steen, V. M., Andreassen, O. A., & Le Hellard, S. (2018). Recently evolved human-specific methylated regions are enriched in schizophrenia signals. *BMC Evolutionary Biology, 18*(1), 63. https://doi.org/10.1186/s12862-018-1177-2

Bayer, T. A., Falkai, P., & Maier, W. (1999). Genetic and non-genetic vulnerability factors in schizophrenia: the basis of The "two hit hypothesis". *Journal of Psychiatric Research, 33*(6), 543–548. https://doi.org/10.1016/s0022-3956(99)00039-4

Blanchard, N., Dunay, I. R., & Schlüter, D. (2015). Persistence of toxoplasma gondii in the central nervous system: A fine-tuned balance between the parasite, the brain and the immune system. *Parasite Immunology, 37*(3), 150–158. https://doi.org/10.1111/pim.12173

Bleuler, E. (1911). *Dementia praecox oder die Gruppe der Schizophrenien*. Deutike.

Blight, O., Díaz-Mariblanca, G. A., Cerdá, X., & Boulay, R. (2016). A proactive–reactive syndrome affects group success in an ant species. *Behavioral Ecology, 27*(1), 118–125. https://doi.org/10.1093/beheco/arv127

Brüne, M. (2004). Schizophrenia-an evolutionary enigma? *Neuroscience & Biobehavioral Reviews, 28*(1), 41–53. https://doi.org/10.1016/j.neubiorev.2003.10.002

Brüne, M. (2016). Borderline personality disorder: Why 'fast and furious'? *Evolution, medicine, and public health, 2016*(1), 52–66. https://doi.org/10.1093/emph/eow002

Brüne, M. (2019). Latent toxoplasmosis: host–parasite interaction and psychopathology. *Evolution, Medicine, and Public Health, 2019*(1), 212–213. https://doi.org/10.1093/emph/eoz032

Brüne, M. (2022). Evolution perspectives on schizophrenia spectrum disorders. In R. Abed & P. St John-Smith (Eds.), *Evolutionary psychiatry. Current perspectives on evolution and mental health (pp. 153–168)*. Cambridge University Press.

Brüne, M., Brüne-Cohrs, U., McGrew, W. C., & Preuschoft, S. (2006). Psychopathology in great apes: Concepts, treatment options and possible homologies to human psychiatric disorders. *Neuroscience and Biobehavioral Reviews, 30*(8), 1246–1259. https://doi.org/10.1016/j.neubiorev.2006.09.002

Burns, J. (2007). *The descent of madness: Evolutionary origins of psychosis and the social brain*. Routledge/Taylor & Francis Group.

Cantor-Graae, E., & Selten, J. P. (2005). Schizophrenia and migration: A meta-analysis and review. *The American Journal of Psychiatry, 162*(1), 12–24. https://doi.org/10.1176/appi.ajp.162.1.12

Capitanio, J. P. (2004). Personality factors between and within species. In B. Thierry, M. Singh, & W. Kaumanns (Eds.), *Macaque Societies*. Cambridge University Press.

Cheli, S. (2023). An evolutionary look at oddity and schizotypy: How the rise of social brain informs clinical practice. *New Ideas in Psychology, 68*. https://doi.org/10.1016/j.newideapsych.2022.100993

Cheli, S., Cavalletti, C., Mancini, F., & Goldzweig, G. (2021). What if metacognition is not enough? Its association with delusion may be moderated by self-criticism. *Current Psychology*. https://doi.org/10.1007/s12144-021-02451-7

Cicero, D. C., Jonas, K. G., Li, K., Perlman, G., & Kotov, R. (2019). Common taxonomy of traits and symptoms: Linking schizophrenia symptoms, schizotypy, and normal personality. *Schizophrenia Bulletin, 45*(6), 1336–1348. https://doi.org/10.1093/schbul/sbz005

Crow, T. J. (1990). The continuum of psychosis and its genetic origins. The sixty-fifth Maudsley lecture. *The British Journal of Psychiatry: the Journal of Mental Science, 156*, 788–797. https://doi.org/10.1192/bjp.156.6.788

Crow, T. J. (1999). Commentary on Annett, Yeo et al., Klar, Saugstad and Orr: cerebral asymmetry, language and psychosis--the case for a Homo sapiens-specific sex-linked gene for brain growth. *Schizophrenia Research, 39*(3), 219–231. https://doi.org/10.1016/s0920-9964(99)00076-6

Davies, E. (2007). Developmental aspects of schizophrenia and related disorders: Possible implications for treatment strategies. *Advances in Psychiatric Treatment, 13*(5), 384–391. https://doi.org/10.1192/apt.bp.106.002600

Del Giudice, M. (2010). Reduced fertility in patients' families is consistent with the sexual selection model of schizophrenia and schizotypy. *PLoS One, 5*(12), e16040. https://doi.org/10.1371/journal.pone.0016040

Del Giudice, M. (2015). Attachment in middle childhood: An evolutionary–developmental perspective. *New Directions for Child and Adolescent Development*, 2015(148), 15–30. https://doi.org/10.1002/cad.20101

Del Giudice, M. (2018). *Evolutionary psychopathology: A unified approach*. New York: Oxford University Press.

Del Giudice, M., Booth, T., & Irwing, P. (2012). The distance between Mars and Venus: Measuring global sex differences in personality. *PLoS One, 7*(1), e29265. https://doi.org/10.1371/journal.pone.0029265

Delgado García, G., & García Landa, J. (1979). Reactivity of the intradermal test with toxoplasmosis in schizophrenic patients. *Revista Cubana de Medicina Tropical, 31*, 225–231.

Dunbar, R. I. (2009). The social brain hypothesis and its implications for social evolution. *Annals of Human Biology, 36*(5), 562–572. https://doi.org/10.1080/03014460902960289

Dunbar, R. I. (2022). *How religion evolved: And why it endures*. Pelican Books.

Edmundson, M., & Kwapil, T. R. (2013). A five-factor model perspective of schizotypal personality disorder. In T. A. Widiger & P. T. Costa Jr. (Eds.), *Personality disorders and the five-factor model of personality* (pp. 147–161). American Psychological Association. https://doi.org/10.1037/13939-010

Ellis, B. J., Boyce, W. T., Belsky, J., Bakermans-Kranenburg, M. J., & van IJzendoorn, M. H. (2011). Differential susceptibility to the environment: An evolutionary-neurodevelopmental theory. *Development and Psychopathology, 23*, 7–28. https://doi.org/10.1017/s0954579410000611

Ettinger, U., Meyhöfer, I., Steffens, M., Wagner, M., & Koutsouleris, N. (2014). Genetics, cognition, and neurobiology of schizotypal personality: a review of the overlap with schizophrenia. *Frontiers in Psychiatry, 5*, 18. https://doi.org/10.3389/fpsyt.2014.00018

Figueredo, A. J., Vásquez, G., Brumbach, B. H., Sefcek, J. A., Kirsner, B. R., & Jacobs, W. J. (2005). The K-factor: Individual differences in life history strategy. *Personality and Individual Differences, 39*(8), 1349–1360. https://doi.org/10.1016/j.paid.2005.06.009

Flegr, J. (2007). Effects of toxoplasma on human behavior. *Schizophrenia Bulletin, 33*(3), 757–760. https://doi.org/10.1093/schbul/sbl074

Flint, J., & Munafò, M. (2014). Schizophrenia: Genesis of a complex disease. *Nature, 511*(7510), 412–413. https://doi.org/10.1038/nature13645

Garwood, L., Dodgson, G., Bruce, V., & McCarthy-Jones, S. (2015). A preliminary investigation into the existence of a hypervigilance subtype of auditory hallucination in people with psychosis. *Behavioral and Cognitive Psychotherapy, 43*, 52–62. https://doi.org/10.1017/S1352465813000714

Glenn, A. L., Kurzban, R., & Raine, A. (2011). Evolutionary theory and psychopathy. *Aggression and Violent Behavior, 16*(5), 371–380. https://doi.org/10.1016/j.avb.2011.03.009

Gosling, S. D., & John, O. P. (1999). Personality dimensions in non-human animals: A cross-species review. *Current Directions in Psychological Science, 8*, 69–75. https://doi.org/10.1111/1467-8721.00017

Gregory, M. D., Eisenberg, D. P., Hamborg, M., Kippenhan, J. S., Kohn, P., Kolachana, B., Dickinson, D., & Berman, K. F. (2021). Neanderthal-derived genetic variation in living humans relates to schizophrenia diagnosis, to psychotic symptom severity, and to dopamine synthesis. *American Journal of Medical Genetics. Part B, Neuropsychiatric Genetics: The Official Publication of the International Society of Psychiatric Genetics, 186*(5), 329–338. https://doi.org/10.1002/ajmg.b.32872

Haeffel, G. J., Jeronimus, B. F., Fisher, A. J., Kaiser, B. N., Weaver, L. J., Vargas, I., Goodson, J. T., Soyster, P. D., & Lu, W. (2022). The hierarchical taxonomy of psychopathology (HiTOP) is not an improvement over the DSM. *Clinical Psychological Science, 10*(2), 285–290. https://doi.org/10.1177/21677026211068873

Keller, M. C., & Miller, G. (2006). Resolving the paradox of common, harmful, heritable mental disorders: Which evolutionary genetic models work best?. *The Behavioral and Brain Sciences, 29*(4), 385–452. https://doi.org/10.1017/S0140525X06009095

Keyes, K., Eaton, N., Krueger, R., Skodol, A., Wall, M., Grant, B., et al. (2013). Thought disorder in the meta-structure of psychopathology. *Psychological Medicine, 43*(8), 1673–1683. https://doi.org/10.1017/S0033291712002292

King, J. E., Weiss, A., & Farmer, K. H. (2005). A chimpanzee (*pan troglodytes*) analogue of cross-national generalization of personality structure: Zoological parks and an African sanctuary. *Journal of Personality, 73*, 389–410. https://psycnet.apa.org/doi/10.1111/j.1467-6494.2005.00313.x

Kotov, R., Jonas, K. G., Carpenter, W. T., Dretsch, M. N., Eaton, N. R., Forbes, M. K., Forbush, K. T., Hobbs, K., Reininghaus, U., Slade, T., South, S. C., Sunderland, M., Waszczuk, M. A., Widiger, T. A., Wright, A. G. C., Zald, D. H., Krueger, R. F., Watson, D., & Workgroup, H. T. O. P. U. (2020). Validity and utility of hierarchical taxonomy of psychopathology (HiTOP): I. Psychosis superspectrum. *World psychiatry: official journal of the World Psychiatric Association (WPA), 19*(2), 151–172. https://doi.org/10.1002/wps.20730

Kozbelt, A., Kaufman, S. B., Walder, D. J., Ospina, L. H., & Kim, J. U. (2014). The evolutionary genetics of the creativity-psychosis connection. In J. C. Kaufman (Ed.), *Creativity and mental illness* (pp. 102–132). Cambridge University Press.

Ku, B. S., Compton, M. T., Walker, E. F., & Druss, B. G. (2021). Social fragmentation and schizophrenia: A systematic review. *The Journal of Clinical Psychiatry, 83*(1), 21r13941. https://doi.org/10.4088/JCP.21r13941

Kwapil, T. R., & Barrantes-Vidal, N. (2015). Schizotypy: Looking back and moving forward. *Schizophrenia Bulletin, 41*(Suppl 2), S366–S373. https://doi.org/10.1093/schbul/sbu186

Lilienfeld, S. O., Gershon, J., Duke, M., Marino, L., & de Waal, F. B. (1999). A preliminary investigation of psychopathic personality (psychopathy) in chimpanzees (pan troglodytes*). Journal of Comparative Psychology, 113*, 365–375. https://psycnet.apa.org/doi/10.1037/0735-7036.113.4.365

Linscott, R. J., & van Os, J. (2013). An updated and conservative systematic review and meta-analysis of epidemiological evidence on psychotic experiences in children and adults: On the pathway from proneness to persistence to dimensional expression across mental disorders. *Psychological Medicine, 43*(6), 1133–1149. https://doi.org/10.1017/S0033291712001626

Luhrmann, T. M., Padmavati, R., Tharoor, H., & Osei, A. (2015). Differences in voice-hearing experiences of people with psychosis in the U.S.A., India and Ghana: Interview-based study. *The British Journal of Psychiatry: the Journal of Mental Science, 206*(1), 41–44. https://doi.org/10.1192/bjp.bp.113.139048

Luyten, P., & Fonagy, P. (2015). The neurobiology of mentalizing. *Personality Disorders: Theory, Research, and Treatment, 6*(4), 366–379. https://doi.org/10.1037/per0000117

McGrath, J. J., Saha, S., Al-Hamzawi, A., Alonso, J., Bromet, E. J., Bruffaerts, R., Caldas-de-Almeida, J. M., Chiu, W. T., de Jonge, P., Fayyad, J., Florescu, S., Gureje, O., Haro, J. M., Hu, C., Kovess-Masfety, V., Lepine, J. P., Lim, C. C., Mora, M. E., Navarro-Mateu, F., Ochoa, S., et al. (2015). Psychotic experiences in the general population: A cross-National Analysis Based on 31,261 respondents from 18 countries. *JAMA Psychiatry, 72*(7), 697–705. https://doi.org/10.1001/jamapsychiatry.2015.0575

Mealey, L. (1995). The sociobiology of sociopathy: An integrated evolutionary model. *The Behavioral and Brain Sciences, 18*, 523–599. https://psycnet.apa.org/doi/10.1017/S0140525X00039595

Meehl, P. E. (1962). Schizotaxia, schizotypy, schizophrenia. *American Psychologist, 17*(12), 827–838. https://doi.org/10.1037/h0041029

Michalska da Rocha, B., Rhodes, S., Vasilopoulou, E., & Hutton, P. (2018). Loneliness in Psychosis: A Metaanalytical Review. *Schizophrenia Bulletin, 44*(1), 114–125. https://doi.org/10.1093/schbul/sbx036

Millon, T. (2011). Classifying personality disorders: An evolution-based alternative to an evidence-based approach. *Journal of Personality Disorders, 25*(3), 279–304. https://doi.org/10.1521/pedi.2011.25.3.279

Mittal, V. A., Dhruv, S., Tessner, K. D., Walder, D. J., & Walker, E. F. (2007). The relations among putative biorisk markers in schizotypal adolescents: Minor physical anomalies, movement abnormalities, and salivary cortisol. *Biological Psychiatry, 61*(10), 1179–1186. https://doi.org/10.1016/j.biopsych.2006.08.043

Moorman, E. L., & Samuel, D. B. (2018). Representing schizotypal thinking with dimensional traits: A case for the five factor schizotypal inventory. *Psychological Assessment, 30*(1), 19–30. https://doi.org/10.1037/pas0000497

Nettle, D. (2001). *Strong imagination: Madness, creativity and human nature*. Oxford University Press.

Owen, M. J., Craddock, N., & Jablensky, A. (2007). The genetic deconstruction of psychosis. *Schizophrenia Bulletin, 33*, 905–911. https://doi.org/10.1093/schbul/sbm053

Pedersen, C. B., Antonsen, S., Timmermann, A., Pedersen, M. G., Ejlskov, L., Horsdal, H. T., Agerbo, E., Webb, R. B., Raaschou-Nielsen, O., Sigsgaard, T., Sabel, C. E., Fan, C.-C., & Thompson, W. K. (2022). Urban-rural differences in schizophrenia risk: Multilevel survival analyses of individual- and Neighborhood-level indicators, Urbanicity and population density in a Danish National Cohort. *Open, 3*(1), sgab056. https://doi.org/10.1093/schizbullopen/sgab056

Petrocchi, N., & Cheli, S. (2019). The social brain and heart rate variability: Implications for psychotherapy. *Psychology and Psychotherapy, 92*(2), 208–223. https://doi.org/10.1111/papt.12224

Poirotte, C., Kappeler, P. M., Ngoubangoye, B., Bourgeois, S., Moussodji, M., & Charpentier, M. J. (2016). Morbid attraction to leopard urine in toxoplasma-infected chimpanzees. *Current Biology: CB, 26*(3), R98–R99. https://doi.org/10.1016/j.cub.2015.12.020

Polimeni, J. (2012). *Shamans among us. Schizophrenia, shamanism and the evolutionary origins of religion*. EvoEbooks.

Poortinga, Y. H., & Van Hemert, D. A. (2001). Personality and culture: Demarcating between the common and the unique. *Journal of Personality, 69*(6), 1033–1060. https://doi.org/10.1111/1467-6494.696174

Price, J. S., & Stevens, A. (1998). The human male socialisation strategy set: Cooperation, defection, individualism, and schizotypy. *Evolution and Human Behavior, 19*, 58–70. https://doi.org/10.1016/S1090-5138(97)00105-0

Pryluk, R., Kfir, Y., Gelbard-Sagiv, H., Fried, I., & Paz, R. (2019). A Tradeoff in the neural code across regions and species. *Cell, 176*(3), 597–609.e18. https://doi.org/10.1016/j.cell.2018.12.032

Shaner, A., Miller, G., & Mintz, J. (2004). Schizophrenia as one extreme of a sexually selected fitness indicator. *Schizophrenia Research, 70*(1), 101–109. https://doi.org/10.1016/j.schres.2003.09.014

Smeland, O. B., Frei, O., Dale, A. M., & Andreassen, O. A. (2020). The polygenic architecture of schizophrenia - rethinking pathogenesis and nosology. *Nature Reviews. Neurology, 16*(7), 366–379. https://doi.org/10.1038/s41582-020-0364-0

Stevens, A., & Price, J. (1996). *Evolutionary psychiatry. A new beginning*. Routledge.

Tienari, P., Wynne, L. C., Sorri, A., Lahti, I., Läksy, K., Moring, J., Naarala, M., Nieminen, P., & Wahlberg, K. E. (2004). Genotype-environment interaction in schizophrenia-spectrum disorder. Long-term follow-up study of Finnish adoptees. *The British Journal of Psychiatry: the Journal of Mental Science, 184*, 216–222. https://doi.org/10.1192/bjp.184.3.216

Tinbergen, N. (1963). On aims and methods of ethology. *Zeitschrift für Tierpsychologie., 20*(4), 410–433. https://doi.org/10.1111/j.1439-0310.1963.tb01161.x

Torrey, E. F., Torrey, B. B., & Burton-Bradley, B. G. (1974). The epidemiology of schizophrenia in Papua New Guinea. *American Journal of Psychiatry, 131*, 567–573.

Torrey, E. F., Bartko, J. J., Lun, Z. R., & Yolken, R. H. (2007). Antibodies to toxoplasma gondii in patients with schizophrenia: A meta-analysis. *Schizophrenia Bulletin, 33*(3), 729–736. https://doi.org/10.1093/schbul/sbl050

Trofimova, I., Robbins, T. W., Sulis, W. H., & Uher, J. (2018). Taxonomies of psychological individual differences: Biological perspectives on millennia-long challenges. *Philosophical Transactions of the Royal Society of London. Series B, Biological Sciences, 373*(1744), 20170152. https://doi.org/10.1098/rstb.2017.0152

Troisi, A. (2005). The concept of alternative strategies and its relevance to psychiatry and clinical psychology. *Neuroscience and Biobehavioral Reviews, 29*(1), 159–168. https://doi.org/10.1016/j.neubiorev.2004.06.012

Trubetskoy, V., Pardiñas, A. F., Qi, T., Panagiotaropoulou, G., Awasthi, S., Bigdeli, T. B., Bryois, J., Chen, C. Y., Dennison, C. A., Hall, L. S., Lam, M., Watanabe, K., Frei, O., Ge, T., Harwood, J. C., Koopmans, F., Magnusson, S., Richards, A. L., Sidorenko, J., Wu, Y., et al. (2022). Mapping genomic loci implicates genes and synaptic biology in schizophrenia. *Nature, 604*(7906), 502–508. https://doi.org/10.1038/s41586-022-04434-5

Uher, J., & Asendorpf, J. B. (2008). Personality assessment in the great apes: Comparing ecologically valid behavior measures, behavior ratings, and adjective ratings. *Journal of Research in Personality, 42*, 821–838. https://psycnet.apa.org/doi/10.1016/j.jrp.2007.10.004

Varese, F., Smeets, F., Drukker, M., Lieverse, R., Lataster, T., Viechtbauer, W., Read, J., van Os, J., & Bentall, R. P. (2012). Childhood adversities increase the risk of psychosis: A meta-analysis of patient-control, prospective- and cross-sectional cohort studies. *Schizophrenia Bulletin, 38*(4), 661–671. https://doi.org/10.1093/schbul/sbs050

Verbeke, L., & De Clercq, B. (2014). Integrating oddity traits in a dimensional model for personality pathology precursors. *Journal of Abnormal Psychology, 123*(3), 598–612. https://doi.org/10.1037/a0037166

Wolf, M., van Doorn, G. S., Leimar, O., & Weissing, F. J. (2007). Life-history trade-offs favour the evolution of animal personalities. *Nature, 447*(7144), 581–584. https://doi.org/10.1038/nature05835

Wood, L., & Irons, C. (2016). Exploring the associations between social rank and external shame with experiences of psychosis. *Behavioural and Cognitive Psychotherapy, 44*(5), 527–538. https://doi.org/10.1017/S1352465815000570

Xu, K., Schadt, E. E., Pollard, K. S., Roussos, P., & Dudley, J. T. (2015). Genomic and network patterns of schizophrenia genetic variation in human evolutionary accelerated regions. *Molecular Biology and Evolution, 32*(5), 1148–1160. https://doi.org/10.1093/molbev/msv031

Yeo, R. A., Gangestad, S. W., Edgar, C., & Thoma, R. (1999). The evolutionary genetic underpinnings of schizophrenia: The developmental instability model. *Schizophrenia Research, 39*(3), 197–206. https://doi.org/10.1016/s0920-9964(99)00074-2

Zimmer, A., Youngblood, A., Adnane, A., Miller, B. J., & Goldsmith, D. R. (2021). Prenatal exposure to viral infection and neuropsychiatric disorders in offspring: A review of the literature and recommendations for the COVID-19 pandemic. *Brain, Behavior, and Immunity, 91*, 756–770. https://doi.org/10.1016/j.bbi.2020.10.024

Zimmermann, J., Widiger, T. A., Oeltjen, L., Conway, C. C., & Morey, L. C. (2022). Developing preliminary scales for assessing the HiTOP detachment Spectrum. *Assessment, 29*(1), 75–87. https://doi.org/10.1177/10731911211015313

Zwir, I., Del-Val, C., Hintsanen, M., Cloninger, K. M., Romero-Zaliz, R., Mesa, A., Arnedo, J., Salas, R., Poblete, G. F., Raitoharju, E., Raitakari, O., Keltikangas-J¨arvinen, L., de Erausquin, G. A., Tattersall, I., Lehtim¨aki, T., & Cloninger, C. R. (2022). Evolution of genetic networks for human creativity. *Molecular Psychiatry, 27*(1), 354–376. https://doi.org/10.1038/s41380-021-01097-y

Chapter 3
Conceptualization of Schizotypy Within the Hierarchical Taxonomy of Psychopathology and Other Nosologies

Charlie C. Su and David C. Cicero

Schizotypy within the Hierarchical Taxonomy of Psychopathology and other nosologies refers to traits or symptoms similar to schizophrenia, but in a diminished form, and it represents a risk for the development of schizophrenia-spectrum disorders (Meehl, 1962). Schizophrenia-spectrum disorders are thought to exist on a continuum with subclinical psychotic-like experiences on one end of the spectrum and full-blown psychosis on the other (Kwapil & Barrantes-Vidal, 2015). Modern conceptualizations of schizotypy suggest that it is multidimensional and composed of at least three dimensions, including positive, negative, and disorganized schizotypy (Kwapil et al., 2018; Raine et al., 1994). Positive schizotypy includes delusion-like and hallucination-like experiences, commonly termed magical ideation and perceptual aberration, respectively (Chapman, 1966; Chapman & Chapman, 1980). Negative schizotypy is similar to the negative symptoms of schizophrenia and is commonly operationally defined as physical and social anhedonia (Chapman et al., 1976). Disorganized schizotypy is similar to disorganized symptoms of schizophrenia and includes odd and unusual thoughts, speech, and behavior (Hewitt & Claridge, 1989).

Although similar to many constructs used clinically (e.g., schizotypal personality disorder and attenuated psychosis syndrome), schizotypy is primarily a research construct and does not explicitly appear in traditional or alternative taxonomies of psychopathology. However, the conceptualization of schizotypy and related constructs is well represented in these systems. This chapter explores how schizotypy compares to the operationalization of related constructs in the Diagnostic and Statistical Manual of Mental Disorders (DSM-5-TR; American Psychiatric Association, 2022), International Classification of Diseases (ICD-11; World Health

C. C. Su · D. C. Cicero (✉)
University of North Texas, Denton, TX, USA
e-mail: Charliesu@my.unt.edu; David.cicero@unt.edu

S. Cheli, P. H. Lysaker (eds.), *A Dimensional Approach to Schizotypy*,
https://doi.org/10.1007/978-3-031-41788-7_3

Organization, 2022), and Hierarchical Taxonomy of Psychopathology (HiTOP; Kotov et al., 2017).

Schizotypy and the Diagnostic and Statistical Manual of Mental Disorders

The Diagnostic and Statistical Manual of Mental Disorders (DSM) is widely adopted as the gold-standard reference for psychopathology in the United States (Maj, 2015). The lack of a unifying nosology for mental health syndromes prior to 1950 motivated researchers and clinicians to standardize diagnostic criteria with the goal of guiding case conceptualization, treatment planning, and further research. Since the first edition was published in 1952 (American Psychiatric Association, 1952), the DSM has had an incontrovertible influence in myriad settings, including research, clinical, forensic, and educational. The DSM-5 (American Psychiatric Association, 2013) was recently updated to the DSM-5-TR (American Psychiatric Association, 2022) with changes in diagnostic entities, diagnostic criteria and specifiers, and terminology. However, changes to descriptions for relevant schizotypy constructs are minimal, and while the current chapter makes references to the DSM-5-TR, the discussion remains consistent with the DSM-5. The term "schizotypy" is not listed anywhere within the DSM-5-TR, but many of the constructs related to schizotypy are represented within its pages.

As previously described, schizotypy conceptualizes psychosis as a spectrum ranging from subclinical symptoms to frank psychosis. By definition, subclinical symptoms are not explicitly included in the main body (i.e., Section II) of the DSM. Thus, the schizotypy conceptualization is broader than described in the DSM because it extends past the diagnosable syndromes into lower ends of the spectrum (Kwapil & Barrantes-Vidal, 2015; Lenzenweger, 2006). The DSM defines the key features of psychotic disorders as delusions, hallucinations, disorganized thinking (formal thought disorder), grossly disorganized or abnormal motor behavior, and negative symptoms. The DSM-5-TR outlines schizophrenia-spectrum disorders mostly in the Schizophrenia Spectrum and Other Psychotic Disorders chapter of Section II in increasing severity. Diagnoses include delusional disorder, brief psychotic disorder, schizophreniform disorder, schizophrenia, schizoaffective disorder, psychotic disorders secondary to other conditions (i.e., substance use and other medical conditions), and catatonia. These diagnoses roughly correspond to the high end of multidimensional schizotypy (Kwapil & Barrantes-Vidal, 2015).

A schizotypal personality disorder (PD) is cross-listed in the Personality Disorders and Schizophrenia Spectrum and Other Psychotic Disorders chapters, reflecting the finding that schizotypal traits and schizophrenia symptoms are on a common continuum (Linscott & van Os, 2010). Individuals with schizotypal PD endorse pervasive and persistent patterns of social and interpersonal difficulties and eccentric cognitive patterns, but their symptom presentations are insufficient in severity to meet the criteria for frank psychosis. The primary difference between schizotypy and schizotypal PD is that a diagnosis of schizotypal PD does not necessarily imply a risk for the development of frank psychosis (Lenzenweger, 2006).

While the diagnostic categories in Section II include many constructs similar to schizotypy, Section III (Emerging Measures and Models) offers two conceptualizations that are more closely aligned with schizotypy. These include attenuated psychosis syndrome (APS) and the alternative model of personality disorders (AMPD). The diagnosis of attenuated psychosis syndrome grew out of decades of research into risk for schizophrenia, including schizotypy research (Woods et al., 2010). Emerging research suggests that identifying and intervening with people at risk for psychosis could delay the onset, improve the course, and possibly prevent the onset of psychosis (e.g., Fusar-Poli et al., 2019). Thus, the main purpose of this diagnosis is to identify and appropriately treat people at risk for psychosis. The syndrome is marked by attenuated psychotic symptoms that are distressing and have a recent onset or exacerbation but are not severe enough to meet criterion A for schizophrenia.

Attenuated psychosis syndrome is similar to schizotypy in that assessment for both aim to identify people at risk for psychosis. However, there are major differences in how these are operationalized. First, schizotypy research is built on the idea that the majority of people with schizotypy will not ultimately develop schizophrenia over the course of their lifetimes (Kwapil & Barrantes-Vidal, 2015; Meehl, 1990). Thus, if the assessment of schizotypy was 100% accurate, still only 10% of those identified would develop schizophrenia. In contrast, the APS approach aims to identify individuals who are at imminent risk for psychosis (e.g., within 6 months to 2 years). If this approach was 100% accurate, everyone identified as at-risk would develop schizophrenia in the absence of preventative treatment. As a result, schizotypy screening aims to identify people in the premorbid stage, while APS assessment aims to identify people in the prodromal stage who are already beginning to experience symptoms (Addington et al., 2015).

Another critical difference between schizotypy and APS is that schizotypy is primarily a research tool, but APS is also a clinical tool used as a diagnosis. People identified as having schizotypy in research studies are typically recruited from the general population, but individuals with APS are typically treatment-seeking individuals and recruited from clinics (Debbané et al., 2015). Previous research comparing the approaches has corroborated these differences. In a sample of undergraduates, over 70% of individuals identified as having schizotypy met criterion A for APS in that they had at least one clinically significant attenuated psychotic symptom (Cicero et al., 2014). However, nearly all of these individuals either did not experience significant distress as a result of their symptoms or did not have an onset or exacerbation of symptoms in the last 6 months as required for an APS diagnosis. Thus, the schizotypy approach identifies similar symptoms to the APS approach but also identifies a much wider group of individuals whose experiences are similar in some ways and different in others.

The second aspect of Section III in the DSM that is consistent with schizotypy is the Alternative Model of Personality Disorders (AMPD). The AMPD is a new conceptualization of personality disorders, which defines them dimensionally based on levels of maladaptive personality traits, including five domains (i.e., psychoticism, detachment, antagonism, constraint, and negative affectivity) and twenty-five facets within these five domains. HiTOP, discussed below, was designed in a similar manner, with thought disorder, detachment, antagonistic externalizing, disinhibited externalizing, and internalizing spectra mapping directly onto these domains (Kotov et al., 2017). Thus, multidimensional schizotypy is represented in the AMPD primarily in the psychoticism (positive and disorganized schizotypy) and detachment (negative schizotypy) domains in the same way that it is represented in HiTOP. The psychoticism domain includes three pathological personality traits, including cognitive and perceptual dysregulation, unusual beliefs and experiences, and eccentricity. Thus, cognitive and perceptual dysregulation and eccentricity correspond to disorganized schizotypy, and unusual beliefs and experiences correspond to positive schizotypy. Several of the detachment personality traits correspond to aspects of negative schizotypy, including restricted affectivity, withdrawal, intimacy avoidance, anhedonia, and suspiciousness.

Schizotypy and the International Classification of Diseases

In contrast to the ubiquitous use of the DSM nosology in clinical research, the World Health Organization's (WHO) International Classification of Diseases (ICD) system is far more commonly used in clinical practice across international settings (Clark et al., 2017). ICD diagnoses often provide the basis for the provision of medical services, facilitating healthcare access for individuals who meet diagnostic criteria. Trends in healthcare (e.g., more structured administrative demands of services, electronic record-keeping, and evidence-based practices) promote the increased integration of the ICD with clinical processes. The primary objective for the ICD is similar to the DSM—matching clinical syndromes to evidence-based treatment (Clark et al., 2017).

The ICD-11, published in 2022, is the most recent iteration and encompasses revisions that prioritize global applicability, empirical evidence, and clinical utility. The Mental, Behavioural or Neurodevelopmental Disorders chapter (MBND) of the ICD-11's Clinical Descriptions and Diagnostic Guidelines version provides detailed descriptions and codes that guide clinicians in diagnosing and treating psychopathology. Similar to the most recent DSM editions, the ICD-11 shifts toward dimensional assessments of psychopathology by specifying course and symptom qualifiers that aim to address longitudinal instability and prognostic invalidity of clinical diagnoses. The ICD-11's organization of personality disorders signals a paradigm shift from a categorical to a dimensional approach. The diagnostic categories of specific personality disorders outlined in previous ICD editions have been replaced by an all-inclusive code for personality pathology. In addition to specifiers for symptom severity, personality functioning for an individual is assessed in the ICD-11 across five domains (i.e., negative affectivity, dissociality, anankastia, detachment, and disinhibition), which corresponds well with the DSM's AMPD. Notably, psychoticism is not included as a trait in the ICD because these traits relate to schizotypal disorder, which is not considered a personality disorder in the ICD.

The Schizophrenia, Schizotypal and Delusional Disorders subchapter in the ICD-10 was renamed the Schizophrenia or Other Primary Psychotic Disorders subchapter, diagnostic criteria for schizophrenia-spectrum disorders were updated, and schizophrenia subtypes were eliminated. Disorders outlined within this subchapter vary in severity among six symptom domains (i.e., positive symptoms, negative symptoms, depressive mood symptoms, manic mood symptoms, psychomotor symptoms, and cognitive symptoms) and are largely homologous to the DSM-5-TR's schizophrenia-spectrum disorders.

The symptoms defining schizotypal PD in the DSM are included in schizotypal disorder in the ICD-11. Despite the similarity in symptoms and descriptions, the theoretical differences between schizotypal *personality* disorder and schizotypal disorder are substantial. As mentioned, the DSM includes schizotypal PD in both the psychotic disorders section and the personality disorders section. The ICD, in comparison, explicitly states that the primary difference between schizophrenia and schizotypal disorder is the severity of the symptoms, which implies a psychosis continuum and is consistent with the quasi- and fully-dimensional models of schizotypy (Handest & Parnas, 2005). Moreover, the ICD asserts that schizotypal disorder has a chronic and stable course and that individuals with the diagnosis rarely develop schizophrenia. However, several studies have shown that people with schizotypal disorder are more likely to develop schizophrenia (e.g., Nordentoft et al., 2006)

Schizotypy and the Hierarchical Taxonomy of Psychopathology

The Hierarchical Taxonomy of Psychopathology (Kotov et al., 2017) is an international consortium of psychopathology nosologists that aims to improve upon traditional diagnostic systems, such as the DSM and ICD. As shown in Fig. 3.1 (Forbes & Wright, 2020), the General Factor of Psychopathology (p-factor) is at the top of the hierarchy and represents the commonality of all psychopathology. Under the p-factor are three superspectra, including the psychosis, externalizing, and internalizing superspectra (Kotov et al., 2020; Krueger et al., 2021; Watson et al., 2022).[1] The next level comprises six spectra, including thought disorder, detachment, internalizing, antagonistic externalizing, disinhibited externalizing, and somatoform. Below the spectra are subfactors and dimensional syndromes, followed by homogenous symptom components and maladaptive traits. The bottom level includes individual signs, symptoms, and maladaptive behaviors. Figure 3.1 also shows a link between the HiTOP model and traditional diagnoses in the DSM.

[1] The official working model does not include the psychotic and internalizing superspectra, but these superspectra have been proposed in a series of manuscripts (Kotov et al., 2020; Watson et al., 2022).

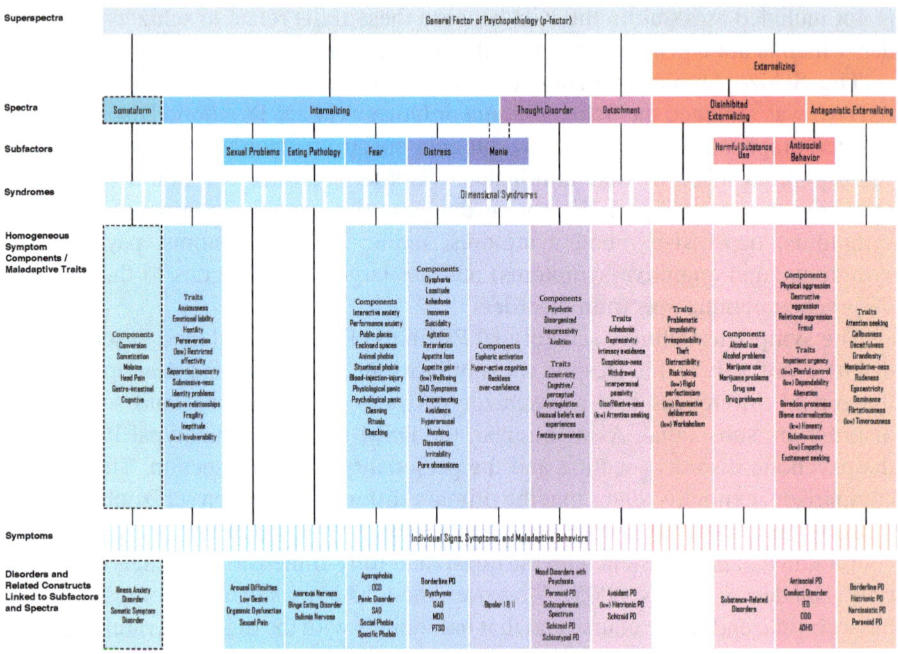

Official HiTOP Figure. This figure depicts the full current official HiTOP framework. Dashed lines indicate dimensions included as provisional aspects of the framework. This figure is published under creative commons by 4.0 by Miri Forbes and Aidan Wright. The model is continuously updated and available at https://osf.io/gds3n

Abbreviations: ADHD, attention-deficit/hyperactivity disorder; GAD, generalized anxiety disorder; IED, intermittent explosive disorder; MDD, major depressive disorder; OCD, obsessive–compulsive disorder; ODD, oppositional defiant disorder; PD, personality disorder; PTSD, posttraumatic stress disorder; SAD, separation anxiety disorder.

Fig. 3.1 Official HiTOP Working Model (Published under creative commons 4.0 by Miri Forbes and Aidan Wright)

A key similarity between schizotypy and HiTOP is that both represent an attempt to deal with the well-known limitations of traditional nosologies. These limitations include (a) heterogeneity in symptoms among people diagnosed with the same disorder, (b) excessive comorbidity among disorders, (c) arbitrary borders between what is considered psychopathology and what is considered normal, and (d) inability to account for subthreshold cases, among others. HiTOP addresses these limitations by accounting for psychopathology dimensionally and hierarchically, which are the two cardinal features of the model.

Schizotypy is broadly consistent with both of these features. It is a narrower construct than HiTOP in that it explains only psychosis-spectrum psychopathology, while HiTOP attempts to explain all manifestations of psychopathology. However, schizotypy and HiTOP deal with the heterogeneity of psychosis-spectrum pathology in a similar manner. Schizotypy can also be conceptualized as having a hierarchical structure with a general schizotypy factor at the top, followed by positive, negative, disorganized schizotypy factors and specific signs and symptoms at the bottom of the hierarchy. The psychosis superspectrum in HiTOP is similar to the general schizotypy factor, and the thought disorder and detachment spectra are similar to positive and negative schizotypy, respectively. The thought disorder spectrum is sometimes confused with "formal thought disorder," which is characterized by disordered thinking and speech (Kerns & Berenbaum, 2003). Within HiTOP, the symptoms associated with formal thought disorder are termed "disorganization" and located on the thought disorder spectrum. Thus, multidimensional schizotypy fits well with this model; constructs comprising positive and disorganized schizotypy are included in thought disorder, and constructs comprising negative schizotypy are included on the detachment spectrum. These similarities are a result of decades of research into the heterogeneity of schizotypy and psychotic-spectrum psychopathology influencing the conceptualization of the HiTOP model.

The hierarchical organization of HiTOP addresses the first two limitations of other diagnostic systems (i.e., heterogeneity among people diagnosed with the same disorder and excessive comorbidity seen in categorical systems). Similar to psychopathology more broadly, schizotypy includes a wide variety of seemingly disparate symptoms that co-occur more often than would be expected if the symptoms represent distinct disorders with distinct causes (Krueger & Markon, 2006). For example, Meehl's original checklist included anhedonia, ambivalence, body image aberrations, cognitive slippage, flat affect, magical ideation, deflated self-esteem, and narcissism, among many other features (Meehl, 1973). Contemporary researchers describe this constellation of symptoms as multidimensional, including positive, negative, and disorganized symptoms, all under the umbrella of schizotypy. Within HiTOP, this heterogeneity is captured by levels of thought disorder and detachment traits and symptoms, rather than a diagnosis such as schizophrenia. Comorbidity is also built into the system so that symptoms that often co-occur are grouped together on the same spectra (Kotov et al., 2021). For example, avoidant and schizoid personality disorders are often comorbid in clinical and general population samples (Sanislow et al., 2012), and the symptoms of both disorders would be included on the detachment spectrum in HiTOP.

Schizotypy is broadly consistent with the dimensional structure of HiTOP, but there is some debate about whether it is better understood as a categorical taxon or a dimensional individual difference variable (Mason, 2014). These approaches are referred to as the quasi-dimensional and fully-dimensional models, respectively. Dating back to Paul Meehl (1962), the quasi-dimensional model posits that there is a discrete taxon with a prevalence rate of about 10% of the population, and that individuals within that taxon vary dimensionally from subclinical symptoms through frank psychosis. Ten percent of people within the taxon develop full-blown schizophrenia, resulting in a prevalence rate of 1% for schizophrenia in the general population (Meehl, 1962). This categorical conceptualization was based, in part, on his hypothesis that schizophrenia-spectrum pathology is caused by a single gene called "schizogene" (Meehl, 1990). Phenotypic expressions of this gene then interacted with environmental factors to determine whether the individual would decompensate into schizophrenia or maintain less severely expressed schizotypy. He later revised his theory to suggest that schizotypy is caused by several genes (i.e., polygenic potentiators), which is closer to the current consensus that schizophrenia is related to many different genes (e.g., Giegling et al., 2017; Kato et al., 2022). Indeed, several studies aiming to resolve this debate have concluded that schizotypy is taxonic, with prevalence estimates similar to Meehl's original conjecture of 10% (Golden & Meehl, 1979; Korfine & Lenzenweger, 1995; Rawlings et al., 2008).

In contrast, the fully-dimensional model posits that schizotypy is continuously distributed throughout the population (Grant et al., 2018). This approach is more consistent with HiTOP, which clearly conceptualizes the psychosis spectrum in the same way. Evidence that psychosis is continuous has mounted in the 60 years since Meehl originally presented his theory. For example, psychotic and psychotic-like symptoms have been shown to exist in the general population at much higher rates than would be expected if schizotypy were a discrete entity with approximately a 10% prevalence rate (Hanssen et al., 2005; Linscott & van Os, 2010). The dimensional approach is also consistent with the etiological evidence, which has failed to find specific genes or biomarkers with strong enough effects to produce a taxon (Collins et al., 2012; Nelson et al., 2013). Moreover, schizotypy has been shown to have the same multidimensional structure as schizophrenia (Vollema & van den Bosch, 1995) and to be related to the same genes (Walter et al., 2016), cognitive and social-cognitive deficits (Miller & Lenzenweger, 2012), social and environmental factors (O'Hare et al., 2022), and neuroanatomical abnormalities (Mittal et al., 2007; van der Meer et al., 2013). Thus, decades of research show that schizotypy has a dimensional relationship with frank psychosis.

Dimensional models ameliorate the other two limitations of traditional nosologies, including the inability to account for subthreshold cases and the artificial boundary between disorder and non-disorder. Under HiTOP, individuals are given scores on dimensional traits and symptoms rather than present/absent diagnoses (Kotov et al., 2017). Categorical decisions about treatment still need to be made (e.g., level of care and whether to treat at all), but these decisions are typically made based on distress and impairment, in addition to symptom severity. Subthreshold symptoms are accounted for in the system in the same manner because a dichotomy is not made between disorder and non-disorder. The fully dimensional approach to schizotypy deals with both of these issues in the same manner; symptoms are quantified on a spectrum, and people are not dichotomized by schizotypy presentation (Kwapil & Barrantes-Vidal, 2015).

The quasi-dimensional model of schizotypy, by definition, contradicts this basic tenet of HiTOP by drawing a distinction between people in the schizotypy taxon and everyone else. This presents an issue with case-control design research or what researchers have termed the psychometric high-risk approach (Lenzenweger, 1994). In this approach, participants are typically identified as having high schizotypy based on their scores on self-report measures, such as the Magical Ideation, Perceptual Aberration, and Revised Social Anhedonia Scales (Kwapil, 1998). These participants are then compared to a group of participants with moderate-to-low scores on these measures. This approach creates a similar problem to the DSM and ICD systems because people near the boundary are categorized into different groups despite little substantive differences between individuals.

Despite the considerable differences in theory between HiTOP and the quasi-dimensional approach to schizotypy, both systems stress the importance of subthreshold cases. The key similarity between HiTOP and both approaches to schizotypy is that they account for far more psychopathology than just individuals meeting the criteria for DSM or ICD diagnoses, such as schizophrenia and schizotypal (personality) disorder. Although schizotypy researchers aim to "carve nature at its joints" (i.e., separate disorder from non-disorder), schizotypy is primarily a research tool, and these categorizations do not have the same real-world impact that a clinical diagnosis would have in a treatment setting.

As mentioned, both the quasi- and fully-dimensional schizotypy approaches recognize that psychosis exists on a spectrum (Mason, 2014), and schizotypy researchers tend to focus on the lower end of the spectrum (Kwapil & Barrantes-Vidal, 2015). Within HiTOP, the difference in severity is arguably conceptualized as symptoms versus traits, with symptoms representing the more severe end of the spectrum and traits representing the less severe end. Recent research suggests that psychoticism traits and psychotic symptoms are part of the same spectrum in large samples of people with chronic serious mental illness (Cicero et al., 2019). In this study, a factor model in which positive schiztoypy loaded with psychotic symptoms fit better than a factor model in which positive schizotypy formed a separate factor distinct from symptoms. Moreover, the same was true for negative schizotypy, which loaded alongside negative symptoms and (low) extraversion on a negative factor.

The fully dimensional model allows for the possibility of "happy" or "benign" schizotypes who are high on the positive dimension but low on the negative and disorganized dimensions (Mohr & Claridge, 2015). Happy/benign schizotypes experience the traits and symptoms associated with positive schizotypy in a pleasant way, such as creativity or openness to experience. Indeed, studies have consistently shown that positive schizotypy is associated with increased creativity (Acar & Sen, 2013). This idea has historically been controversial, with some researchers suggesting that all aspects of schizotypy are experienced as distressing (e.g., Lenzenweger, 2018). However, many people with lived experience of psychosis-spectrum disorders report experiences similar to the happy schizotypy model. For example, the Hearing Voices Network is an international movement led by people who experience auditory hallucinations and includes the possibility of benign or adaptive positive symptoms as one of its core principles (Styron et al., 2017). Happy/benign schizotypy is consistent with the HiTOP model and AMPD because these individuals would have high scores on the thought disorder (HiTOP) and psychoticism (AMPD) dimensions but low scores on the detachment domain (both models). Moreover, happy schizotypes have low levels of impairment, which is rated separately in HiTOP. In contrast, this cannot be accounted for with Section II DSM constructs because these constructs are heterogenous and defined by a combination of positive, negative, and disorganized symptoms.

Although the term "schizotypy" does not appear in Fig. 3.1 or in any official HiTOP figures, all constructs considered to be part of schizotypy are captured within the model. The thought disorder spectrum within HiTOP includes symptoms of DSM/ICD syndromes such as schizophrenia, schizoaffective disorder, schizotypal (personality) disorder, and mood disorders with psychotic features, among others. The next level includes homogeneous symptom components and maladaptive traits such as psychotic symptoms (e.g., hallucinations, delusions, and cognitive distortions), disorganization (e.g., incoherent and tangential speech, illogical or circumstantial thinking, and unusual behavior or appearance), inexpressivity (e.g., decreased expression of emotion including alogia, limited vocal intonation, flat or blunted affect, and poor eye contact), and avolition (i.e., lack of motivation to engage in goal-directed behavior, maintain relationships or work, and self-care and hygiene). These symptoms represent the severe end of the schizotypy spectrum.

The conceptualization of schizotypy is most closely represented with the maladaptive traits within HiTOP. Positive, negative, and disorganized schizotypy are each composed of multiple traits and symptoms, and maladaptive traits on the thought disorder spectrum in HiTOP closely correspond to positive and disorganized schizotypy. Positive schizotypy is conceptualized within HiTOP as unusual beliefs (i.e., the tendency to hold unfounded and irrational thoughts, beliefs, and ideas about the world) and unusual experiences (i.e., perceptual distortions that do not correspond to reality, aberrant salience, and dissociation or detachment from reality, one's surroundings, or oneself). The constructs correspond closely to magical ideation and perceptual aberration, respectively. Moreover, cognitive-perceptual dysregulation (i.e., uncommon or unusual thought processes, such as dissociative experiences, derealization, and depersonalization) and fantasy proneness (e.g., inclination to excessively daydream, fantasize, and become engrossed in one's thoughts and experiences) are both part of the thought disorder spectrum in HiTOP and positive schizotypy. Disorganized schizotypy is similar to eccentricity in HiTOP, which is defined as strange, unusual, or bizarre appearance, behavior, speech, or thought. A related construct, cognitive slippage, is commonly seen as part of disorganized schizotypy and is included within the thought disorder spectrum of HiTOP (Gooding et al., 2001).

Negative schizotypy includes several different traits, such as social anhedonia, physical anhedonia, constricted affect, and reduced emotional expression. Within HiTOP, these are defined as social withdrawal (i.e., avoidance of interpersonal interactions and a preference for being alone that is underscored by a genuine disinterest in interacting with others), romantic disinterest (i.e., a general lack of interest in, desire for, and enjoyment of sex, eroticism, and interpersonal intimacy), anhedonia (i.e., general deficits in positive emotions and energy levels, with diminished experience of joy and excitement), emotional detachment (i.e., the tendency to be emotionally distant and reserved), and (low) exhibitionism (i.e., preference for not being the center of attention or drawing the attention of others). In summary, positive and disorganized schizotypy are well-represented in the thought disorder spectrum of HiTOP, and negative schizotypy is represented in the detachment domain.

Two other constructs that commonly co-occur with schizotypy are paranoia/suspiciousness and mania. However, it is presently unclear where they fit within both HiTOP and schizotypy. Within HiTOP, suspiciousness is provisionally located within the detachment domain (Kotov et al., 2017), reflecting the influence of the Alternative Model of Personality Disorders, which also subsumes suspiciousness within detachment (American Psychiatric Association, 2022). At the same time, most factor analytic studies of schizotypy have found that suspiciousness forms a separate factor distinct from positive, negative, and disorganized schizotypy (e.g., Cicero & Kerns, 2010a or b; Stefanis et al., 2004). Thus, it is unclear whether suspiciousness belongs to the detachment or thought disorder domain. Alternatively, some research has suggested that suspiciousness does not belong with schizotypy at all and instead belongs with antagonism (Lynam & Widiger, 2001).

Mania is provisionally included in both the thought disorder and internalizing domains in HiTOP, and a work group was established specifically to determine its placement (Kotov et al., 2021). Kraepelin originally proposed a dichotomy between dementia praecox (i.e., what is now called schizophrenia) and manic depression (i.e., what is now called bipolar disorder; Kendler, 1986). However, researchers have debated whether his dichotomy is accurate for more than 100 years since its conception. Hypomania, a milder form of mania, often co-occurs with schizotypy (Kwapil et al., 2000). Although, factor analytic studies on schizotypy have generally found that mania forms a separate factor from positive schizotypy (Hua & Kerns, 2018; Preti et al., 2015). Similarly, research has been mixed on whether dissociation is distinct from or a part of positive schizotypy (Cicero & Kerns, 2010b; Watson, 2003). Within HiTOP, dissociation has been tentatively hypothesized to be part of the psychosis superspectrum, but the official model (see Fig. 3.1) places dissociation in the distress subfactor of the internalizing spectrum. Future work will clarify where these constructs belong within the HiTOP model.

Summary and Conclusions

Despite the term "schizotypy" not appearing in the DSM, the ICD, or HiTOP, the conceptualization of schizotypy is well represented in these diagnostic systems. As mentioned, schizotypy has two primary characteristics, including being a description of traits and symptoms similar to schizophrenia but in a diminished form and representing a risk for the development of schizophrenia. All three diagnostic systems include descriptive constructs that are similar to positive, negative, and disorganized schizotypy. Moreover, all three systems recognize at least some degree of dimensionality in the constructs. However, HiTOP best captures the dimensional nature of schizotypy and the emphasis on subthreshold cases, while the attenuated psychosis syndrome in the DSM best captures the psychosis proneness aspect of schizotypy.

References

Acar, S., & Sen, S. (2013). A multilevel meta-analysis of the relationship between creativity and schizotypy. *Psychology of Aesthetics, Creativity, and the Arts, 7*(3), 214–228. https://doi.org/10.1037/a0031975

Addington, J., Liu, L., Buchy, L., Cadenhead, K. S., Cannon, T. D., Cornblatt, B. A., Perkins, D. O., Seidman, L. J., Tsuang, M. T., & Walker, E. F. (2015). North American Prodrome

Longitudinal Study (NAPLS 2): The prodromal symptoms. *The Journal of Nervous and Mental Disease, 203*(5), 328–335.
American Psychiatric Association. (1952). *Diagnostic and statistical manual of mental disorders (1st ed.).*
American Psychiatric Association. (2013). *Diagnostic and statistical manual of mental disorders* (5th ed.). https://doi.org/10.1176/appi.books.9780890425596
American Psychiatric Association (Ed.). (2022). *Diagnostic and statistical manual of mental disorders: DSM-5-TR* (Fifth edition, text revision). American Psychiatric Association Publishing.
Chapman, J. (1966). The early symptoms of schizophrenia. *The British Journal of Psychiatry, 112*(484), 225–251.
Chapman, L. J., & Chapman, J. P. (1980). Scales for rating psychotic and psychotic-like experiences as continua. *Schizophrenia Bulletin, 6*(3), 477–489.
Chapman, L. J., Chapman, J. P., & Raulin, M. L. (1976). Scales for physical and social anhedonia. *Journal of Abnormal Psychology, 85*, 374–382. https://doi.org/10.1037/0021-843x.85.4.374
Cicero, D. C., & Kerns, J. G. (2010a). Multidimensional factor structure of positive schizotypy. *Journal of Personality Disorders, 24*(3), 327–343. https://doi.org/10.1521/pedi.2010.24.3.327
Cicero, D. C., & Kerns, J. G. (2010b). Can disorganized and positive schizotypy be discriminated from dissociation? *Journal of Personality, 78*(4), 1239–1270. https://doi.org/10.1111/j.1467-6494.2010.00649.x
Cicero, D. C., Martin, E. A., Becker, T. M., Docherty, A. R., & Kerns, J. G. (2014). Correspondence between psychometric and clinical high risk for psychosis in an undergraduate population. *Psychological Assessment, 26*(3), 901–915. https://doi.org/10.1037/a0036432
Cicero, D. C., Jonas, K. G., Li, K., Perlman, G., & Kotov, R. (2019). Common taxonomy of traits and symptoms: Linking schizophrenia symptoms, schizotypy, and normal personality. *Schizophrenia Bulletin*. https://doi.org/10.1093/schbul/sbz005
Clark, L. A., Cuthbert, B., Lewis-Fernández, R., Narrow, W. E., & Reed, G. M. (2017). Three approaches to understanding and classifying mental disorder: *ICD-11, DSM-5*, and the National Institute of Mental Health's Research Domain Criteria (RDoC). *Psychological Science in the Public Interest, 18*(2), 72–145. https://doi.org/10.1177/1529100617727266
Collins, A. L., Kim, Y., Sklar, P., & International Schizophrenia Consortium, O'Donovan, M. C., & Sullivan, P. F. (2012). Hypothesis-driven candidate genes for schizophrenia compared to genome-wide association results. *Psychological Medicine, 42*(3), 607–616. https://doi.org/10.1017/S0033291711001607
Debbané, M., Eliez, S., Badoud, D., Conus, P., Flückiger, R., & Schultze-Lutter, F. (2015). Developing psychosis and its risk states through the lens of schizotypy. *Schizophrenia Bulletin, 41*(suppl 2), S396–S407.
Forbes, M. K., & Wright, A. G. C. (2020, November 02). *Official HiTOP working model* [Figure]. Open Science Framework. https://osf.io/gds3n
Fusar-Poli, P., Sullivan, S. A., Shah, J. L., & Uhlhaas, P. J. (2019). Improving the detection of individuals at clinical risk for psychosis in the community, primary and secondary care: An integrated evidence-based approach. *Frontiers in Psychiatry, 10*(774). https://doi.org/10.3389/fpsyt.2019.00774
Giegling, I., Hosak, L., Mössner, R., Serretti, A., Bellivier, F., Claes, S., Collier, D. A., Corrales, A., DeLisi, L. E., Gallo, C., Gill, M., Kennedy, J. L., Leboyer, M., Maier, W., Marquez, M., Massat, I., Mors, O., Muglia, P., Nöthen, M. M., et al. (2017). Genetics of schizophrenia: A consensus paper of the WFSBP task force on genetics. *The World Journal of Biological Psychiatry: The Official Journal of the World Federation of Societies of Biological Psychiatry, 18*(7), 492–505. https://doi.org/10.1080/15622975.2016.1268715
Golden, R. R., & Meehl, P. E. (1979). Detection of the schizoid taxon with MMPI indicators. *Journal of Abnormal Psychology, 88*, 217–233.
Gooding, D. C., Tallent, K. A., & Hegyi, J. V. (2001). Cognitive slippage in schizotypic individuals. *Journal of Nervous and Mental Disease, 189*, 750–756.

Grant, P., Green, M. J., & Mason, O. J. (2018). Models of Schizotypy: The importance of conceptual clarity. *Schizophrenia Bulletin, 44*(suppl_2), S556–S563. https://doi.org/10.1093/schbul/sby012

Handest, P., & Parnas, J. (2005). Clinical characteristics of first-admitted patients with ICD-10 schizotypal disorder. *British Journal of Psychiatry, 187*(S48), s49–s54. https://doi.org/10.1192/bjp.187.48.s49

Hanssen, M., Bak, M., Bijl, R., Vollebergh, W., & van Os, J. (2005). The incidence and outcome of subclinical psychotic experiences in the general population. *The British Journal of Clinical Psychology, 44*(Pt 2), 181–191. https://doi.org/10.1348/014466505X29611

Hewitt, J. K., & Claridge, G. S. (1989). The factor structure of schizotypy in a normal population. *Personality and Individual Differences, 10*, 323–329.

Hua, J. P. Y., & Kerns, J. G. (2018). Differentiating positive schizotypy and mania risk scales and their associations with spontaneous eye blink rate. *Psychiatry Research, 264*, 58–66. https://doi.org/10.1016/j.psychres.2018.03.068

Kato, H., Kimura, H., Kushima, I., Takahashi, N., Aleksic, B., & Ozaki, N. (2022). The genetic architecture of schizophrenia: Review of large-scale genetic studies. *Journal of Human Genetics*, 1–8. https://doi.org/10.1038/s10038-022-01059-4

Kendler, K. S. (1986). Kraepelin and the differential diagnosis of dementia praecox and manic-depressive insanity. *Comprehensive Psychiatry, 27*(6), 549–558. https://doi.org/10.1016/0010-440X(86)90059-3

Kerns, J. G., & Berenbaum, H. (2003). The relationship between formal thought disorder and executive functioning component processes. *Journal of Abnormal Psychology, 112*, 339–352. https://doi.org/10.1037/0021-843x.112.3.339

Korfine, L., & Lenzenweger, M. F. (1995). The taxonicity of schizotypy: A replication. *Journal of Abnormal Psychology, 104*(1), 26–31.

Kotov, R., Krueger, R. F., Watson, D., Achenbach, T. M., Althoff, R. R., Bagby, R. M., Brown, T. A., Carpenter, W. T., Caspi, A., Clark, L. A., Eaton, N. R., Forbes, M. K., Forbush, K. T., Goldberg, D., Hasin, D., Hyman, S. E., Ivanova, M. Y., Lynam, D. R., Markon, K., et al. (2017). The Hierarchical Taxonomy of Psychopathology (HiTOP): A dimensional alternative to traditional nosologies. *Journal of Abnormal Psychology, 126*(4), 454–477. https://doi.org/10.1037/abn0000258

Kotov, R., Jonas, K. G., Carpenter, W. T., Dretsch, M. N., Eaton, N. R., Forbes, M. K., Forbush, K. T., Hobbs, K., Reininghaus, U., Slade, T., South, S. C., Sunderland, M., Waszczuk, M. A., Widiger, T. A., Wright, A. G. C., Zald, D. H., Krueger, R. F., Watson, D., & HiTOP Utility Workgroup. (2020). Validity and utility of Hierarchical Taxonomy of Psychopathology (HiTOP): I. Psychosis superspectrum. *World Psychiatry, 19*(2), 151–172. https://doi.org/10.1002/wps.20730

Kotov, R., Krueger, R. F., Watson, D., Cicero, D. C., Conway, C. C., DeYoung, C. G., Eaton, N. R., Forbes, M. K., Hallquist, M. N., Latzman, R. D., Mullins-Sweatt, S. N., Ruggero, C. J., Simms, L. J., Waldman, I. D., Waszczuk, M. A., & Wright, A. G. C. (2021). The Hierarchical Taxonomy of Psychopathology (HiTOP): A quantitative nosology based on consensus of evidence. *Annual Review of Clinical Psychology, 17*, 83–108. https://doi.org/10.1146/annurev-clinpsy-081219-093304

Krueger, R. F., & Markon, K. E. (2006). Reinterpreting comorbidity: A model-based approach to understanding and classifying psychopathology. *Annual Review of Clinical Psychology, 2*, 111–133.

Krueger, R. F., Hobbs, K. A., Conway, C. C., Dick, D. M., Dretsch, M. N., Eaton, N. R., Forbes, M. K., Forbush, K. T., Keyes, K. M., Latzman, R. D., Michelini, G., Patrick, C. J., Sellbom, M., Slade, T., South, S. C., Sunderland, M., Tackett, J., Waldman, I., Waszczuk, M. A., et al. (2021). Validity and utility of Hierarchical Taxonomy of Psychopathology (HiTOP): II. Externalizing superspectrum. *World Psychiatry, 20*(2), 171–193. https://doi.org/10.1002/wps.20844

Kwapil, T. R. (1998). Social anhedonia as a predictor of the development of schizophrenia-spectrum disorders. *Journal of Abnormal Psychology, 107*, 558–565. https://doi.org/10.1037/0021-843X.107.4.558

Kwapil, T. R., & Barrantes-Vidal, N. (2015). Schizotypy: Looking back and moving forward. *Schizophrenia Bulletin, 41*(Suppl 2), S366–S373. https://doi.org/10.1093/schbul/sbu186

Kwapil, T. R., Miller, M. B., Zinser, M. C., Chapman, L. J., Chapman, J., & Eckblad, M. (2000). A longitudinal study of high scorers on the hypomanic personality scale. *Journal of Abnormal Psychology, 109*, 222–226.

Kwapil, T. R., Gross, G. M., Silvia, P. J., Raulin, M. L., & Barrantes-Vidal, N. (2018). Development and psychometric properties of the Multidimensional Schizotypy Scale: A new measure for assessing positive, negative, and disorganized schizotypy. *Schizophrenia Research, 193*, 209–217. https://doi.org/10.1016/j.schres.2017.07.001

Lenzenweger, M. F. (1994). Psychometric high-risk paradigm, perceptual aberrations, and schizotypy: An update. *Schizophrenia Bulletin, 20*(1), 121–135.

Lenzenweger, M. F. (2006). Schizotaxia, schizotypy, and schizophrenia: Paul E. Meehl's blueprint for the experimental psychopathology and genetics of schizophrenia. *Journal of Abnormal Psychology, 115*, 195–200. https://doi.org/10.1037/0021-843X.115.2.195

Lenzenweger, M. F. (2018). Schizotypy, Schizotypic psychopathology, and schizophrenia: Hearing echoes, leveraging prior advances, and probing new angles. *Schizophrenia Bulletin, 44*(Suppl 2), S564–S569. https://doi.org/10.1093/schbul/sby083

Linscott, R. J., & van Os, J. (2010). Systematic reviews of categorical versus continuum models in psychosis: Evidence for discontinuous subpopulations underlying a psychometric continuum. Implications for DSM-V, DSM-VI, and DSM-VII. *Annual Review of Clinical Psychology, 6*, 391–419. https://doi.org/10.1146/annurev.clinpsy.032408.153506

Lynam, D. R., & Widiger, T. A. (2001). Using thc five-factor model to represent the DSM-IV personality disorders: An expert consensus approach. *Journal of Abnormal Psychology, 110*, 401–412.

Maj, M. (2015). The media campaign on the DSM-5: Recurring comments and lessons for the future of diagnosis in psychiatric practice. *Epidemiology and Psychiatric Sciences, 24*(3), 197–202. https://doi.org/10.1017/S2045796014000572

Mason, O. J. (2014). The duality of Schizotypy: Is it both dimensional and categorical? *Frontiers in Psychiatry, 5*, 134. https://doi.org/10.3389/fpsyt.2014.00134

Meehl, P. E. (1962). Schizotaxia, schizotypy, and schizophrenia. *American Psychologist, 17*, 827–838.

Meehl, P. E. (1973). *Manual for use with checklist of schizotypic signs*.

Meehl, P. E. (1990). Toward an integrated theory of schizotaxia, schizotypy, and schizophrenia. *Journal of Personality Disorders, 4*, 1–99.

Miller, A. B., & Lenzenweger, M. F. (2012). Schizotypy, social cognition, and interpersonal sensitivity. *Personality Disorders: Theory, Research, and Treatment, 3*(4), 379–392. https://doi.org/10.1037/a0027955

Mittal, V. A., Dhruv, S., Tessner, K. D., Walder, D. J., & Walker, E. F. (2007). The relations among putative biorisk markers in schizotypal adolescents: Minor physical anomalies, movement abnormalities, and salivary cortisol. *Biological Psychiatry, 61*(10), 1179–1186. https://doi.org/10.1016/j.biopsych.2006.08.043

Mohr, C., & Claridge, G. (2015). Schizotypy—Do not worry, it is not all worrisome. *Schizophrenia Bulletin, 41 Suppl 2*(Suppl 2), S436–S443. https://doi.org/10.1093/schbul/sbu185

Nelson, M. T., Seal, M. L., Pantelis, C., & Phillips, L. J. (2013). Evidence of a dimensional relationship between schizotypy and schizophrenia: A systematic review. *Neuroscience & Biobehavioral Reviews, 37*(3), 317–327.

Nordentoft, M., Thorup, A., Petersen, L., Ohlenschlaeger, J., Melau, M., Christensen, T. Ø., Krarup, G., Jørgensen, P., & Jeppesen, P. (2006). Transition rates from schizotypal disorder to psychotic disorder for first-contact patients included in the OPUS trial. A randomized clinical trial of integrated treatment and standard treatment. *Schizophrenia Research, 83*(1), 29–40. https://doi.org/10.1016/j.schres.2006.01.002

O'Hare, K., Watkeys, O., Whitten, T., Dean, K., Laurens, K. R., Tzoumakis, S., Harris, F., Carr, V. J., & Green, M. J. (2022). Cumulative environmental risk in early life: Associations with Schizotypy in childhood. *Schizophrenia Bulletin*, sbac160. https://doi.org/10.1093/schbul/sbac160

Preti, A., Corrias, I., Gabbrielli, M., Lai, V., Muratore, T., Pintus, E., Pintus, M., Sanna, S., Scanu, R., Tronci, D., Vellante, M., Siddi, S., Petretto, D. R., & Carta, M. G. (2015). The independence of schizotypy from affective temperaments—A combined confirmatory factor analysis of SPQ and the short TEMPS-A. *Psychiatry Research, 225*(1–2), 145–156. https://doi.org/10.1016/j.psychres.2014.10.027

Raine, A., Reynolds, C., Lencz, T., Scerbo, A., Triphon, N., & Kim, D. (1994). Cognitive-perceptual, interpersonal, and disorganized features of schizotypal personality. *Schizophrenia Bulletin, 20*, 191–201.

Rawlings, D., Williams, B., Haslam, N., & Claridge, G. (2008). Taxometric analysis supports a dimensional latent structure for schizotypy. *Personality and Individual Differences, 44*(8), 1640–1651. https://doi.org/10.1016/j.paid.2007.06.005

Sanislow, C. A., da Cruz, K., Gianoli, M. O., & Reagan, E. (2012). Avoidant personality disorder, traits, and type. In *The Oxford handbook of personality disorders* (pp. 549–565). Oxford University Press. https://doi.org/10.1093/oxfordhb/9780199735013.013.0025

Stefanis, N. C., Smyrnis, N., Avramopoulos, D., Evdokimidis, I., Ntzoufras, I., & Stefanis, C. N. (2004). Factorial composition of self-rated schizotypal traits among young males undergoing military training. *Schizophrenia Bulletin, 30*(2), 335–350.

Styron, T., Davidson, L., & Utter, L. (2017). The hearing voices network: Initial lessons and future directions for mental health professionals and systems of care. *Psychiatric Quarterly, 88*(4), 769–785. https://doi.org/10.1007/s11126-017-9491-1

van der Meer, L., Groenewold, N. A., Pijnenborg, M., & Aleman, A. (2013). Psychosis-proneness and neural correlates of self-inhibition in theory of mind. *PLoS One, 8*(7), e67774. https://doi.org/10.1371/journal.pone.0067774

Vollema, M. G., & van den Bosch, R. J. (1995). The multidimensionality of schizotypy. *Schizophrenia Bulletin, 21*(1), 19–31. https://doi.org/10.1093/schbul/21.1.19

Walter, E. E., Fernandez, F., Snelling, M., & Barkus, E. (2016). Genetic consideration of schizotypal traits: A review. *Frontiers in Psychology, 7*. https://doi.org/10.3389/fpsyg.2016.01769

Watson, D. (2003). Investigating the construct validity of the dissociative taxon: Stability analyses of normal and pathological dissociation. *Journal of Abnormal Psychology, 112*(2), 298–305.

Watson, D., Levin-Aspenson, H. F., Waszczuk, M. A., Conway, C. C., Dalgleish, T., Dretsch, M. N., Eaton, N. R., Forbes, M. K., Forbush, K. T., Hobbs, K. A., Michelini, G., Nelson, B. D., Sellbom, M., Slade, T., South, S. C., Sunderland, M., Waldman, I., Witthöft, M., Wright, A. G. C., et al. (2022). Validity and utility of Hierarchical Taxonomy of Psychopathology (HiTOP): III. Emotional dysfunction superspectrum. *World Psychiatry, 21*(1), 26–54. https://doi.org/10.1002/wps.20943

Woods, S. W., Walsh, B. C., Saksa, J. R., & McGlashan, T. H. (2010). The case for including Attenuated Psychotic Symptoms Syndrome in DSM-5 as a psychosis risk syndrome. *Schizophrenia Research, 123*(2–3), 199–207. https://doi.org/10.1016/j.schres.2010.08.012

World Health Organization. (2022). *International Classification of Diseases Eleventh Revision (ICD-11).*

Chapter 4
Psychosocial Functioning in Schizotypy: Potential Links to Social, Cognitive, and Affective Processes

Kyle S. Minor, Jessica L. Mickens, Madisen T. Russell, Sophia C. Koesterer, Ceouna M. Hegwood, and Danielle B. Abel

Introduction

From the clothes we wear to the topics we discuss, the desire to connect with others drives human behavior. Some people, however, have difficulty making these connections. Deficits in social functioning are a core feature of schizophrenia and other psychotic disorders. These deficits extend to those high in schizotypy (Abu-Akel et al., 2018), a group at greater risk for psychotic and other psychopathological disorders (Gooding et al., 2005). Deficits in social functioning are distressing, as they are linked to lower quality of life (Minor & Cohen, 2010) and cited by people with schizophrenia as a primary treatment target (Shumway et al., 2003).

Those high in schizotypy have shown deficits across various social behaviors: they endorse fewer prosocial behaviors on self-report scales (Luther et al., 2023), make more errors on laboratory-based theory of mind tasks (Wastler & Lenzenweger, 2021), and are less likely to socialize in daily life (Minor et al., 2020). Many potential explanations have been given as to why those high in schizotypy experience deficits in social functioning. Yet, there is not a prevailing consensus in the literature.

This chapter aims to increase understanding of why deficits in social functioning occur in people high in schizotypy. To begin, we summarize findings from schizotypy studies and focus on how methods used to assess schizotypy and social functioning can lead to discrepant—or even conflicting—results. Then, we discuss four

K. S. Minor (✉)
Department of Psychology, Indiana University- Purdue University Indianapolis, Indianapolis, IN, USA

IUPUI School of Science, Indianapolis, IN, USA
e-mail: ksminor@iupui.edu

J. L. Mickens · M. T. Russell · S. C. Koesterer · C. M. Hegwood · D. B. Abel
Department of Psychology, Indiana University- Purdue University Indianapolis, Indianapolis, IN, USA

S. Cheli, P. H. Lysaker (eds.), *A Dimensional Approach to Schizotypy*, https://doi.org/10.1007/978-3-031-41788-7_4

potential explanations to help clarify why social functioning deficits occur. Each explanation focuses on deficits in other social, cognitive, or affective processes, including (1) social skills deficits, (2) cognitive deficits, (3) anticipated pleasure deficits, and (4) emotion regulation deficits. Note that these explanations are not mutually exclusive nor do they encompass all theories provided across the literature. Each is compelling, however, and has the potential to increase our understanding about the mechanisms underlying social functioning deficits in schizotypy. Finally, we discuss how the field can better understand social deficits in the future.

Social Functioning Deficits in Schizotypy: What We Know So Far

Deficits in social functioning are typically in the small to moderate effect size range when those high in schizotypy are compared to those low in schizotypy (Aghvinian & Sergi, 2018; Dinzeo et al., 2018; Minor et al., 2018)—less severe than the large differences found in schizophrenia (Abel & Minor, 2021)—and the size frequently depends on how schizotypy and social functioning are assessed. Regarding measurement of schizotypy, a significant hurdle is the heterogeneity of schizotypy traits. Thus, researchers typically examine schizotypy in one of two ways: by combining all schizotypy traits into a total score (i.e., general approach) or separating traits into individual factors (i.e., specific approach).

Using a general approach, researchers have observed links between increased affective reactivity and worse social functioning (Marggraf et al., 2019), found those high in schizotypy show less activation in the prefrontal cortex when presented with social rejection photographs (Premkumar et al., 2012), and seen people high in schizotypy exhibit increased atypical semantic activation when speaking (Minor & Cohen, 2012). Although this general approach has shown that social deficits occur across schizotypy broadly, a common criticism is that it fails to account for the significant heterogeneity found in schizotypy.

Implementing an approach where relationships between social functioning and individual schizotypy factors are examined can address this criticism. To do so, researchers separate schizotypy scales into multiple sets of traits (positive, negative, disorganized) to determine how each trait is related to social processes within a single study. For example, Kwapil et al. (2012) observed that people high in both positive and negative schizotypy reported wanting to be alone when they were around others, but this feeling was moderated by different constructs (anxiety in positive schizotypy, decreased positive affect in negative schizotypy). The ability to compare differences between schizotypy traits (and how processes affect these differences) within studies is a major advantage of this approach.

Across studies, differences have been observed in the strength of associations between specific schizotypy traits and social processes. In line with findings in schizophrenia, negative schizotypy traits show the strongest associations with social functioning and have demonstrated relationships with reduced social engagement, decreased social interest, and greater defeatist performance beliefs (Dinzeo et al., 2018; Kwapil et al., 2012; Luther et al., 2016). There is also evidence that positive and disorganized traits are associated with worse social functioning. For example, positive traits have shown associations with decreased resilience to social stressors (Zyla & Lenzenweger, 2022), whereas disorganized traits are related to increased negative affect and disorganization in daily life (Kwapil et al., 2020).

The method used to assess social functioning also matters when testing associations between schizotypy and social functioning. Cohen et al. (2014) have described a paradox within schizotypy research where deficits are often in line with those found in schizophrenia on subjective scales, but objective measures show much smaller—sometimes negligible—differences. Springfield and Pinkham (2020) extended this paradox to social functioning, finding those high in schizotypy showed significant differences on a self-report scale but did not differ from those low in schizotypy on a performance-based role-play task. Thus, researchers must take methodology into account when describing relationships between social functioning and schizotypy.

To date, there is strong evidence that people high in schizotypy show deficits in social functioning. The strength of this relationship depends, however, on the methods used to assess schizotypy and social functioning. It is critical for researchers to identify processes that explain why those high in schizotypy exhibit impaired social functioning. In the following sections, we discuss four explanations with support from schizophrenia and schizotypy studies (see Table 4.1).

Explanation 1: Social Skills Deficits

From the social literature, the first potential explanation centers on social skills deficits observed across the schizophrenia-spectrum. When people with schizophrenia interact with others, we know they have more interpersonal conflicts than healthy controls (Weittenhiller et al., 2021) and spend less time engaged in substantive conversations (Abel et al., 2021). It is thought that social skills deficits contribute to impaired social functioning because: (1) others are less likely to pursue interactions when someone displays lower social competence and (2) lower social competence impairs one's motivation to interact with others. An entire field of treatment has been designed to help those with schizophrenia improve their social skills; these treatments generally produce small to moderate improvements in social functioning (Turner et al., 2018).

There is also evidence that social skills deficits extend to people with Schizotypal Personality Disorder (SPD). On a simulated role-play task, Waldeck and Miller (2000) observed people with SPD exhibited more deficits in social skills compared to a control group. These deficits were observed despite those with SPD exhibiting similar performance to controls on a multiple-choice task where they identified appropriate social responses. Much like in schizophrenia, a recent systematic review

Table 4.1 Overview of four potential explanations for social skills deficits

Potential explanation	Domain	Findings in schizotypy	Overview of deficit in relation to social functioning	Example of how deficit can affect social functioning in Schizotypy
Social skills deficits	Social	Those high in schizotypy have deficits in a variety of social skills, including less ability to connect in social situation and less engagement in conversations.	Deficits in social skills can lead to lower social functioning due to impaired abilities in connecting with others.	Despite being around others as much as their peers, a person high in schizotypy relies more on "small talk" and rarely discusses personally meaningful topics. In turn, they have difficulty developing friendships.
Cognitive deficits	Cognitive	Those high in schizotypy exhibit deficits in neurocognitive, social cognitive, and metacognitive functioning. The evidence is strongest for social cognitive and metacognitive deficits.	Deficits in cognition can lead to impaired information processing in social situations. Social cognitive and metacognitive deficits specifically refer to social processing.	In a social situation, a person high in schizotypy has difficulty taking their conversational partner's perspective or integrating information from their past conversations and applying it to the current interaction.
Anticipated pleasure	Cognitive, affective	Those high in schizotypy generally show deficits in anticipating pleasure for social, but not in non-social, situations. In-the-moment pleasure is typically not impaired.	Deficits in anticipated pleasure can lead to decreased motivation to pursue social activities and less engagement in activities when one is involved in them.	A person high in schizotypy turns down an invitation to a social outing because they do not anticipate having fun (even though they liked the last outing). Over time, this leads to fewer meaningful social connections.
Emotion regulation	Affective	Those high in schizotypy exhibit greater negative affect and less positive affect and are also more likely to implement maladaptive emotion regulation strategies.	Deficits in emotion regulation can lead to more net negative emotion in social situations, as well as a greater likelihood of using maladaptive strategies in these situations.	When interacting in a group, a person high in schizotypy experiences more negative emotion than the rest of the group, uses expressive suppression to avoid sharing feelings, and leaves the interaction without engaging.

highlighted how social skills training appears to be an effective intervention for those with SPD (Kirchner et al., 2018) and multiple studies suggest social skills training leads to better outcomes in people with SPD when paired with other treatments (McClure et al., 2019; Nordentoft et al., 2006).

Compared to other points on the schizophrenia-spectrum, less is known about the social skills of people high in schizotypy. However, it seems social skills deficits occur even in the absence of impairment in other key areas. For example, cognitive impairment is known to have an important role in social functioning deficits (see Explanation 2). However, Aghvinian and Sergi (2018) observed people high in schizotypy report broad deficits in social functioning on subjective scales even when their neurocognitive and social-cognitive performance is intact.

Social skills deficits have also been observed outside of self-report scales in schizotypy. Using audio files from daily life, Minor et al. (2018, 2020) observed those high in schizotypy were just as likely as those low in schizotypy to be around others but significantly less likely to engage in substantive conversations or active socialization. Thus, what separates those with schizotypy from their peers is not a lack of social opportunities. Rather, it could be that their social skills are not as developed, leading to more small talk and less active engagement in conversations. In turn, lower quality interactions could result in less meaningful social connection and drive the social functioning deficits found in schizotypy.

It is clear social skills deficits occur across the schizophrenia-spectrum and contribute to social functioning deficits. Although research is sparse in schizotypy, studies illustrate the presence of social skills deficits in SPD and people reporting high schizotypy traits. Social skills training is an evidence-based treatment for people with schizophrenia, and there is support for its use paired with other treatments in SPD. Liberman and Robertson (2005) implemented a randomized pilot social skills training in high school students with high levels of schizotypy. Following 8 weeks, those randomized to the intervention showed significant improvements in social domains that were maintained 1 year post-intervention. This suggests social skills training could be an effective treatment for people high in schizotypy and help to reduce the social deficits found in these cohorts. However, more studies are needed to determine the efficacy of this treatment in schizotypy.

Explanation 2: Cognitive Deficits

The cognitive literature offers a second explanation for the social deficits observed in schizotypy. Impairments in a wide range of cognitive functioning have been observed across the schizophrenia-spectrum. Here, we focus on three related, but distinct, domains where impairment has been found: neurocognition, social cognition, and metacognition. Adequate neurocognition is considered a building block for other cognitive processes; it is an essential limiting factor for effective social-cognitive and metacognitive performance (Minor et al., 2015).

Approximately 80% of people with schizophrenia show neurocognitive deficits (McCleery & Nuechterlein, 2018) and these deficits are a better predictor of social functioning than psychotic symptoms (Green, 1996). However, the presence of neurocognitive deficits in schizotypy has been debated: a meta-analysis showed deficits are relatively small in these cohorts and some domains are not significantly affected (Chun et al., 2017). An example of the debate on neurocognition's role comes from the cognitive load literature in schizotypy. Studies often compare performance in standard and cognitive load conditions, with the cognitive load condition introducing stimuli designed to reduce the cognitive resources available for a task (Minor et al., 2016). Marggraf and colleagues (2019) used this paradigm to test semantic coherence—an indicator of how clearly one communicates. Past studies have shown that semantic coherence is compromised in those with schizotypy (Minor et al., 2011). However, Marggraf and colleagues (2019) found no differences in semantic coherence across either standard or cognitive load conditions.

Impairments in social cognition are clearer in schizotypy and inherently related to social functioning. Social cognitive impairments reflect problems in processes (e.g., emotion recognition, theory of mind) needed to draw social inferences about others (Green et al., 2008). These deficits appear to be strongly associated with disorganized and negative traits, but associations have been shown—and not shown—with all schizotypy traits (see Cowan et al., 2018). Regarding social functioning, social cognitive deficits influence one's ability to perform social tasks by compromising abilities in core social areas. For example, if one misidentifies an emotion being expressed or cannot take the perspective of their social partner, they may inadequately respond to them in an interaction.

Metacognitive deficits in schizotypy have also been found (Chan et al., 2015), with the strongest relationships observed with negative traits (Davis et al., 2020). Metacognition is defined as an individual's capacity to form complex representations of themselves and others and to use that knowledge effectively (Ayala et al., 2023; Lysaker et al., 2020). In relation to social functioning, metacognitive deficits may place a ceiling on one's ability to form complex ideas about theirs and others place in the world leading to reduced empathy (Bonfils et al., 2019), social networks (Masse et al., 2020), and communication abilities (Myers et al., 2023). In turn, this reduces potential for intimate social relationships (Lysaker et al., 2022). A recent study by Luther et al. (2023) found negative schizotypy traits mediated the relationship between metacognition and social functioning in a nonclinical sample. This supports the view that negative traits are a key to explaining how metacognitive impairments result in social functioning deficits in schizotypy.

In sum, the evidence for the role of cognitive deficits in explaining social functioning deficits in those high in schizotypy is mixed. The strongest evidence appears to be in support of social cognition and metacognition; notably, negative schizotypy traits have an important role in explaining social impairments for both types of cognition. Several well-established treatments have shown varying degrees of promise in people on the schizophrenia-spectrum, including cognitive remediation (Eack et al., 2009), social cognitive training (Kurtz et al., 2016), metacognitive therapy (Minor et al., 2022), and combinations of these approaches (Friedman-Yakoobian et al., 2019). To our knowledge, none of these treatments have been implemented in those high in schizotypy to target social functioning.

Explanation 3: Anticipated Pleasure Deficits

Another possible explanation for social deficits in schizotypy focuses on the finding that people with schizophrenia report significant differences from controls when asked to forecast pleasure (Strauss & Gold, 2012), but between-group differences are not found in consummatory, or "in-the-moment," pleasure (Cohen & Minor, 2010). There is evidence that this finding extends to social stimuli. For example, people with schizophrenia have reported reduced social reward valuation (Catalano et al., 2018) and reduced anticipated pleasure when asked to rate social games (Campellone & Kring, 2018), whereas a recent meta-analysis found only small differences in consummatory pleasure—with negligible differences in standardized laboratory experiments (Abel et al., 2023).

Deficits in anticipated pleasure can impact social functioning in critical ways. If one does not anticipate enjoying a social activity, they will be less motivated when social opportunities are presented. This can lead to lower social participation and less engagement when socializing. The mechanisms behind the observed disconnect between anticipated and consummatory pleasure in schizophrenia are unclear, but it has led to questions about the true nature of hedonic deficits in the disorder (Strauss & Gold, 2012). Is what we are observing anhedonia, is it an issue with predicting future emotion, or does it reflect problems simulating positive emotions when reflecting on past experiences (or some combination of these explanations)? The answer to these questions may help us understand social functioning deficits across the schizophrenia-spectrum.

Although anticipated deficits are found in people with schizophrenia, there is some evidence they may not be present in those high in schizotypy (Yan et al., 2019). Visser et al. (2020) recent meta-analysis compared self-reported anticipated and consummatory pleasure in those high and low in schizotypy. Compared to those low in schizotypy, participants high in schizotypy exhibited small deficits in consummatory pleasure and small to moderate deficits in anticipated pleasure. Those with more negative traits exhibited lower anticipated pleasure scores than those high in positive traits. Significant differences were not found, however, when comparing differences in anticipated to consummatory pleasure across groups. This suggests the temporal discrepancy might not be present in schizotypy when subjective ratings are used.

Evidence for anticipated deficits in schizotypy is stronger in the context of social situations (Moore et al., 2019). In a study of over 2000 Chinese university students, Zhang et al. (2020) observed that deficits in anticipated social pleasure were a specific feature of schizotypy. Again, negative schizotypy traits showed strong correlations with low anticipated social pleasure. Other schizotypy studies have also found evidence of reduced anticipated positive emotion in social, but not in non-social, conditions (Yan et al., 2019). Using ecological momentary assessment, Zhang et al. (2022) found negative traits predicted lower levels of anticipated emotions in positive social situations, providing additional support for a social-specific deficit for those high in schizotypy (Alfimova et al., 2021; Moore et al., 2019).

Although differences between subjective consummatory and anticipated pleasure were not observed in a meta-analysis (Visser et al., 2020), multiple studies have shown deficits in anticipated pleasure for social stimuli using laboratory and real-world methodologies (Alfimova et al., 2021; Moore et al., 2019; Zhang et al., 2022). Thus, deficits in anticipated pleasure do appear to be present for those high in schizotypy—particularly those with negative traits—and these findings are most robust for social stimuli.

Explanation 4: Emotion Regulation Deficits

The final explanation comes from the affective literature and centers on deficits in emotion regulation. Emotion regulation refers to a series of processes that dictate how one shapes, manages, and expresses their emotions (Gross, 2014). Those with schizophrenia exhibit problems at multiple stages of the emotion regulation process (Bartolomeo et al., 2022; Raugh and Strauss, 2021). Relatedly, there is evidence that people with schizophrenia experience co-activation of negative emotion whenever positive emotion is experienced (Strauss et al., 2018). This could impact social functioning in important ways. For example, one experiences lower net enjoyment during socialization if they feel high levels of negative emotion in addition to positive emotion, which could make them less motivated to pursue the social activity in the future.

Compared to those low in schizotypy, people high in schizotypy demonstrate increased negative emotion (Horan et al., 2008; Minor et al., 2018) and decreased positive emotion (Kwapil et al., 2020; Schwartz et al., 2022) in response to a range of stimuli. In a study analyzing real-world audio files, our team observed a greater proportion of negative emotion words used during social interactions in a high schizotypy group (Minor et al., 2018). A follow-up study found that although positive affect increased in social situations for those low in schizotypy, it remained unchanged in the high schizotypy group (Minor et al., 2020). These findings could suggest those low in schizotypy may be motivated to pursue future social activities given the increased positive affect they experience, whereas those high in schizotypy may lack this motivation based on their greater use of negative emotion words and absence of an increase in positive emotion during social situations.

Going beyond affect, there is also clear evidence of a link between schizotypy traits and the use of emotion regulation strategies. Common emotion regulation strategies include expressive suppression (tendency to reduce behavioral expressions of emotion), cognitive reappraisal (tendency to change emotional responses by reframing thoughts), and perspective taking (tendency to see situations from another's point of view). The relationships between negative schizotypy traits and these strategies appear strongest: negative traits show medium to large relationships with expressive suppression (Gunn & Donahue, 2022; Henry et al., 2009; Li et al., 2019), small to large relationships with cognitive reappraisal (Guo et al., 2021; Li et al., 2019), and small relationships with perspective taking (Gunn & Donahue, 2022).

There is also evidence of links between positive and disorganized traits with emotion regulation strategies. Positive schizotypy traits have demonstrated small to medium relationships with expressive suppression (Gunn & Donahue, 2022; Guo et al., 2021; Li et al., 2019), but negligible relationships with cognitive reappraisal (Gunn & Donahue, 2022; Guo et al., 2021), and perspective taking (Guo et al., 2021). Fewer studies have examined relationships between disorganized symptoms and emotion regulation strategies, but some evidence shows medium correlations with expressive suppression and small correlations with perspective taking (Gunn & Donahue, 2022). These findings are important for understanding social functioning because each of these emotion regulation strategies enhances one's ability to manage and control negative emotions—which those high in schizotypy experience at greater rates—when interacting with others. In turn, adaptive emotion regulation may make one more effective in their social interactions and more likely to pursue them in the future.

Identifying emotional abnormalities and discrepancies in emotion regulation strategies is important; targeting these irregularities via therapy, however, could potentially help those high in schizotypy improve their social functioning. There is evidence that people high in positive schizotypy attend to negative emotion more frequently than those low in schizotypy, whereas those high in negative schizotypy attend less to positive emotion (Lai et al., 2021). This suggests that identifying people's unique patterns in attending to emotion and helping them understand their use of emotion regulation strategies and how these strategies impact social functioning could be beneficial in improving social functioning in schizotypy.

Integration, Implications, and Summary

The four explanations provided here give a framework for why those high in schizotypy experience deficits in social functioning (Fig. 4.1). Although each explanation is discussed individually, there is a clear overlap between them. People high in schizotypy exhibit deficits in each of these four processes, and there is compelling evidence that each can lead to social impairment. Identifying how (and for whom) overlap occurs is key for furthering our understanding of how social deficits manifest in schizotypy. For example, someone high in negative schizotypy could display deficits in metacognition and anticipated pleasure, and may rely on expressive suppression as an emotion regulation strategy. In this instance, treatment may initially target anticipated versus experienced social pleasure while also discussing how expressive suppression can be maladaptive in some social situations. Long-term goals could include implementing more adaptive emotion regulation strategies and developing their metacognitive abilities to improve their understanding of how to

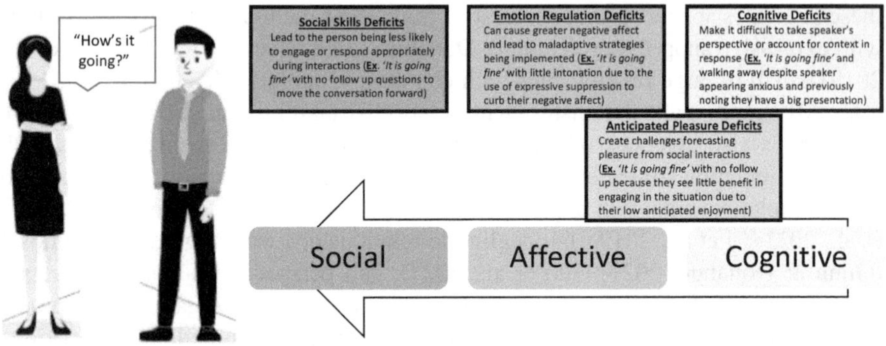

Fig. 4.1 Example of how potential explanations can impact social functioning in those high in schizotypy

integrate information about themselves and others across a range of social situations. The treatment approach outlined here would differ in someone high in positive schizotypy who may exhibit deficits in social skills and their use of cognitive reappraisal. Although both people experience social functioning deficits, the mechanisms underlying those deficits should lead to different treatment approaches.

This chapter outlined four potential explanations for the social functioning deficits found in those high in schizotypy. We first covered the importance of accounting for how schizotypy and social functioning are measured given that different methodologies often lead to different results. Then, we focused on findings across the schizophrenia and schizotypy literatures in relation to our four potential explanations. These explanations covered several social, cognitive, and affective processes. They included deficits found in schizotypy in social skills, cognitive abilities, anticipated pleasure, and emotion regulation. Future work should seek to integrate these explanations by testing how much each contributes to the social functioning deficits found in those high in schizotypy. Doing so will help us better understand causal mechanisms and how to treat social impairments in schizotypy.

References

Abel, D. B., & Minor, K. S. (2021). Social functioning in schizophrenia: Comparing laboratory-based assessment with real-world measures. *Journal of Psychiatric Research, 138*, 500–506.

Abel, D. B., Salyers, M. P., Wu, W., Monette, M., & Minor, K. S. (2021). Quality versus quantity: Determining real-world social functioning deficits in schizophrenia. *Psychiatry Research, 301*, 113980.

Abel, D.B., Rand, K.L., Salyers, M.P., Myers, E.J., Mickens, J.L., & Minor, K.S. (2023). Do people with schizophrenia enjoy social activities as much as everyone else? A meta-analysis of consummatory social pleasure. *Schizophrenia Bulletin.*

Abu-Akel, A., Baxendale, L., Mohr, C., & Sullivan, S. (2018). The association between schizotypal traits and social functioning in adolescents from the general population. *Psychiatry Research, 270*, 895–900.

Aghvinian, M., & Sergi, M. J. (2018). Social functioning impairments in schizotypy when social cognition and neurocognition are not impaired. *Schizophrenia Research: Cognition, 14*, 7–13.

Alfimova, M. V., Lezheiko, T., Plakunova, V., & Golimbet, V. (2021). Relationships between schizotypal features, trait anticipatory and consummatory pleasure, and naturalistic hedonic states. *Motivation and Emotion, 45*, 649–600.

Ayala, A., Mickens, J. L., Myers, E. J., Abel, D. B., Hegwood, C. M., Davis, B. J., Lysaker, P. H., & Minor, K. S. (2023). Metacognitive beliefs and metacognitive capacity: Do they assess related phenomena? *Journal of Nervous and Mental Disease*.

Bartolomeo, L. A., Raugh, I. M., & Strauss, G. P. (2022). Deconstructing emotion regulation in schizophrenia: The nature and consequences of abnormalities in monitoring dynamics. *Schizophrenia Research, 240*, 135–142.

Bonfils, K. A., Lysaker, P. H., Minor, K. S., & Salyers, M. P. (2019). Metacognition, personal distress, and performance-based empathy in schizophrenia. *Schizophrenia Bulletin, 45*, 19–26.

Campellone, T. R., & Kring, A. M. (2018). Anticipated pleasure for positive and negative social interaction outcomes in schizophrenia. *Psychiatry Research, 259*, 203–209.

Catalano, L. T., Heerey, E. A., & Gold, J. M. (2018). The valuation of social rewards in schizophrenia. *Journal of Abnormal Psychology, 127*, 602–611.

Chan, C. C., Spencer, C. C., West, C., Viegas, C., & Bedwell, J. S. (2015). Metacognitive processes in psychometrically defined schizotypy. *Psychiatry Research, 230*, 279–286.

Chun, C. A., Barrantes-Vidal, N., Sheinbaum, T., & Kwapil, T. R. (2017). Expression of schizophrenia-spectrum personality traits in daily life. *Personality Disorders: Theory, Treatment, and Research, 8*, 64–74.

Cohen, A. S., & Minor, K. S. (2010). Emotional experience in patients with schizophrenia revisited: Meta-analysis of laboratory studies. *Schizophrenia Bulletin, 36*, 143–150.

Cohen, A. S., Auster, T. L., MacAulay, R. K., & McGovern, J. E. (2014). The paradox of schizotypy: Resemblance to prolonged severe mental illness in subjective but not objective quality of life. *Psychiatry Research, 217*, 185–190.

Cowan, T., Le, T. P., & Cohen, A. S. (2018). Social cognition and schizotypy. In K. Lewandowski & A. Moustafa (Eds.), *Social cognition in psychosis* (pp. 71–88). Academic Press.

Davis, B. J., Firmin, R. L., Lysaker, P. H., Salyers, M. P., McGrew, J., & Minor, K. S. (2020). An investigation of metacognition in schizotypy: Evidence of linkage with negative traits. *Translational Issues in Psychological Science, 6*, 81–91.

Dinzeo, T. J., Serna, V. C., Pujji, S. D., & Sledjeski, E. M. (2018). The relationship of categorical and phonological verbal fluency to negative schizotypy and social functioning in a non-clinical sample. *Cognitive Neuropsychiatry, 23*, 43–57.

Eack, S. M., Greenwald, D. P., Hogarty, S. S., Cooley, S. J., DiBarry, A. L., Montrose, D. M., & Keshavan, M. S. (2009). Cognitive enhancement therapy for early-course schizophrenia: Effects of a two-year randomized controlled trial. *Psychiatric Services, 60*, 1468–1476.

Friedman-Yakoobian, M., Parrish, E. M., Thomas, A., Lesser, R., Gnong-Granato, A., Each, S., & Keshavan, M. S. (2019). An integrated neurocognitive and social-cognitive treatment for youtth at clinical high risk for psychosis: Cognition for learning and for understanding everyday social situations (CLUES). *Schizophrenia Research, 208*, 55–59.

Gooding, D. C., Tallent, K. A., & Matts, C. W. (2005). Clinical status of at-risk individuals 5 years later: Further validation of the psychometric high-risk strategy. *Journal of Abnormal Psychology, 114*, 170–175.

Green, M. F. (1996). What are the functional consequences of neurocognitive deficits in schizophrenia? *American Journal of Psychiatry, 153*, 321–330.

Green, M. F., Penn, D. L., Bentall, R., Carpenter, W. T., Gaebel, W., Gur, R. C., Kring, A. M., Park, S., Silverstein, S. M., & Heinssen, R. (2008). Social cognition in schizophrenia: An NIMH workshop on definitions, assessment, and research opportunities. *Schizophrenia Bulletin, 34*, 1211–1220.

Gross, J. J. (2014). Emotion regulation: Conceptual and empirical foundations. In JJ Gross (Ed.), *Handbook of emotion regulation* pp. 3–20.

Gunn, C. K., & Donahue, J. J. (2022). Intra- and interpersonal emotion regulation strategies and schizotypic personality characteristics. *Journal of Psychopathology and Behavioral Assessment, 44*, 950–961.

Guo, X., Wang, Y., & Chan, R. C. K. (2021). Mediating role of emotion regulation in the relationship between schizotypy and empathy. *PsyCh Journal, 11*, 335–343.

Henry, J. D., Green, M. J., Restuccia, C., de Lucia, A., Rendell, P. G., McDonald, S., & Grisham, J. R. (2009). Emotion dysregulation and schizotypy. *Psychiatry Research, 166*, 116–124.

Horan, W. P., Blanchard, J. J., Clark, L. A., & Green, M. F. (2008). Affective traits in schizophrenia and schizotypy. *Schizophrenia Bulletin, 34*(5), 856–874.

Kirchner, S. K., Roeh, A., Nolden, J., & Hasan, A. (2018). Diagnosis and treatment of schizotypal personality disorder: Evidence from a systematic review. *NPJ Schizophrenia, 3*, 20.

Kurtz, M. M., Gagen, E., Rocha, N. B. F., Machado, S., & Penn, D. L. (2016). Comprehensive treatments for social cognitive deficits in schizophrenia: A critical review and effect-size analysis of controlled studies. *Clinical Psychology Review, 43*, 80–89.

Kwapil, T. R., Brown, L. H., Silvia, P. J., Myin-Germeys, I., & Barrantes-Vidal, N. (2012). The expression of positive and negative schizotypy in daily life: An experience sampling study. *Psychological Medicine, 42*, 2555–2566.

Kwapil, T. R., Kemp, K. C., Mielock, A., Sperry, S. H., Chun, C. A., Gross, G. M., & Barrantes-Vidal, N. (2020). Association of multidimensional schizotypy with psychotic-like experiences, affect, and social functioning in daily life: Comparable findings across samples and schizotypy measures. *Journal of Abnormal Psychology, 129*, 492–504.

Lai, J., Snyder, M. E., Vijayakumar, K. S. O. M., Bailey, D. H., & Martin, E. A. (2021). Shared and unique affective abnormalities in schizotypy dimensions. *PsyCh Journal, 11*, 149–162.

Li, L. Y., Karcher, N. R., Kerns, J. G., Fung, C. K., & Martin, E. A. (2019). The subjective-objective deficit paradox in schizotypy extends to emotion regulation and awareness. *Journal of Psychiatric Research, 111*, 160–168.

Liberman, R. P., & Robertson, M. J. (2005). A pilot, controlled skills training study of schizotypal high school students. *Verhaltenstherapie, 15*, 176–180.

Luther, L., Salyers, M. P., Firmin, R. L., Marggraf, M. P., Davis, B., & Minor, K. S. (2016). Additional support for the cognitive model of schizophrenia: Evidence of elevated defeatist performance beliefs in schizotypy. *Comprehensive Psychiatry, 68*, 40–47.

Luther, L., Hochheiser, J., Wiesepape, C., & Lysaker, P. H. (2023). Negative schizotypy mediates the relationship between metacognition and social functioning in a nonclinical sample. *Journal of Nervous and Mental Diseases, 211*, 74–78.

Lysaker, P. H., Minor, K. S., Lysaker, J. T., Hasson-Ohayon, I., Bonfils, K., Hochheiser, J., & Vohs, J. L. (2020). Metacognitive function and fragmentation in schizophrenia: Relationship to cognition, self-experience and developing treatments. *Schizophrenia Research Cognition, 19*.

Lysaker, P. H., Holm, T., Kukla, M., Wiespape, C., Faith, L., Musselman, A., & Lysaker, J. T. (2022). Psychosis and the challenges to narrative identity and the good life: Advances from research on the integrated model of metacognition. *Journal of Research on Personality, 100*, 104267.

Marggraf, M. P., Davis, B. J., Hardin, K. L., Abplanalp, S. J., Haller, J. A., DeCrescenzo, P., & Minor, K. S. (2019). Speech production and disorganization in schizotypy: Investigating the role of cognitive and affective systems. *Journal of Psychiatric Research, 114*, 11–16.

Masse, M., Paquin, K., Lysaker, P. H., & Lecomte, T. (2020). Evolution of social networks in early psychosis. *Psychosis, 12*, 222–233.

McCleery, A., & Nuechterlein, K. H. (2018). Cognitive impairment in psychotic illness: Prevalence, profile of impairment, developmental course, and treatment considerations. *Dialogues in Clinical Neuroscience, 21*, 239–248.

McClure, M. M., Graff, F., Triebwasser, J., Perez-Rodriguez, M., Rosell, D. R., Koenigsberg, H., Hazlett, E. A., Siever, L. J., Harvey, P. D., & New, A. S. (2019). Guanfacine augmentation of a combined intervention of computerized cognitive remediation therapy and social skills training for schizotypal personality disorder. *American Journal of Psychiatry, 176*, 307–314.

Minor, K. S., & Cohen, A. S. (2010). Affective reactivity of speech disturbances in schizotypy. *Journal of Psychiatric Research, 44*, 99–105.

Minor, K. S., & Cohen, A. S. (2012). The role of atypical semantic activation and stress in odd speech: Implications for individuals with psychometrically defined schizotypy. *Journal of Psychiatric Research, 46*, 1231–1236.

Minor, K. S., Cohen, A. S., Weber, C. R., & Brown, L. A. (2011). The relationship between atypical semantic activation and odd speech in schizotypy across emotionally evocative conditions. *Schizophrenia Research, 126*, 144–149.

Minor, K. S., Marggraf, M. P., Davis, B. J., Luther, L., Vohs, J. L., Buck, K. D., & Lysaker, P. H. (2015). Conceptual disorganization weakens links in cognitive pathways: Disentagnling neurocognition, social cognition, and metacognition in schizophrenia. *Schizophrenia Research, 169*, 153–158.

Minor, K. S., Marggraf, M. P., Davis, B. J., Mehdiyoun, N. F., & Breier, A. (2016). Affective systems induce formal thought disorder in early-stage psychosis. *Journal of Abnormal Psychology, 125*, 537–542.

Minor, K. S., Davis, B. J., Marggraf, M. P., Luther, L., & Robbins, M. L. (2018). Words matter: Implementing the electronically activated recorder in schizotypy. *Personality Disorders: Theory, Research, and Treatment, 9*, 133–143.

Minor, K. S., Hardin, K. L., Beaudette, D. M., Waters, L. C., White, A. L., Gonzenbach, V., & Robbins, M. L. (2020). Social functioning in schizotypy: How affect influences social behavior in daily life. *Journal of Clinical Psychology, 76*, 2212–2221.

Minor, K. S., Marggraf, M. P., Davis, B. J., Mickens, J. L., Abel, D. B., Robbins, M. L., Buck, K. D., Wiehe, S. E., & Lysaker, P. H. (2022). Personalizing interventions using real-world interactions: Implementing symptoms and social functioning in schizophrenia with tailored metacognitive therapy. *Journal of Consulting and Clinical Psychology, 90*, 18–28.

Moore, M. M., Chan, R. C. K., Huang, J., & Martin, E. A. (2019). Affective forecasting and accuracy in social anhedonia: Predicted and experienced emotion for a social interaction. *Journal of Clinical Psychology, 75*, 1684–1700.

Myers, E. J., Abel, D. B., Hardin, K. L., Bettis, R. J., Beard, A. M., Salyers, M. P., Lysaker, P. H., & Minor, K. S. (2023). Mild vs. moderate: How behavioral speech measures predict metacognitive capacity across different levels of formal thought disorder. *Journal of Psychiatric Research, 157*, 43–49.

Nordentoft, M., Thorup, A., Petersen, L., Ohlenschlaeger, J., Melau, M., Christensen, T. O., Krarup, G., Jorgensen, P., & Jeppesen, P. (2006). Transition rates from schizotypal personality disorder to psychotic disorder for first-contact patients in the OPUS trial: A randomized clinical trial of integrated treatment and standard treatment. *Schizophrenia Research, 83*, 29–40.

Premkumar, P., Ettinger, U., Inchley-Mort, S., Sumich, A., Williams, S. C. R., Kuipers, E., & Kumari, V. (2012). Neural processing of social rejection: The role of schizotypal personality traits. *Human Brain Mapping, 33*, 695–706.

Raugh, I. M., & Strauss, G. P. (2021). Deconstructing emotion regulation in schizophrenia: The nature and consequences of abnormalities at the identification stage. *European Archives of Psychiatry and Clinical Neuroscience, 272*, 1061–1071.

Schwartz, E. K., Le, T. P., & Cohen, A. S. (2022). Sharing positive events: Ecological momentary assessment of emotion regulation via social capitalization in schizotypy. *Psychiatry Research, 308*, 114377.

Shumway, M., Saunders, T., Shern, D., Pines, E., Downs, A., Burbine, T., & Beller, J. (2003). Preferences for schizophrenia treatment outcomes among public policy makers, consumers, families, and providers. *Psychiatric Services, 54*, 1124–1128.

Springfield, C. R., & Pinkham, A. E. (2020). Introspective accuracy for social competence in psychometric schizotypy. *Cognitive Neuropsychiatry, 25*, 57–70.

Strauss, G. P., & Gold, J. M. (2012). A new perspective on anhedonia in schizophrenia. *American Journal of Psychiatry, 169*, 364–373.

Strauss, G. P., Ruiz, I., Dickinson, E. K., & Visser, K. H. (2018). The role of negative emotion abnormalities in anhedonic symptoms of schizophrenia. In S. Sangha & D. Foti (Eds.), *Neurobiology of abnormal emotion and motivated behaviors: Integrating animal and human research, 259–276*. Elsevier Academic Press.

Turner, D. T., McGlanaghy, E., Cuijpers, P., van der Gaag, M., Karyotaki, E., & MacBeth, A. (2018). A meta-analysis of social skills training and related interventions for psychosis. *Schizophrenia Bulletin, 44*, 475–491.

Visser, K. F., Chapman, H. C., Ruiz, I., Raugh, I. M., & Strauss, G. P. (2020). A meta-analysis of self-reported anticipatory and consummatory pleasure in the schizophrenia-spectrum. *Journal of Psychiatric Research, 121*, 68–81.

Waldeck, T. L., & Miller, L. S. (2000). Social skills deficits in schizotypal personality disorder. *Psychiatry Research*, 237–246.

Wastler, H. M., & Lenzenweger, M. F. (2021). Cognitive and affective theory of mind in positive schizotypy: Relationship to schizotypal traits and psychosocial functioning. *Journal of Personality Disorders, 35*, 538–553.

Weittenhiller, L. P., Mikhail, M. E., Mote, J., Campellone, T. R., & Kring, A. M. (2021). What gets in the way of social engagement in schizophrenia? *World Journal of Psychiatry, 11*, 13–26.

Yan, C., Lui, S. S. Y., Zou, C., Zhou, F., Cheung, E. F. C., Shum, D. H. K., & Chan, R. C. K. (2019). Anticipatory pleasure for future rewards is attenuated in patients with schizophrenia but not in individuals with schizotypal traits. *Schizophrenia Research, 206*, 118–126.

Zhang, R., Wang, Y., Yang, Z., Li, Y., Wang, Y., Cheung, E. F. C., Shun, D. H. K., Yang, T., Barkus, E. J., & Chan, R. C. K. (2020). Network structure of anticipatory pleasure and risk features: Evidence from a large college sample. *PsyCh Journal, 9*, 223–233.

Zhang, R., Yang, T., Chen, S., Cheung, E. F. C., Barkus, E., & Chan, R. C. K. (2022). Subclinical psychopathology and affective forecasting: Role of in-the-moment feelings. *PsyCh Journal, 11*, 317–326.

Zyla, H. O., & Lenzenweger, M. F. (2022). Resilience and psychosocial functioning in schizotypy. *Personality Disorders: Theory, Research, and Treatment, 13*, 654–661.

Chapter 5
Schizotypal Disorder: Phenomenological Perspectives on Diagnosis, Psychopathology, and Psychotherapy

Borut Škodlar and Mads Gram Henriksen

A Brief History of the Evolution of the Diagnosis of Schizotypal Disorder

Schizotypal personality disorder became a formal diagnosis in the DSM-III (APA, 1980) and later in ICD-10 (WHO, 1992). DSM-III marks the entry of the so-called operational revolution in psychiatry, that is, the operational diagnostic manuals define mental disorders on polythetic diagnostic criteria instead of on prototypal descriptions as in the pre-operational diagnostic manuals (e.g., DSM-II and ICD-9). In DSM-III and subsequent versions, schizotypal personality disorder is considered a *personality disorder* and listed among these in the diagnostic manual. Still, it is believed to bear a psychopathological and genetic kinship to schizophrenia. This kinship is more pronounced in ICD-10 (WHO, 1992), where schizotypal disorder (F21) is *not* considered a personality disorder but rather a syndrome, listed among the psychotic disorders, immediately after schizophrenia (F20) in ICD-10 and after schizoaffective disorder in ICD-11. In ICD, schizotypal disorder is thus more explicitly considered a part of the schizophrenia spectrum. One apparent difference between the DSM-III+ and ICD-10 constructs is the diagnostic criterion of "occasional transient quasi-psychotic episodes" for schizotypal disorder in ICD-10. Although no corresponding criterion can be found in DSM-III+, DSM-5 specifies in the text description that these patients "may experience transient psychotic episodes

B. Škodlar (✉)
University Psychiatric Clinic Ljubljana and Medical Faculty, University of Ljubljana, Ljubljana, Slovenia
e-mail: borut.skodlar@psih-klinika.si

M. G. Henriksen
Mental Health Center Amager, University Hospital of Copenhagen and Center for Subjectivity Research, Department of Communication, Faculty of Humanities, University of Copenhagen, Copenhagen, Denmark

S. Cheli, P. H. Lysaker (eds.), *A Dimensional Approach to Schizotypy*,
https://doi.org/10.1007/978-3-031-41788-7_5

(lasting minutes to hours)" (APA, 2013, p.657; cf. APA, 1980, p.312). In ICD-11, the difference between schizotypal disorder and schizophrenia boils down to intensity or duration of symptoms. Here, transient psychotic symptoms are allowed to last <1 month in schizotypal disorder, adding further weight to the concept of schizophrenia spectrum. This nosological change matches the findings of a recent study that explored patients, who initially were diagnosed with schizotypal disorder and who later were re-diagnosed with schizophrenia (Nordgaard et al., 2021). The study found no substantial changes in psychopathology and concluded that instead of witnessing a true "transition" from one disorder (schizotypal disorder) to another (schizophrenia), the diagnostic change was rather due to dimensional fluctuations within the same condition (a schizophrenia spectrum disorder).

Interestingly, this development in ICD-11 was foreshadowed in the original concept of "schizotype," which was introduced by Rado as an abbreviation for the "schizophrenic phenotype" (Rado, 1953, p.410). Rado believed that beneath the overt psychotic symptoms of schizophrenia there were specific, enduring psychodynamic traits that were characteristic of the schizotype, and he designated these core traits the "schizotypal organization." Rado (1953) proposed that the symptomatic expressions of the underlying schizotypal organization could manifest in different degrees of severity, depending on combinations of inherited deficiencies ("integrative pleasure deficiency" and "proprioceptive diathesis") and the person's adaptive capacities: *compensated* cases (resembling schizoidia), *decompensated* cases (resembling pseudoneurotic schizophrenia), and *disintegrated* cases (schizophrenic psychosis) (cf. Parnas et al., 2005, p.15). Meehl (1962), building on Rado's work, introduced the concept of schizotaxia to designate a "neural integrative deficit" (synaptic slippage), which, in his view, developed into the schizotypal organization. Neither Rado nor Meehl believed that a schizotypal organization necessarily followed a pattern of symptomatic progression. In other words, many persons with a schizotypal organization will remain *compensated* throughout their life and never *decompensate* into pseudoneurotic symptomatic pictures or *disintegrate* into schizophrenia. Their work emphasized the importance of a continuity of disorders of schizophrenia—an idea that to some extent already had been anticipated in the literature. For example, Bleuler, who introduced the concept of schizophrenia, also described "latent schizophrenia," not as a subtype of schizophrenia, but as a way in which schizophrenia also may manifest: "It is extremely important to recognize that they [the symptoms] exist in varying degrees and shadings on the entire scale from pathological to normal; also the milder cases, the latent schizophrenics with far less manifest symptoms, are many times more common than the overt, manifest cases (Bleuler, 1950, p. 13)." Other scholars coined other concepts to try to delimit such "latent" or "borderline" conditions, which typically were characterized by the presence of Bleulerian fundamental symptoms of schizophrenia but without pronounced psychotic symptoms or severe deteriorations of personality—e.g., "ambulatory schizophrenias" (Zilboorg, 1941, 1957), "borderline schizophrenia" (Kety et al., 1968a, b; Vanggaard, 1979; Spitzer et al., 1979), "pseudoneurotic schizophrenia" (Hoch & Polatin, 1949; Hoch & Catell, 1959), "the psychotic character" (Frosch, 1964), and, of course, the "schizotype" (Rado, 1953; Meehl, 1962) (for a discussion of the distinction between schizotypal disorder and borderline personality disorder, see Zandersen et al., 2019).

The conceptual and empirical basis for the diagnosis of schizotypal (personality) disorder came from clinical studies like those mentioned above, describing attenuated forms of schizophrenia, and from family studies exploring characteristic traits of schizophrenia in biological relatives of patients with schizophrenia (Kendler, 1985).[1] The US-DK adoption studies are especially important in this context as they found a distribution of disorders related to schizophrenia in biological families of patients with schizophrenia, which led to the emergence of "the *schizophrenia spectrum* of disorders" (Kety et al., 1968a, b, p. 353; our emphasis). The concept of *schizophrenia spectrum disorders* has since been validated (e.g., Kendler et al., 1995; Bigdeli et al., 2014), documenting a shared vulnerability in this spectrum that may manifest in different ways and with varying severity.

Finally, we will mention two sets of prospective psychopathological studies, which further corroborate the idea of a shared vulnerability to schizophrenia spectrum disorder. The first is the US-DK high-risk prospective study (Mednick et al., 1987), which examined 207 children of mothers with schizophrenia and found that i.a. inappropriate emotional rapport and subtle formal thought disorders in adolescence (age 15) before illness onset predicted an adult diagnostic outcome within the schizophrenia spectrum (i.e., schizophrenia, non-affective psychosis, and schizotypal disorder). In the New York high-risk project (Erlenmeyer-Kimling et al., 1993), childhood attentional dysfunction was found to be related to anhedonia, social isolation, and psychosis in persons at risk of schizophrenia. Other studies, exploring the subjective dimension and, more specifically, anomalous self-experiences (viz. self-disorders), found that high levels of non-psychotic self-disorders significantly predicted a later diagnosis within the schizophrenia spectrum in patients initially diagnosed outside the schizophrenia spectrum (Parnas et al., 2011; Koren et al., 2020).

Given the common difficulty in grasping these subtle, non-psychotic experiential alterations (self-disorders), we first offer a general description of some of the self-disorders that research in phenomenological psychopathology in the last decades consistently has found to hyper-aggregate in schizophrenia spectrum disorders (i.e., schizophrenia, non-affective psychosis, and schizotypal disorder) but not in other mental disorders or healthy controls (Henriksen et al., 2021). Then we present a rich clinical vignette, contextualizing some of these experiential alterations within the lifeworld and life history of a patient with schizotypal disorder. In the final section, we present concrete psychotherapeutic strategies, informed by phenomenological research on self-disorders, for treating schizotypal disorder.

[1] Several classical psychiatrists also described various peculiarities or eccentricities in some of the relatives of patients with schizophrenia (or dementia praecox), and they applied different concepts to articulate such traits, most importantly in our context, "schizoidia" (Bleuler)—for details, see Parnas et al. (2005, p. 6–7).

Inner Experiential Situation

In this section, we describe some common contours of the inner world in schizophrenia spectrum disorders and then turn toward the experiences of a single patient with schizotypal disorder. To this end, we draw upon the first author's longstanding clinical work with patients with schizophrenia spectrum disorders and the second author's work of anomalous self-experiences in schizophrenia spectrum disorders.

The inner experiential situation in schizophrenia spectrum disorders is often pervaded by profound and enduring anxiety (Henriksen et al., 2010). While anxiety is a diagnostically non-specific symptom, occurring across disorders (Mølstrøm et al., 2020), the specificity of anxiety in schizophrenia spectrum disorders comes to the fore when considered in the context of other symptoms and the overall psychopathological Gestalt in which it occurs (Nielsen, 2023). Typically, anxiety is not bound to specific objects but exhibits a much more diffuse and general character (described as pan-anxiety in classical literature), sometimes intensifying into social phobia and/or panic attacks. Often, anxiety is deeply connected to interactions with others—for example, anxiety may be related to perplexity and enduring problems with understanding the implicit rules of social interaction (Blankenburg, 1971), paranoid ideation (e.g., fear of being harmed or exploited by others), primary self-reference (e.g., an inexplicable feeling of being the center of attention), and transitivism (i.e., experiences of frail or permeable self/other boundaries). A recent study (Nielsen, 2023) summarized key structural forms of social anxiety in schizophrenia spectrum disorders under the headings of anxiety about losing uniqueness, fusion anxiety, and engulfment (Laing, 1977), arguing that sociality as such in this spectrum may be perceived as an ontological threat.

Frequently, these forms of anxiety are reflected in the patient's social engagement, for example, in tendencies toward social withdrawal or isolation. In fact, many patients report a hermit-like lifestyle with a tendency to stay in the shadow of social world as a bystander and distant observer, and they may be inclined to adopt what Sass called "a truth-taking stare," that is, a distant, highly reflective, observational stance (Sass, 1990). In this context, it is important to emphasize that these patients usually do not simply withdraw. Very often, they are tormented by their social difficulties and they have a deep longing for interpersonal connection and a need to partake in the social world, while, at the same time, balancing their need to be alone and keep the social world at a distance (Nilsson et al., 2019). This paradoxicality in social relatedness has i.a. been described as "a distanced dependency" (Matussek, 1959) and "positive withdrawal" (Corin, 1990).

The distance to the social world is also reflected in emotional experiences, described by some patients as if there is a "buffer" or "glass-wall" between them and others or the world (Vodušek et al., 2014). Some patients describe it as diminished sense of being present in the world or as decreased affectability by events occurring in the social world. Many struggle with feelings of emptiness or inner void (Zandersen & Parnas, 2019), numbness, or not being able to establish a firmly embodied and attuned contact with others. Such negatively experienced emotions may be associated with certain pessimistic or nihilistic self- or world-views.

Some patients with schizotypal disorder report intensely reflecting upon and analyzing social encounters, both prior to (e.g., analyzing all possible directions a conversation may take), during (e.g., minutely observing everything), and after social encounters (sometimes causing many sleepless nights) (Rosenbaum et al., 2019). Sleep disturbance and altered or reversed day-and-night rhythms are frequent triggers for exacerbation of symptoms and a reason for a low quality of life in these patients (Ferrarelli, 2021). Various disturbances in the flow of thoughts are also common, for example, thought pressure, thought block, spatialization of thoughts (e.g., thoughts may acquire physical properties and be felt to be located to specific parts of the head or moving around in a certain felt pattern), and pseudo-obsessions (i.e., intrusions, often with a disturbing pictorial content, which are not immediately resisted and which occur with lack of insight) (Rasmussen & Parnas, 2022).

Closely intertwined with the experiences and feelings described above is a profound sense of existential solitude, i.e., a feeling of being markedly different (ontologically different) from others or simply "wrong" (Parnas & Henriksen, 2014, p. 253). Very often such feelings have been present since childhood and persist across changing social contexts. Another important part of the experiential situation of our schizotypal patients is a felt openness to "another presence," for example, something or someone in their own proximity (i.e., *Anwesenheit*) or within themselves (i.e., an alterity or otherness that shines from within). In some cases, the latter materializes as a kind of breakthrough into deeper or hidden dimensions of reality and sometimes such insights may acquire a delusional elaboration (Stephensen et al., 2023).

Finally, there are many other important experiential aspects of the clinical picture of schizotypal disorder, which we have not mentioned here, including introspective alienation, depersonalization, derealization, autoscopic phenomena, perceptualization of inner speech, and various perceptual disorders, for example, heightened sensitivity and responsivity to perceptual stimuli such as colors, light, noise, and sounds.

Clinical Vignette[2]

A 37-year-old patient, translator by profession, was hospitalized for the first time due to a brief psychotic episode, when he was 20. In the following years, he had four further hospitalizations at the ages of 27, 28, 33, and 36, always suffering from a short-lasting, acute psychotic episode, which resolved within 1–2 days. In all of these occasions, he was admitted to the hospital, and after an extensive period of sleep, he reported a distanced and critical stance toward his psychotic experiences and interpretations. In each of these instances,

[2] We would like to cordially thank our patient, who kindly shared his experiences with us, allowed us to write about them, read them, and corrected them linguistically.

except for the last one, where he attended a ritual of walking on burning coals, which induced a psychotic experience, he had used marijuana and was usually sleepless for several nights before the onset of psychotic insight and delusions. One of these psychotic episodes led to life-endangering behavior, where he attempted to jump through the window of his apartment on the fourth floor after the hidden nature of the universe, composed of particles and energy, was revealed to him. However, the window glass and blinds stopped him, so that he did not fall down, but was only cut by the glass. His inner motivation for the jump was extreme boredom after everything had been revealed and made understandable for him. He could expect nothing more from this life and death, he thought, was only a passage, an unimportant moment in one's life. In the other four psychotic episodes, he also experienced an insight into the true nature of the universe, but his acts or behaviors there were not dangerous. Within each psychotic episode, he experienced fear of annihilation, fear of being dissolved into nothingness and of being forgotten forever.

As a child, he rarely wept and was always silent on one side, and hyperactive and disinhibited on the other side. He remembers feeling unpopular and excluded from the company of classmates in primary school without noticing why. He thinks it might have been because he was very direct in his communication. In fourth grade, at the age of 11 or 12, he realized that he risked not having friends if something did not change. He started observing and analyzing others that were popular and he imitated their behavior. He took notes on how to behave to be socially acceptable, since he needed to make efforts to acquire self-evidence in communication. He developed a "false identity," a picture of what he thought others would like and he was successful with that. In secondary school, at the age of 17 or 18, he stopped with this adjusted behavior, because, through a computer game, he met others who had similar interests and humor, being ironic and cynical about everything. With them, he didn't need to compromise his tendency for nonconventional behavior, which has resided in him for as long as he remembers. He nonetheless still felt insecure and had low self-esteem due to the experience of threatening excommunication.

His parents divorced when he was 14. He lived with his mother and maintained contact with his father. After his brother was born, when he was 5, he felt that the mother's care completely shifted to his brother, and that everybody expected him to be grown up.

He described himself as a reader and gamer, sports were never his thing. He could play computer games for hours, if not the whole day. He describes himself as a cynic, who has seen enough of interpersonal contacts. They are uneasy for him and he has a tendency to withdraw. When he is among people, he is always on the lookout, but he has a capacity to create a distance from himself and to observe himself from a third-person perspective. He uses this capacity to bring changes to his life.

He started studying, but he felt disgust about everything: the subject matter, the professors, and everybody there. Soon afterward, he experienced his first psychotic episode and after a year he entered another faculty, where he felt there were too many dogmas, and he was not attracted to the study. Both studies, that is the common ground, were extremely boring and unattractive for him. His thoughts were wandering and he was not mentally present. Boredom was a big issue for him in his teenage years. He was always looking for escapes such as computer games, fantasy card games, and books, where he could be fully present and alive. He often felt that life has no meaning and no quality that could attract him. He wouldn't say he had difficulties with concentration, but he simply wasn't there; he wasn't interested. He has always preferred nighttime, when it is quiet and nobody is around. He finds the silence and the smell of the night wonderful. Staying awake during the day and sleeping at night has always been a problem for him, making it difficult for him to function.

Other people and feelings of being rejected by them have been the major organizing theme for him since his childhood and remain to be such. He describes that he always had difficulties with his directness and potential inappropriateness of his statements or actions, and he still faces this problem, even though he managed to find friends with similar open, direct, and nonchalant way of interacting with each others, joking, or being cynical about things. Other people easily make him nervous and irritable, quarrelsome with a tendency to interrupt them during conversations. He had a long-lasting interest in mystical themes, magical forces, epic battles, and archetypal heroes, but he feels he lost contact with these themes through materialism and nihilism of everyday life. He experiences psychotic episodes as breakthroughs of mystical themes into the consciousness, accompanied by a simultaneous absolute confirmation of their existence. He reports that he would not choose not to experience psychotic and insightful states, but that experiencing them is a double-edged sword. For him, they serve as a kind of existential compass in life; he considers them to be both a burden and a blessing. He is convinced that many people, doctors included, think of them as part of insanity but, for him, these experiences are much more than that.

Psychotherapeutic Implications

Psychotherapy of patients with schizotypal disorder is a very interesting, but also sometimes challenging and long journey. It consists, like a good psychotherapeutic process for any mental disorder, in an insight-inducing, supportive, psycho-educative, and socially re-educative process (Stone, 1985). It needs to address the patients' basic human need to be understood in their individuality of living with certain difficulties and opportunities, stemming from or related to the mental disorder from which they suffer. These patients must be approached and understood within a humane, non-judgmental, containing, holding, and supportive therapeutic environment (Bion, 1962; Winnicott, 1965), which provides a space for calming down from overwhelming anxiety, a place for strengthening one's sense of self and identity, and for augmenting meta-cognitive capacities (Lysaker et al., 2018) and mentalization (Allen et al., 2008) that are related to affect regulation and stability of functioning (Pedersen et al., 2014).

Patients with schizotypal disorder, as we saw in the previous sections, like patients with schizophrenia, often become anxiously paralyzed in social situations and risk taking a distanced, hyperreflective, overanalyzing, and/or paranoid stance. This swinging between social paralysis or frozenness, on the one hand, and isolation with deepfelt longing for social connectedness, on the other hand, is often a primary source of their personal suffering. Psychotherapy needs to address this socially related anxiety or uneasiness and try to alleviate it as one of its main goals. Notably, psychotherapeutic goals are always collaboratively determined and agreed upon between the patient and the therapist in their therapeutic alliance (Safran & Muran, 2000). The therapist's *modus operandi,* with a genuine interest, phenomenological openness, and unconditional positive regard (Rogers, 1957) of the patient, facilitates the above-mentioned environment and thus a corrective emotional experience for the patient (Knight, 2005). With phenomenological openness, we mean adopting a position of "staying with" the patient's experience and resisting premature interpretations of these experiences until a broad and clear picture of them has emerged (Škodlar & Henriksen, 2019). Such insights into the patient's experience are of great diagnostic and therapeutic importance, as they may help us to understand what the patient is going through experientially and existentially. They can also reinforce the contact with a therapist who, in addition to providing a good emotional experience and a safe haven for the patient, can also offer the possibility of translating between the patient's experience and the world of other people. Encouraged and empowered by safety and positive emotional experiences, the patient may become more autonomous with enhanced sense of agency and belonging, meaning and hope, and with increased capacities for coping and adapting, which are all milestones on the path of personal recovery (Davidson, 2003).

Immersing ourselves in the experience of the patient with schizotypal disorder leads us through different areas and aspects of their experience and existence. First, we make ourselves available to the patient to share his difficult feelings of anxiety, which are frequently triggered at every turn and across many situations. The patient may tell us how, alongside his anxiety, he has endless wonderings and ruminations about the many details and little things he notices in social situations or life in general. It is important, at this point, *not* to question the patient about *why* he believes he is having such thoughts or where these thoughts come from, because, at this early point in the psychotherapeutic process, the patient may often inhabit a hyperreflective stance and, by asking such questions, we risk inviting further hyperreflection, which potentially may flare-up existing symptoms (Škodlar et al., 2013; Arnfred et al., 2018). Instead, we need to strengthen the patient's sense of stability, embodiment, and selfhood, which often reduces and calms down hyper-reflection and ruminations.

Relaxation methods like progressive muscle relaxation, autogenic training, abdominal breathing, yoga, and especially mindfulness (Chadwick, 2019), are, in our experience, all very useful methods for reducing hyper-reflection and becoming more firmly embodied and in touch with one's own body, emotions, and experiences. Group or individual therapeutic sessions are helpful for familiarizing patients with such bodywork or relaxation methods. It is very important that the patients get their own live experience with these exercises and their effects, and then discuss these experiences with the therapist or are accompanied by the therapist during the exercises. In this way, patients will be better able to cope with unusual bodily sensations and learn not to reflect too much on them and instead adopt a more accepting and "letting go" attitude toward such experiences. As described earlier, patients with schizotypal disorder tend to adopt a hyperreflective stance, and experiences occurring in the practice of bodywork and relaxation methods may occasion interpretations, which, again, may distract the patient from becoming more embodied and in touch with their own body, emotions, and experience. This risks reinforcing the very symptoms (e.g., hyper-reflection or feelings of disembodiment) that these relaxation methods are trying to treat and provide relief from (Nelson et al., 2009). Patients who experience loose ego boundaries (transitivism), which is typically felt as very disturbing, may, in our experience, profit greatly from weighted duvets, which help them feel the boundary of their own body and feel more wholly demarcated.

Extravagancies or personal idiosyncrasies, that is, peculiarities in behavior, interests, activities, ignorance of social rules, humor, or outward appearance, which are a relatively frequent accompaniment of schizotypal disorder, should also be addressed therapeutically. It is important to explore what the intrinsic motivation is for such features, how patients experience them from the inside, what they mean to them, and what, if anything, they would like to do about them. It is always important to look at the overall meaning that a particular detail of the patient's life has for him or her, and, of course, to remember that it is their life to lead.

Due to the nature of their experience and the persistence of their problems, patients with schizotypal disorder risk sometimes seeing life as empty, worthless, unattractive and ultimately not worthy of living. Ambivalence and suicidality are therefore frequent companions on their life journey (Škodlar, 2007). Psychotherapy is one of the few opportunities they have to talk about these difficult aspects of their lives and, according to research, it is also one of the few protective factors against suicide for them (Škodlar et al., 2008). The therapist must always bear this in mind.

Many patients with schizotypal disorder report being able to see every situation from multiple perspectives, often at the same time. The problem herein is that often no single one of these perspectives can simply be relied on and taken for granted (Blankenburg, 1971; Henriksen et al., 2010), providing a common ground between them and others. At times, usually when they are tense, irritated, or emotionally distressed, they may experience a transient psychotic experience, where one of the multiple perspectives ossifies and overrides the others. For example, one of our patients with schizotypal disorder felt that his cousin's wedding was staged for him.

A few days after the wedding, this interpretation gave way, and he no longer believed his cousin's wedding had any particular reference to him.

Some patients with schizotypal disorder, including the patient we have presented here, experience a mystical perspective on life and often find it very meaningful. Their great openness to different perspectives, which often appears to be linked to their weakened sense of embodiment and indwelling in the world, can, in our experience, sometimes swing in either genuinely mystical or psychotic directions. Thorough therapeutic conversations about these personally significant experiences are extremely important for the patients, and they may help with prevention of slips into psychosis as well as sustain the possibility for mystical experiences to be cultivated and integrated into the patient's life (Škodlar & Ciglenečki, 2017).

Finally, it is also very important to discover all that is beautiful, stimulating, and inspiring, while exploring the inner landscapes of our patients, that is, to discover with them what they like to do and what makes them happy and fulfilled. To find their strengths, talents, hobbies, and things or occupations that have brought them joy in the past. In our experience, they are often interested in philosophy and religion, many like to work in different artistic fields, are interested in some areas or aspects of science, exercise or sport, reading or gaming. Discussions on these topics can be very stimulating for them, exploring together with a therapist their strong sides, which are uninhibited by the mental disorder. It can also be destigmatizing and stimulating to discuss famous people with the patients; people, who in some way are or have been confronted by something like the problems facing them. They may find encouragement, inspiration, and hope through such conversations and readings.

Returning now to our clinical vignette, we can see in the course of our patient's treatment a number of characteristics for the treatment of schizotypal disorder. Prior to his first psychotic episode, he had not received treatment, and after the psychotic episodes, he discontinued the low-dose antipsychotic that he had been prescribed. Thus, he has not been receiving antipsychotic therapy for most of the time.

During each of his psychotic episodes, he was hospitalized for a few days in a psychiatric intensive care unit and then discharged. After the second psychotic episode, he was referred to our Unit for Psychotherapy for Psychoses at the University Psychiatric Clinic Ljubljana, where he has been involved in psychiatric-psychotherapeutic treatment. He has always liked to come to the sessions, discuss his experiences and the therapist's responses. Far more important to him than the treatment of his symptoms or problems were the conversations about how everything he had experienced had brought him to a new understanding of the world. He liked to reflect about universal topics, existential questions, and meanings, and he had read a lot about these themes. This was most likely one of the strongest reasons for why he stayed in contact with the therapist and in psychotherapy. He did not think he had any major mental problem, the psychotic episodes were all brief and transitory, and they even had a positive value for him. Even if he felt that he did not need more serious therapy, he nonetheless liked to come and talk about the outlook on life, about consciousness and its transformations, and about the meaning of life as a whole.

While being treated in our psychotherapy unit, he positively evaluated individual psychotherapeutic sessions. In therapy sessions, apart from the aforementioned global themes, he also discussed the relationship with his parents, their divorce, and emotional consequences of the birth of his brother. At the same time, he profited from discussing everyday life and situations with other people in the unit: communication strategies, signs and symbols, meanings and common-sense aspects of statements, gestures, behaviors, and humor. He recognized that he has struggled with these areas since his childhood.

In groups, according with his basic vulnerability, he had difficulties finding common ground and common themes with other patients. He experienced himself as a "patchwork," not belonging anywhere, and for this reason, he tended to be alone. If he didn't agree with others in the group, he withdrew or did not speak. In the psychoeducation group, he expressed that he recognized himself in almost every aspect of vulnerability to psychosis. With recognition and naming of his vulnerabilities within the horizon of self-disorders, for example, how he felt different from others and how he was unable to come to terms with the taken-for-granted aspects of communication and behavior between people, he was able to better understand his life situation and his enduring problems in interactions with others, which had been with him since childhood.

He did not consider his psychotic experiences as morbid or as profoundly interfering with his life. On the contrary, he considered them a motivation for further struggles in life, exploring new opportunities and insights. He was attracted and vitalized, as we have already said, by discussing existential and mystical themes. Experiencing psychotic and spiritual insights altogether gave him a momentum to be active in life, and it has helped him away from a more passive position, with self-pity for being ill and incapable of functioning, to a more active position, striving for existential meaning and further insights.

The psychotherapeutic process has offered him an opportunity to express his whole experience of himself and his views on life, and to affirm and encourage him in his efforts to understand himself and his vulnerabilities better. Through the conversations, he was better able to identify and integrate those parts of his relationships to other people and things in the world that were different, special, and unusual. As he gradually felt more secure and more confident, these vulnerabilities and his struggles with them eventually softened, and he discovered more positive aspects in relationships and found it easier to feel part of them and of belonging to this world in general.

References

Allen, J. G., Fonagy, P., & Bateman, A. (2008). *Mentalizing in clinical practice*. American Psychiatric Publishing.

APA: American Psychiatric Association. (1980). *Diagnostic and statistical manual of mental disorders, third edition (DSM-III)*. APA.

APA: American Psychiatric Association. (2013). *Diagnostic and statistical manual of mental disorders* (5th ed.). APA.

Arnfred, S. M., Møller, P., & Davidsen, A. S. (2018). Approaching patients with hyperreflectivity and perplexity: An empirical qualitative investigation. *Trends in Psychiatry and Psychotherapy, 40*(3), 216–225.

Bigdeli, T. B., Bacanu, S. A., Webb, B. T., Walsh, D., O'Neill, F. A., Fanous, A. H., et al. (2014). Molecular validation of the schizophrenia spectrum. *Schizophrenia Bulletin, 40*, 60–65.

Bion, W. R. (1962). *Learning from experience*. Karnac.

Blankenburg, W. (1971). *Der Verlust der natürlichen Selbstverständlichkeit*. Enke.

Bleuler, E. (1950). Dementia praecox or the group of schizophrenias. International Universities Press.

Chadwick, P. (2019). Mindfulness for psychosis: A humanising therapeutic process. *Current Opinion in Psychology, 28*, 317–320.

Corin, E. E. (1990). Facts and meaning in psychiatry. An anthropological approach to the lifeworld of schizophrenics. *Culture, Medicine, and Psychiatry, 14*, 153–188.

Davidson, L. (2003). *Living outside mental illness: Qualitative studies of recovery in schizophrenia*. New York University Press.

Erlenmeyer-Kimling, L., Cornblatt, B. A., Rock, D., Roberts, S., Bell, M., & West, A. (1993). The New York high-risk project: Anhedonia, attentional deviance, and psychopathology. *Schizophrenia Bulletin, 19*(1), 141–153.

Ferrarelli, F. (2021). Sleep abnormalities in schizophrenia: State of the art and next steps. *American Journal of Psychiatry, 178*(10), 903–913.

Frosch, J. (1964). The psychotic character: Clinical psychiatric considerations. *Psychiatric Quarterly, 38*(1), 81–96.

Henriksen, M. G., Škodlar, B., Sass, L. A., & Parnas, J. (2010). Autism and perplexity: A qualitative and theoretical study of basic subjective experiences in schizophrenia. *Psychopathology, 43*(6), 357–368.

Henriksen, M. G., Raballo, A., & Nordgaard, J. (2021). Self-disorders and psychopathology: A systematic review. *Lancet Psychiatry, 8*(11), 1001–1012.

Hoch, P. H., & Cattell, J. P. (1959). The diagnosis of pseudoneurotic schizophrenia. *Psychiatric Quaterly, 33*(1), 17–43.

Hoch, P. H., & Polatin, P. (1949). Pseudoneurotic forms of schizophrenia. *Psychiatric Quaterly, 23*(2), 248–276.

Kendler, K. S. (1985). Diagnostic approaches to schizotypal personality disorder: A historical perspective. *Schizophrenia Bulletin, 11*(4), 538–553.

Kendler, K. S., Neale, M. C., & Walsh, D. (1995). Evaluating the spectrum concept of schizophrenia in the Roscommon family study. *American Journal of Psychiatry, 152*(5), 749–754.

Kety, S. S., Rosenthal, D., Wender, P. H., & Schulsinger, F. (1968a). Mental illness in the biological and adoptive families of adopted schizophrenics. In D. Rosenthal & S. S. Kety (Eds.), *Transmission of schizophrenia* (pp. 345–362). Pergamon Press.

Kety, S. S., Rosenthal, D., Wender, P. H., & Schulsinger, F. (1968b). The types and prevalence of mental illness in the biological and adoptive families of adopted schizophrenics. *Journal of Psychiatric Research, 6*, 345–362.

Knight, Z. G. (2005). The use of 'corrective emotional experience' and the search for the bad object in psychotherapy. *American Journal of Psychiatry, 59*, 30–41.

Koren, D., Tzivoni, Y., Schalit, L., et al. (2020). Basic self-disorders in adolescence predict schizophrenia spectrum disorders in young adulthood: A 7-year follow-up study among non-psychotic help-seeking adolescents. *Schizophrenia Research, 216*, 97–103.

Laing, R. D. (1977). *The divided self. An existential study in sanity and madness*. Penguin.

Lysaker, P. H., Hamm, J. A., Hasson-Ohayon, I., Pattison, M. L., & Leonhardt, B. L. (2018). Promoting recovery from severe mental illness: Implications from research on metacognition and metacognitive reflection and insight therapy. *World Journal of Psychiatry, 8*(1), 1–11.

Matussek, P. (1959). Die Angst in der schizophrenen Psychose. *Zeitschrift für Psycho- somatische Medizin, 6*(1), 10–15.

Mednick, S. A., Parnas, J., & Schulsinger, F. (1987). The Copenhagen High-Risk Project, 1962–1986. *Schizophrenia Bulletin, 13*, 485–495.

Meehl, P. E. (1962). Schizotaxia, schizotypy, schizophrenia. *American Psychologist, 17*(12), 827–838.
Mølstrøm, I. M., Henriksen, M. G., & Nordgaard, J. (2020). Differential-diagnostic confusion and non-specificity of affective symptoms and anxiety: An empirical study of first-admission patients. *Psychiatry Research, 291*. https://doi.org/10.1016/j.psychres.2020.113302
Nelson, B., Sass, L. A., & Škodlar, B. (2009). The phenomenological model of psychotic vulnerability and its possible implications for psychological interventions in the ultra-high risk ('prodromal') population. *Psychopathology, 42*(5), 283–292.
Nielsen, K. M. (2023). Social anxiety in schizophrenia: The specificity of the unspecific. *Philosophical Psychology*. https://doi.org/10.1080/09515089.2023.2177143
Nilsson, L. S., Urfer Parnas, A., & Nordgaard, J. (2019). Social life in the schizophrenia spectrum: A phenomenological study of five patients. *Psychopathology, 52*(4), 232–239.
Nordgaard, J., Handest, R., Henriksen, M. G., Vollmer-Larsen, A., Handest, P., & Parnas, J. (2021). "Transition" to schizophrenia or fluctuations within the same disorder? *Psychopathology, 54*(5), 253–261.
Parnas, J., & Henriksen, M. G. (2014). Disordered self in the schizophrenia spectrum: A clinical and research perspective. *Harvard Review of Psychiatry, 22*(5), 251–265.
Parnas, J., Licht, D., & Bovet, P. (2005). The cluster a personality disorders: A review. In M. Maj, H. S. Akiskal, J. E. Mezzich, & A. Okasha (Eds.), *Personality disorders (WPA series: Evidence and experience in psychiatry)* (Vol. 8, pp. 1–74). Wiley.
Parnas, J., Raballo, A., Handest, P., Jansson, L., Vollmer-Larsen, A., & Saebye, D. (2011). Self-experience in the early phases of schizophrenia: 5-year follow-up of the Copenhagen Prodromal Study. *World Psychiatry, 10*, 200–204.
Pedersen, S. H., Poulsen, S., & Lunn, S. (2014). Affect regulation: Holding, containing and mirroring. *International Journal of Psychoanalysis, 95*(5), 843–864.
Rado, S. (1953). Dynamics and classification of disordered behavior. *American Journal of Psychiatry, 110*(6), 406–416.
Rasmussen, A. R., & Parnas, J. (2022). What is obsession? Differentiating obsessive-compulsive disorder and the schizophrenia spectrum. *Schizophrenia Research, 243*, 1–8.
Rogers, C. R. (1957). The necessary and sufficient conditions of therapeutic personality change. *Journal of Consulting and Clinical Psychology, 21*, 95–103.
Rosenbaum, B., Henriksen, M. G., & Škodlar, B. (2019). Self-disorders in psychosis: A possible integrative concept of phenomenology and psychoanalysis. In G. Foresti & C. Eizirik (Eds.), *Psychoanalysis and psychiatry: Partners and competitors in the mental health field* (pp. 203–216). Routledge.
Safran, J. D., & Muran, J. C. (2000). *Negotiating the therapeutic alliance*. Guilford Publications.
Sass, L. A. (1990). The truth-taking-stare: A Heideggerian interpretation of a schizophrenic world. *Journal of Phenomenological Psychology, 21*(2), 121–149.
Škodlar, B. (2007). Spüre mein Leben nicht mehr. Bitte, für mich entscheiden. In J. Schlimme (Ed.), *Unentschiedenheit und Selbsttötung. Vergewisserungen der Suizidalität* (pp. 175–190). Göttingen, Germany.
Škodlar, B., & Ciglenečki, J. (2017). Multiple orientations within the worldviews in psychosis and mysticism: Relevance for psychotherapy. *Discipline filosofiche, 27*(1), 189–200.
Škodlar, B., & Henriksen, M. A. (2019). Toward a phenomenological psychotherapy for schizophrenia. *Psychopathology, 52*(2), 1–9.
Škodlar, B., Tomori, M., & Parnas, J. (2008). Subjective experience and suicidal ideation in schizophrenia. *Comprehensive Psychiatry, 49*(5), 482–488.
Škodlar, B., Henriksen, M. G., Sass, L. A., Nelson, B., & Parnas, J. (2013). Cognitive-behavioral therapy for schizophrenia: A critical evaluation of its theoretical framework from a clinical-phenomenological perspective. *Psychopathology, 46*, 249–265.
Spitzer, R. L., Endicott, J., & Gibbon, M. (1979). Crossing the border into borderline personality and borderline schizophrenia: The development of criteria. *Archives of General Psychiatry, 36*(1), 17–24.

Stephensen, H., Urfer-Parnas, A., & Parnas, J. (2023). Double bookkeeping in schizophrenia spectrum disorder: An empirical-phenomenological study. *European Archives of Psychiatry and Clinical Neuroscience*. https://doi.org/10.1007/s00406-023-01609-7

Stone, M. (1985). Schizotypal personality: Psychotherapeutic aspects. *Schizophrenia Bulletin, 11*, 576–589.

Vanggaard, T. (1979). *Borderlands of sanity: Neurosis, schizophrenic borderline states, atypical endogenous depression*. Munksgaard.

Vodušek, V., Parnas, J., Tomori, M., & Škodlar, B. (2014). The phenomenology of emotion experience in first-episode psychosis. *Psychopathology, 47*, 252–260.

WHO: World Health Organization. (1992). *The ICD-10 classification of mental and behavioural disorders: Clinical descriptions and diagnostic guidelines*. World Health Organization.

Winnicott, D. W. (1965). From dependence towards independence in the development of the individual. In D. W. Winnicott (Ed.), *The maturational processes and the facilitating environment* (pp. 83–92). Hogarth.

Zandersen, M., & Parnas, J. (2019). Identity disturbance, feelings of emptiness, and the boundaries of the schizophrenia spectrum. *Schizophrenia Bulletin, 45*(1), 106–113.

Zandersen, M., Henriksen, M. G., & Parnas, J. (2019). A recurrent question: What is borderline? *Journal of Personality Disorders, 33*(3), 341–369.

Zilboorg, G. (1941). Ambulatory schizophrenia. *Psychiatry, 4*(2), 149–155.

Zilboorg, G. (1957). Further observations on ambulatory schizophrenias. *American Journal of Orthopsychiatry, 27*(4), 677–682.

Chapter 6
Conceptualization and Assessment of Multidimensional Schizotypy

Neus Barrantes-Vidal and Thomas R. Kwapil

Conceptualization and Assessment of Multidimensional Schizotypy

Current diagnostic systems recognize that schizophrenia is part of a family of etiologically and phenomenologically related disorders (e.g., American Psychiatric Association, 2022). Furthermore, most models recognize that these disorders reflect the most severe manifestations of a continuum of clinical and subclinical impairment (Tandon et al., 2009; van Os et al., 2009), often referred to as *schizotypy*. Thus, schizophrenia can be understood as the most severe manifestation of a continuum of clinical and subclinical impairment. As noted by Kwapil and Barrantes-Vidal (2015), schizotypy provides a *useful* and *unifying* construct for conceptualizing schizophrenia-spectrum psychopathology. Schizotypy is useful in that it provides a basis for understanding the development, expression, trajectory, risk and resilience, and treatment of schizophrenia-spectrum conditions and for characterizing variation in normal behavior. Schizotypy offers a unifying framework in that it encompasses a broad spectrum of conditions including schizophrenia, related psychotic disorders, spectrum personality disorders, the prodrome, and subclinical expressions. Schizotypy allows for the examination of etiological and developmental

N. Barrantes-Vidal
Departament de Psicologia Clínica i de la Salut, Universitat Autònoma de Barcelona, Barcelona, Spain

Centre for Biomedical Research Network on Mental Health (CIBERSAM), Instituto de Salud Carlos III, Barcelona, Spain
e-mail: neus.barrantes@uab.cat

T. R. Kwapil (✉)
Department of Psychology, University of Illinois at Urbana-Champaign, Champaign, IL, USA
e-mail: trkwapil@illinois.edu

S. Cheli, P. H. Lysaker (eds.), *A Dimensional Approach to Schizotypy*,
https://doi.org/10.1007/978-3-031-41788-7_6

pathways that may underlie schizophrenia-spectrum psychopathology. Furthermore, the study of subclinical schizotypy minimizes the confounding effects that complicate the study of patients with schizophrenia, such as medication, stigma, and chronic and disabling symptoms.

Schizotypy and, by extension, schizophrenia are heterogeneous. This heterogeneity is evident at the phenotypic level, as well as at the etiological, developmental, and treatment-response levels. The heterogeneity of schizotypy and schizophrenia can be captured in a common multidimensional structure. Conceptual models and factor analytic studies indicate that positive, negative, and disorganized dimensions underlie schizophrenia (e.g., Lenzenweger & Dworkin, 1996; Liddle, 1987) and these dimensions have been replicated in non-clinically ascertained schizotypy (e.g., Bentall et al., 1989; Christensen et al., 2019; Vollema & van den Bosch, 1995). The positive (or psychotic-like) schizotypy dimension involves disruptions in the content of thought (ranging from odd ideas to delusional beliefs), perceptual abnormalities in all sensory modalities (including illusions and hallucinations), and suspiciousness. The negative (deficit) schizotypy dimension is characterized by diminished experiences including alogia, anergia, avolition, anhedonia, and flattened affect. The disorganized dimension involves disruptions in organizing and expressing thoughts, speech, emotions, and behavior (that range from mild oddities to formal thought disorder and grossly disorganized behavior). Although there is considerable support for a three-factor model of schizotypy and schizophrenia, there is no universal agreement on the number and nature of the dimensions, and other dimensions have been proposed including paranoia and impulsive-nonconformity factors.

The multidimensional structure of schizotypy and schizophrenia provides a useful approach for addressing the heterogeneity of these conditions, enhancing the power and precision of investigations, and informing clinical interventions. The reliable identification and measurement of these dimensions are essential for parsing the heterogeneity of schizotypy and schizophrenia. Treating schizotypy and schizophrenia as a homogenous construct results in a loss of conceptual precision and statistical power for investigating and understanding the origins, development, and expression of these complex conditions. We offer examples of this from three disparate studies examining the expression of multidimensional schizotypy in our own work. In an interview study of the association of positive, negative, and disorganized schizotypy with schizophrenia-spectrum symptoms and impairment, Kemp et al. (2021) reported that using a total score measure of schizotypy accounted for less than half of the variance in interview outcomes than using the three schizotypy dimensions as predictors. Similarly, Sahakyan et al. (2019) examined the association of multidimensional schizotypy with recognition accuracy in a relational memory task. They likewise found that the total schizotypy score accounted for only half of the variance accounted for by the three schizotypy dimensions – and the use of the total score obscured the differential associations of relational memory with positive, negative, and disorganized schizotypy. Kemp et al. (2023) used experience sampling methodology to examine the associations of the schizotypy dimensions with affective dynamics in daily life. The three schizotypy dimensions were associated with markedly different patterns of momentary affective experiences (e.g., negative schizotypy was characterized by diminished intensity and variability of positive affect, whereas disorganized schizotypy was associated with elevated intensity, reactivity, and variability of negative affect) – findings that would have been obscured by treating schizotypy as a unitary construct.

Despite these advantages, the construct of schizotypy has suffered due to a lack of a clear operationalization, including disparate (and sometimes conflicting) conceptualizations in the literature and being used interchangeably with a variety of other descriptors. Nevertheless, schizotypy is an increasingly studied construct with a recent PsychInfo search of the term indicating more than 3000 publications with nearly half of those in the last decade alone. The remainder of the chapter presents a brief review of the history, conceptualization, and assessment of schizotypy, with recommendations for future study.

Origins and History of Schizotypy

The term schizotype was initially coined by Rado (1953) as an abbreviation of "schizophrenic phenotype" to represent a continuum of schizophrenic-like behavioral impairment that may be present across the lifetime. Rado suggested that the liability for schizophrenia was genetically driven and that this vulnerability produced impairment ranging from mild to fully schizophrenic. Meehl (1962, 1964) formally introduced the concept of schizotypy in his landmark 1962 presidential address and his 1964 Checklist of Schizotypic Signs. Meehl's initial model posited that a single dominant "schizogene" produced a neurointegrative defect referred to as schizotaxia that was necessary, although not sufficient, for the development of schizotypy (and by extension, schizophrenia). He described schizotypy as the personality organization that resulted from schizotaxia and conveyed vulnerability for the development of schizophrenia. Meehl's checklist provided detailed descriptions of schizotypic features such as cognitive slippage, anhedonia, and magical ideation. Meehl (1990) significantly updated his original formulation by introducing hypokrisia (a neuronal aberration that characterizes schizotaxia), lessening the role of anhedonia, and expanding the impact of cognitive slippage and the contribution of polygenetic potentiators. Meehl characterized schizotypy as taxonic, suggesting that approximately 10% of the population is schizotypic and that about 10% of schizotypes decompensate into schizophrenia. Lenzenweger (e.g., 2010, 2018) clarified and advanced Meehl's conceptualization that schizotypy is the latent personality organization that conveys liability for schizophrenia. He has supported the role of genetically driven schizotaxia, or neurodevelopmental disruptions, giving rise to schizotypy and argued for the role of secondary biopsychosocial "hits" that exacerbate risk for clinical manifestations.

Meehl's model of schizotypy was rich and integrative (especially when one considers the dominant paradigms in psychiatry and psychology in the early 1960s). His model emphasized (a) genetic heritability of risk for schizophrenia (while recognizing that schizophrenia, per se, is not inherited), (b) that risk for schizophrenia is conveyed by a process of neuromaldevelopment, (c) the essential role of environmental factors (social learning regimes) interacting with genetic and neurodevelopmental risk factors, and (d) the role of an intermediate phenotype (schizotypy) between risk and disease. That said, the model falls short on many specific details. His taxonic formulation of schizotypy was based upon a single-gene model that ultimately has not received support in the literature. Meehl recognized the role of polygenetic potentiators but viewed that the single gene was necessary, albeit not sufficient, for schizophrenia. Likewise, taxometric studies have provided mixed support for a schizotypy taxon. Meehl's conceptualization of the role of environmental factors translating neurally based schizotaxia into schizotypy relied excessively on the largely discredited psychoanalytic concept of the schizophrenogenic mother. Finally, Meehl's conceptualization did not explicitly consider the multidimensional structure of schizotypy – although many of the characteristics in his checklist (e.g., perceptual aberrations, anhedonia) can be understood within a multidimensional framework.

The conceptualization and study of schizotypy also grew out of the field of individual differences with roots going back to Eysenck's (1992) personality trait of psychoticism. Claridge and colleagues (e.g., 1995, 1997) provided a view of schizotypy that built upon dimensional models of personality and psychopathology. This model put forth that schizotypy is fully dimensional in nature and includes adaptive manifestations such as creativity. This fully dimensional approach contrasted with Meehl's "quasi-dimensional" model that represented schizotypy as a forme fruste. Claridge's model proposed that schizotypy results from a combination of genetic, environmental, and personality variations that are normally distributed in the general population. Consistent with Meehl's conceptualization, the fully dimensional model acknowledged dimensionality of schizotypy in the clinical and subclinical ranges but also argued for continuity of schizotypic traits that are part of normal individual differences expressed in the general population. As such, Claridge's model includes both the pathological, quasi-dimensional components, as well as healthy expressions. Claridge and Beech (1995) suggested that schizotypy can be thought of as analogous to trait anxiety that has expressions in the general population, but in its extreme forms, results in clinical disorders. Claridge's original formulation of schizotypy did not overtly present a multidimensional structure; however, using factor analysis in the development of the Oxford-Liverpool Inventory of Feelings (O-LIFE; Mason et al., 1995), they argued for a four-factor structure of schizotypy that included factors mapping onto positive, negative, and disorganized schizotypy.

As with Meehl's model, Claridge's fully dimensional model of schizotypy suffers from several limitations. Claridge conceptualized schizotypy as a normal dimension of personality, which implies that (a) the trait has a relatively normal distribution in the general population, (b) most people fall in middle ranges of the trait, (c) there is meaningful information conveyed along the entire range of the trait, and (d) extremes of the trait tend to be associated with problematic and possibly pathological expressions. However, Claridge and colleagues have not satisfactorily provided support for these issues. Perhaps most concerning are the latter two points. Claridge's model provides explanatory power at the high end (as do most models of schizotypy) in that it gives rise to schizotypic symptoms and schizophrenia-spectrum disorders. He and colleagues also claimed that there are adaptive expressions such as creativity at elevated levels (although not extreme elevations). However, it is unclear what information is provided at the middle levels, low levels, or low extremes of schizotypy and specifically what might be the pathological expressions of low schizotypy. Furthermore, the model that high levels of schizotypy indicate psychosis risk and moderately high levels indicate adaptive expressions only seems to characterize the positive schizotypy (unusual experiences) dimension. It is unclear what the adaptive expressions of moderate levels of negative schizotypy (interpersonal aversiveness) or disorganization might be. Furthermore, given the relatively rare and potentially problematic nature of schizotypic traits, it is not clear that most of the population falls in the middle ranges of such traits.

Current Conceptualization of Schizotypy

Claridge and Meehl's accounts of schizotypy were ground-breaking and provide a powerful foundation; however, both have their significant limitations for currently conceptualizing the construct. As noted by Kwapil and Barrantes-Vidal (2015), we posit that schizotypy is a multidimensional, unifying construct that represents the underlying vulnerability for schizophrenia-spectrum psychopathology that is expressed across a broad range of personality, subclinical, and clinical phenomenology. This model implies that the same etiological, developmental, and phenomenological processes underlie subclinical and clinical manifestations. Thus, schizotypy provides an ideal model for examining these processes and their development. As described above, we believe that a multidimensional conception of schizotypy is an essential aspect of this model and recommend the use of positive, negative, and disorganized symptom dimensions (although we recognize the relevance of identifying and assessing additional dimensions and facets). We also recognize that a lack of overall conceptual clarity and differentiation from similar phenomena present impediments to the utility of schizotypy (Grant et al., 2018). There are numerous terms that are used to describe similar phenomena such as schizotypy, schizotypal personality, psychosis-proneness, psychotic-like experiences, and anomalous experiences, as well as broad labels such as subclinical psychotic symptoms. Furthermore, this terminology has expanded with descriptors of clinically indexed vulnerability for schizophrenia, such as the prodrome, basic symptoms, at-risk mental states for psychosis, and attenuated psychosis syndrome. Although these conditions can enhance our understanding of the etiology and development of schizophrenia-spectrum psychopathology, they often are used interchangeably with schizotypy. The inconsistent definition of schizotypy and assumed interchangeability of terms hinders our ability to integrate findings across studies. Note that the model of schizotypy presented here suggests that the constructs represented by these other terms (e.g., the prodrome) can be considered relatively narrow expressions of the broader schizotypy continuum and often simply represent differences in severity of symptoms. For example, non-disordered schizotypes, prodromal patients, schizotypal personality disordered patients, and psychotic patients may all experience positive symptoms such as erroneous ideas, but in an increasing level of severity from magical ideation to full-blown delusions.

The present model of schizotypy provides a dynamic, multidimensional approach that is not delimited by diagnostic boundaries. It is not intended to replace established diagnostic categories; however, it is suggested that these categories are subsumed within the schizotypy continuum. Thus, schizophrenia, for example, is not conceptualized as a separate condition, but rather as the most extreme expression of schizotypy. It is worth noting that traditional categorical diagnostic systems are increasingly embracing dimensional models of psychopathology (albeit slowly). We recognize that the current conceptualization of schizotypy may not be universally agreed upon, but we argue that it provides a testable framework for understanding a subclinical and clinical continuum of schizophrenia-spectrum psychopathology and for testing hypotheses about etiology, risk, resilience, expression, and treatment of schizophrenia-spectrum conditions.

Assessment of Schizotypy

Our claim that schizotypy is a useful construct is predicated on clear conceptualization *and* psychometrically sound measurement. Historically, schizotypy has been primarily assessed using self-report questionnaires, which offer several notable advantages. These measures can be used to screen large numbers of individuals from the general population, rather than selecting participants based upon clinical status or consanguinity. Schizotypy questionnaires are relatively non-invasive and inexpensive to administer and score, and can be used to screen large numbers of participants at one time. Finally, they can easily be used in conjunction with other measures of risk including family studies.

Psychometric assessment of schizotypy has provided a powerful tool for assessing schizophrenic-like symptoms and impairment. Numerous studies have reported that psychometric schizotypy in non-disordered individuals is associated with psychotic-like (e.g., Gooding et al., 2005), prodromal (e.g., Barrantes-Vidal et al., 2013b), and schizophrenia-spectrum (e.g., Blanchard et al., 2011) symptoms. Furthermore, longitudinal studies (e.g., Chapman et al., 1994; Kwapil, 1998; Lenzenweger, 2021) demonstrated that positive schizotypy predicts the development of psychotic disorders, whereas negative schizotypy predicts the development of schizophrenia-spectrum disorders. Schizotypy is associated with schizophrenic-like patterns of impairment assessed by neurocognition (e.g., Sahakyan & Kwapil, 2016), social cognition (e.g., Cowan et al., 2019), and neuroimaging (e.g., Sahakyan et al., 2021). In addition, schizotypy is associated with normal personality traits (e.g., Kwapil et al., 2018a), impaired attachment (e.g., Sheinbaum et al., 2013), creativity (e.g., Acar & Sen, 2013), and schizophrenic-like symptoms in daily life (e.g., Kwapil et al., 2020; Li et al., 2022).

More than two dozen questionnaire measures have been developed to assess schizotypy. Although there is considerable overlap among these measures, they differ in terms of their conceptual basis, scale development, and number and composition of their factor structure. Among the most widely used of these measures are the Wisconsin Schizotypy Scales (WSS), O-LIFE, Schizotypal Personality Questionnaire (SPQ; Raine, 1991), and Multidimensional Schizotypy Scale (MSS; Kwapil et al., 2018b).

Wisconsin Schizotypy Scales The WSS (e.g., Chapman et al., 1978) refer to a family of measures developed by the Chapmans and their collaborators to assess schizotypic traits drawn largely from Meehl's checklist. The four most widely used scales, including the Perceptual Aberration, Magical Ideation, Physical Anhedonia, and Revised Social Anhedonia Scales, can be used to compute positive and negative schizotypy dimensional scores (Kwapil et al., 2008). The scales range from 30 to 61 true-false items. Winterstein et al. (2011) derived 15-item shortened versions of the scales.

The WSS have good psychometric properties and extensive support for the validity of both the individual scales and their underlying dimensions. The strongest evidence comes from the Chapmans' ten-year longitudinal study that indicated that the Perceptual Aberration and Magical Ideation Scales predicted the development of psychotic disorders (Chapman et al., 1994) and the Revised Social Anhedonia Scale predicted the development of schizophrenia-spectrum disorders (Kwapil, 1998). Kwapil et al. (2013) demonstrated that the positive and negative dimensional scores provided improved prediction over the individual scales. Numerous studies have shown that positive and negative schizotypy, as assessed by the WSS, are associated with schizophrenia-like outcomes and impairment, as demonstrated by interview (e.g., Kwapil et al., 2008), daily life (e.g., Barrantes-Vidal et al., 2013a), and laboratory studies (e.g., Tallent & Gooding, 1999).

Despite strong psychometric properties and demonstrated validity, the WSS have several limitations, primarily regarding the adequacy of their trait coverage. Specifically, the scales do not provide assessment of the disorganized schizotypy dimension, the positive schizotypy factor lacks items assessing paranoia/suspiciousness, and the negative schizotypy factor is largely limited to assessing anhedonia and asociality. Unlike the other three scales, the Physical Anhedonia Scale has not demonstrated good predictive validity for the development of schizophrenia-spectrum disorders. The Revised Social Anhedonia Scale loads primarily on the negative schizotypy factor but tends to cross-load on positive schizotypy, likely reflecting that the scale taps characteristics such as social anxiety and affective dysregulation in addition to negative symptoms. Finally, the scales (especially the anhedonia scales) have numerous items that demonstrate differential item functioning for sex and race.

Oxford-Liverpool Inventory of Feelings and Experiences Bentall et al. (1989) combined 420 items from more than a dozen measures of schizotypy and personality to create the Combined Schizotypal Traits Questionnaire (CSTQ). Mason et al. (1995) subsequently created the 104-item O-LIFE from a factor analysis of the CSTQ. The resulting scale has four factors: unusual experiences, cognitive disorganisation, introvertive anhedonia, and impulsive nonconformity. Mason et al. (2005) developed a 43-item short version.

The O-LIFE and its fully dimensional scales are advantageous in that they measure schizotypy multidimensionally and allow for broad screening of traits in the general population. The O-LIFE has solid psychometric properties and its validity is supported by numerous cross-sectional questionnaire (e.g., Broyd et al., 2019), neurological (Kirschner et al., 2022), and cognitive (e.g., Menjivar Quijano et al., 2022) studies. Thomas et al. (2019) described that the O-LIFE subscales map on well to schizophrenia symptom dimensions. The O-LIFE Unusual Experiences and Impulsive Nonconformity Scales are associated with measures of creativity (e.g., Batey & Furnham, 2008), which is hypothesized to be an adaptive feature of schizotypy (e.g., Mohr & Claridge, 2015).

The unusual experiences and introvertive anhedonia subscales of the O-LIFE largely overlap with the WSS positive and negative schizotypy dimensions. However, contrary to its name, the O-LIFE cognitive disorganization subscale is heavily laden with items tapping neuroticism and social anxiety, rather than disruptions in thought and behavior. Furthermore, there is question of whether Impulsive Nonconformity is a meaningful dimension of schizotypy (e.g., Chapman et al., 1994). Finally, like many of the psychometric assessment measures, the O-LIFE scales lack longitudinal findings demonstrating their relation to the development of schizophrenia-spectrum disorders.

Schizotypal Personality Questionnaire The SPQ was designed to assess schizotypal personality traits in the general population and includes nine subscales based on the diagnostic criteria for schizotypal personality disorder. However, it has been widely used more generally as a measure of schizotypy. The scale contains 74 yes-no items. Raine et al. (1994) indicated that three factors underlie the scales (cognitive-perceptual, interpersonal, and disorganized). Raine and Benishay (1995) subsequently created a 22-item short form of the SPQ (SPQ-B) that produces three factor scores and a total score. The SPQ-B has benefitted from improved psychometric properties in a Likert-scale revision (SPQ-BR; Cohen et al., 2010).

Convergent validity of the SPQ has been demonstrated through its correlations with other schizotypy measures and its relation to interview-based schizotypal personality disorder diagnoses and trait ratings. Raine (1991) indicated that 55% of subjects scoring in the top tenth percentile on the scale met criteria for SPD diagnoses; however, studies have not directly replicated these findings. The SPQ, SPQ-B, and SPQ-BR have demonstrated validity in cross-sectional interview (e.g., Raine, 1991; Raine & Benishay, 1995) questionnaire (e.g., Morrison et al., 2013), psychophysiological (e.g., Prévost et al., 2010) and neurocognitive (e.g., Chun et al., 2013) studies.

The SPQ and its brief scale are advantageous in that they provide a comprehensive self-report measure of schizotypal personality traits that produces continuous factor and subscale scores. That said, some caution should be taken in considering the SPQ as a measure of schizotypy. Schizotypal personality disorder can be understood as a clinical expression of schizotypy and its traits map onto the schizotypy dimensions; however, schizotypy and schizotypal personality disorder are not synonymous. Furthermore, the dimensions assessed by the SPQ only partially map onto typical multidimensional models of schizotypy. The SPQ subscales comprising the cognitive-perceptual factor generally map onto positive schizotypy. However, the subscales assessing the interpersonal factor tend to be saturated with items tapping neuroticism and social anxiety (not typically considered to be characteristic of negative schizotypy), whereas the SPQ disorganization factor appears to broadly assess eccentricity, rather than disorganized schizotypy. Finally, the hypothesized three-factor structure of the SPQ has received only mixed support in the literature (e.g., Gross et al., 2014).

Other commonly used self-report measures of schizotypy tend to tap individual dimensions or symptoms, as opposed to specifically assessing schizotypy. For example, multiple measures assess paranoia, including the Paranoia Checklist (Freeman et al., 2005) and Paranoia Scale (Fenigstein & Vanable, 1992). Several scales assess aberrant beliefs and experiences, such as the Referential Thinking Scale (Lenzenweger et al., 1997), Peters Delusional Inventory (Peters et al., 1999), the Schizotypal Ambivalence Scale (Raulin, 1986), and the Aberrant Salience Inventory (Cicero et al., 2010). In addition, measures of personality pathology such as the Personality Inventory for DSM-5 (PID-5, Krueger et al., 2012) contain subscales or factors that map on, at least in part, to schizotypy. For example, Kemp et al. (2022) provided formulae for computing positive, negative, and disorganized schizotypy factors from the PID-5.

Despite the important contributions produced by studies employing schizotypy questionnaires, these measures suffer from a number of limitations. First, questionnaires often do not map onto current multidimensional conceptualizations of schizotypy. Specifically, some scales fail to assess schizotypy as a multidimensional construct. Furthermore, scales that do so often differ in the number and the content of the factors – and in some cases contain subscales that either do not map onto current conceptual models (e.g., impulsive nonconformity) or do not adequately assess these factors. Likewise, scales that purport to measure the same factor sometimes appear to be measuring different constructs (see Gross et al., 2014). Effective study of schizotypy requires measures that map onto the theoretical model of the construct. The current study of schizotypy is hampered by the use of multiple measures that appear to be measuring differing constructs.

A second limitation reflects that many of the older scales were developed prior to the widespread availability of modern measurement tools, such as IRT and DIF methods, which can improve psychometric properties over and above classical test theory metrics. Many of the extant scales were also developed with relatively small samples often drawn from a single site that lacked diversity. In addition, many of the existing scales employ wording that is outdated, culturally biased, or not globally applicable.

Multidimensional Schizotypy Scale The MSS and companion MSS-Brief (Gross et al., 2018) provide conceptually based, multidimensional questionnaire measures of schizotypy that include subscales assessing positive, negative, and disorganized schizotypy. The MSS contains 77 and the MSS-B contains 38 true-false items. The scales were developed to map onto Kwapil and Barrantes-Vidal's (2015) multidimensional model of schizotypy and to address limitations in extant measures. Scale development involved creation of detailed trait specifications for positive, negative, and disorganized schizotypy, which guided the development of approximately 300 candidate items that were administered to a nationwide derivation sample of over 6000 participants. Item selection was based on classical test theory, IRT, and DIF metrics.

The MSS/MSS-B subscales have good psychometric properties, including internal consistency and test–retest reliability (Kemp et al., 2020). Factor analysis supports the three-factor structure (Kwapil et al., 2018b), although Christensen et al. (2019) indicated that the negative schizotypy factor is characterized by affective and social anhedonia facets. The construct validity of the MSS has been supported by questionnaire (e.g., Kemp et al., 2022), laboratory (e.g., Sahakyan et al., 2019), neuroimaging (Sahakyan et al., 2021) and ambulatory assessment (Kwapil et al., 2020) studies. Interview studies (e.g., Kemp et al., 2021) indicate that all three schizotypy dimensions are associated with impaired functioning. Positive schizotypy is associated with prodromal symptoms and schizotypal and paranoid personality traits, negative schizotypy is associated with negative symptoms, and schizoid and schizotypal traits, and disorganized schizotypy is associated with disorganized schizotypic experiences and depression.

Interview Assessments of Schizotypy Self-report questionnaires provide an efficient screening method for assessing schizotypy. However, such measures can suffer from a variety of biases including participants purposefully over- or under-reporting experiences, not understanding the items or normalizing schizotypic experiences, and lack of awareness. Semi-structured interviews provide a method for obtaining greater detail, assessing context of experiences, providing more fine-grained determination of symptom severity, and ruling out experiences that might be erroneously endorsed on self-report questionnaires. However, the advantages of semi-structured interviews must be balanced by the costs of being time and labor intensive for assessors and participants. In contrast to the wide array of self-report questionnaire measures of schizotypy, there are relatively few semi-structured interviews, and the extant measures were often developed to assess overlapping constructs such as prodromal symptoms or schizophrenia-spectrum personality disorder traits rather than specifically assessing multidimensional schizotypy.

Several interview measures developed to assess prodromal symptoms of psychosis map on well to multidimensional schizotypy, including the Comprehensive Assessment of At-Risk Mental States (Nelson et al., 2014), which provides dimensional ratings of positive symptoms, negative symptoms, cognitive change, emotional disturbance, behavioral change, motor/physical change, and general psychopathology. Similarly, the Structured Interview for Psychosis-Risk Syndromes (McGlashan et al., 2014) offers dimensional ratings of positive, negative, disorganized, and general symptoms. These interviews cover a broad range and severity of schizotypic experiences. The Structured Interview for Schizotypic Symptoms (Kendler et al., 1989) assesses 18 symptom domains including social isolation, suspiciousness, and magical thinking, and five clinical signs. The interview provides a wealth of information relevant to schizotypy and risk for psychosis, but does not map on well to current conceptualizations of schizotypy. A number of interview measures tap individual symptom dimensions. At the present time, there seems to be a clear need for the development of a semi-structured interview that assesses current conceptualizations of multidimensional schizotypy. Such a measure would provide a valuable companion to multidimensional schizotypy questionnaires and a useful measure for both research and clinical practice.

Integrating Multidimensional Schizotypy Across Psychology, Psychiatry, and Neuroscience

In conclusion, schizotypy provides a promising construct for understanding schizophrenia-spectrum psychopathology. The multidimensional structure of schizotypy and schizophrenia, including positive, negative, and disorganized dimensions, offers a useful approach for addressing the heterogeneity of these conditions, enhancing the power and precision of investigations, and informing clinical interventions. Kwapil and Barrantes-Vidal (2015) advocated that the development of clear and testable models and measures of multidimensional schizotypy was essential for understanding the heterogeneity of schizotypy and schizophrenia and for examining their origins, development, and expression. Given the conceptual and measurement achievements of the last decade, we strongly recommend the pursuit of an integrative research approach that examines developmental processes across the range of subclinical and clinical expression of schizotypy. This includes steps such as (a) better integration of current conceptual models and assessments of multidimensional schizotypy with functional and structural neural assessment methods; (b) identifying genetic risk profiles and their modes of action in schizotypy and risk and resilience for clinical disorders; (c) expanded consideration of environmental risk (e.g., stress, trauma, problematic substance use, systemic racism) and protective (e.g., healthy attachment, early intervention) factors and their interactions with genetic and neural factors underlying schizotypy and the development of clinical disorders; (d) enhanced identification of cognitive, neurological, and behavioral endophenotypes that characterize schizotypy broadly defined; and (e) identification and differentiation of the processes that underlie the development, expression, and treatment of the positive, negative, and disorganized dimensions of schizotypy. These endeavors should facilitate the development of interventions that minimize the likelihood of clinical disorders and their impairment. In closing, we strongly advocate that schizotypy offers a unique, useful, and unifying framework for pursuing the origins and development of schizophrenia-spectrum psychopathology.

Acknowledgments Neus Barrantes-Vidal is supported by the ICREA Acadèmia Research Award (Institució Catalana de Recerca i Estudis Avançats) and the Catalan government (Suport als Grups de Recerca, 2021SGR01010).

References

Acar, S., & Sen, S. (2013). A multilevel meta-analysis of the relationship between creativity and schizotypy. *Psychology of Aesthetics, Creativity, and the Arts, 7*, 214–228.

American Psychiatric Association. (2022). *Diagnostic and statistical manual of mental disorders, fifth edition-text revision*. Author.

Barrantes-Vidal, N., Chun, C., Myin-Germeys, I., & Kwapil, T. R. (2013a). Psychometric schizotypy predicts the experience of psychotic-like, paranoid, and negative symptom experiences in daily life. *Journal of Abnormal Psychology, 122*, 1077–1087.

Barrantes-Vidal, N., Gross, G., Sheinbaum, T., Mitjavila, M., Ballespi, S., & Kwapil, T. R. (2013b). Positive and negative schizotypy are associated with prodromal and schizophrenia-spectrum symptoms. *Schizophrenia Research, 145*, 50–55.

Batey, M., & Furnham, A. (2008). The relationship between measures of creativity and schizotypy. *Personality and Individual Differences, 45*, 816–821.

Bentall, R., Claridge, G., & Slade, P. (1989). The multidimensional nature of schizotypal traits: A factor analytic study with normal subjects. *British Journal of Clinical Psychology, 28*, 363–375.

Blanchard, J. J., Collins, L. M., Aghevli, M., Leung, W. W., & Cohen, A. S. (2011). Social anhedonia and schizotypy in a community sample: The Maryland Longitudinal Study of Schizotypy. *Schizophrenia Bulletin, 37*, 587–602.

Broyd, A., Ettinger, U., & Thoma, V. (2019). Thinking dispositions and cognitive reflection performance in schizotypy. *Judgment and Decision making, 14*, 80–90.

Chapman, L. J., Chapman, J. P., & Raulin, M. L. (1978). Body image aberration in schizophrenia. *Journal of Abnormal Psychology, 87*, 399–407.

Chapman, L. J., Chapman, J. P., Kwapil, T. R., Eckblad, M., & Zinser, M. C. (1994). Putatively psychosis-prone subjects ten years later. *Journal of Abnormal Psychology, 103*, 171–183.

Christensen, A. P., Gross, G. M., Golino, H. F., Silvia, P. J., & Kwapil, T. R. (2019). Exploratory graph analysis of the Multidimensional Schizotypy Scale. *Schizophrenia Research, 206*, 43–51.

Chun, C., Minor, K., & Cohen, A. (2013). Neurocognition in psychometrically-defined college schizotypy samples: We are NOT measuring the "right stuff". *Journal of the International Neuropsychological Society, 19*, 1–14.

Cicero, D. C., Kerns, J. G., & McCarthy, D. M. (2010). The aberrant salience inventory: A new measure of psychosis proneness. *Psychological Assessment, 22*, 688–701.

Claridge, G. (1997). Theoretical background issues. In G. Claridge (Ed.), *Schizotypy: Implications for illness and health* (pp. 3–18). Oxford University Press.

Claridge, G., & Beech, T. (1995). Fully and quasi-dimensional constructions of schizotypy. In A. Raine, T. Lencz, & S. Mednick (Eds.), *Schizotypal personality disorder* (pp. 192–216). Cambridge University Press.

Cohen, A. S., Matthews, R. A., Najolia, G. M., & Brown, L. A. (2010). Toward a more psychometrically sound brief measure of schizotypal traits: Introducing the SPQ-brief revised. *Journal of Personality Disorders, 24*, 516–537.

Cowan, T., Le, T. P., & Cohen, A. S. (2019). Social cognition and schizotypy. In K. E. Lewandowski & A. A. Moustafa (Eds.), *Social cognition in psychosis* (pp. 71–88). Academic Press.

Eysenck, H. J. (1992). The definition and measurement of psychoticism. *Personality and Individual Differences, 13*, 757–785.

Fenigstein, A., & Vanable, P. A. (1992). Paranoia and self-consciousness. *Journal of Personality and Social Psychology, 62*, 129–138.

Freeman, D., Garety, P. A., Bebbington, P. E., Smith, B., Rollinson, R., Fowler, D., Kuipers, E., Ray, K., & Dunn, G. (2005). Psychological investigation of the structure of paranoia in a non-clinical population. *British Journal of Psychiatry, 186*, 427–435.

Gooding, D. C., Tallent, K. A., & Matts, C. W. (2005). Clinical status of at-risk individuals 5 years later: Further validation of the psychometric high-risk strategy. *Journal of Abnormal Psychology, 114*, 170–175.

Grant, P., Green, M. J., & Mason, O. J. (2018). Models of schizotypy: The importance of conceptual clarity. *Schizophrenia Bulletin, 44, suppl_2*, S556–S563.

Gross, G. M., Mellin, J., Silvia, P. J., Barrantes-Vidal, N., & Kwapil, T. R. (2014). Comparing the factor structure of the Wisconsin Schizotypy Scales and the Schizotypal Personality Questionnaire. *Personality Disorders: Theory, Research, & Treatment, 5*, 397–405.

Gross, G. M., Kwapil, T. R., Raulin, M. L., Silvia, P. J., & Barrantes-Vidal, N. (2018). The multidimensional Schizotypy scale-brief: Scale development and psychometric properties. *Psychiatry Research, 216*, 7–13.

Kemp, K. C., Gross, G. M., & Kwapil, T. R. (2020). Psychometric properties of the multidimensional schizotypy scale and multidimensional schizotypy scale-brief: Item and scale test-retest reliability and concordance of original and brief forms. *Journal of Personality Assessment, 102*, 508–515.

Kemp, K. C., Bathery, A. J., Barrantes-Vidal, N., & Kwapil, T. R. (2021). Positive, negative, and disorganized schizotypy predict differential patterns of interview-rated schizophrenia-spectrum symptoms and impairment. *Assessment, 28*, 141–152.

Kemp, K. C., Kaczorowski, J. A., Burgin, C. J., Raulin, M. L., Lynam, D. R., Sleep, C., Miller, J. D., Barrantes-Vidal, N., & Kwapil, T. R. (2022). Association of multidimensional schizotypy with PID-5 domains and facets. *Journal of Personality Disorders, 36*, 680–700.

Kemp, K. C., Sperry, S. H., Hernández, L., Barrantes-Vidal, N., & Kwapil, T. R. (2023). Affective dynamics in daily life are differentially expressed in positive, negative, and disorganized schizotypy. *Journal of Psychopathology and Clinical Science, 132*, 110–121.

Kendler, K. S., Lieberman, J. A., & Walsh, D. (1989). The structured interview for Schizotypy (SIS): A preliminary report. *Schizophrenia Bulletin, 15*, 559–571.

Kirschner, M., Hodzic-Santor, B., Antoniades, M., et al. (2022). Cortical and subcortical neuroanatomical signatures of schizotypy in 3004 individuals assessed in a worldwide ENIGMA study. *Molecular Psychiatry, 27*, 1167–1176.

Krueger, R. F., Derringer, J., Markon, K. E., Watson, D., & Skodol, A. E. (2012). Initial construction of a maladaptive personality trait model and inventory for DSM-5. *Psychological Medicine, 42*, 1879–1890.

Kwapil, T. R. (1998). Social anhedonia as a predictor of the development of schizophrenia-spectrum disorders. *Journal of Abnormal Psychology, 107*, 558–565.

Kwapil, T.R., Gross, G.M., Silvia, P.J., & Barrantes-Vidal, N. (2013). Prediction of psychopathology and functional impairment by positive and negative schizotypy in the Chapmans' ten-year longitudinal study. *Journal of Abnormal Psychology, 122*, 807–815.

Kwapil, T. R., & Barrantes-Vidal, N. (2015). Schizotypy: Looking back and moving forward. *Schizophrenia Bulletin, 41*(suppl 2), S366–S373.

Kwapil, T. R., Barrantes-Vidal, N., & Silvia, P. J. (2008). The dimensional structure of the Wisconsin Schizotypy scales: Factor identification and construct validity. *Schizophrenia Bulletin, 34*, 444–457.

Kwapil, T. R., Gross, G. M., Burgin, C. J., Raulin, M. L., Silvia, P. J., & Barrantes-Vidal, N. (2018a). Validity of the multidimensional Schizotypy scale: Associations with schizotypal traits and normal personality. *Personality Disorders: Theory, Research, & Treatment, 9*, 458–466.

Kwapil, T. R., Gross, G. M., Silvia, P. J., Raulin, M. L., & Barrantes-Vidal, N. (2018b). Development and psychometric properties of the Multidimensional Schizotypy Scale: A new measure for assessing positive, negative, and disorganized schizotypy. *Schizophrenia Research, 193*, 209–217.

Kwapil, T. R., Kemp, K. C., Mielock, A., Sperry, S. H., Chun, C. A., Gross, G. M., & Barrantes-Vidal, N. (2020). Association of multidimensional schizotypy with psychotic-like experiences, affect, and social functioning in daily life: Comparable findings across samples and schizotypy measures. *Journal of Abnormal Psychology, 129*, 492–504.

Lenzenweger, M. F. (2010). *Schizotypy and schizophrenia: The view from experimental psychopathology*. Guilford Press.

Lenzenweger, M. F. (2018). Schizotypy, schizotypic psychopathology and schizophrenia. *World Psychiatry, 17*, 25–26.

Lenzenweger, M. F. (2021). Schizotypy 17 years on: Psychotic symptoms in midlife. *Journal of Abnormal Psychology, 130*, 399–412.

Lenzenweger, M. F., & Dworkin, R. (1996). The dimensions of schizophrenia phenomenology: Not one or two, at least three, perhaps four. *British Journal of Psychiatry, 168*, 432–440.

Lenzenweger, M. F., Bennett, M. E., & Lilenfeld, L. R. (1997). The referential thinking scale as a measure of schizotypy: Scale development and initial construct validation. *Psychological Assessment, 9*, 452–463.

Li, L. Y., Schiffman, J., & Martin, E. A. (2022). Affect dynamic signatures of psychosis risk across multiple timescales and contexts. *Clinical Psychological Science, 10*, 960–980.

Liddle, P. F. (1987). The symptoms of chronic schizophrenia: A re-examination of the positive-negative dichotomy. *British Journal of Psychiatry, 151*, 145–151.

Mason, O., Claridge, G., & Jackson, M. (1995). New scales for the assessment of schizotypy. *Personality and Individual Differences, 18*(1), 7–13.

Mason, O., Linney, Y., & Claridge, G. (2005). Short scales for measuring schizotypy. *Schizophrenia Research, 78*, 2–3.

McGlashan, T. H., Walsh, B. C., & Woods, S. W. (2014). *Structured interview for prodromal syndromes*. Yale School of Medicine.

Meehl, P. E. (1962). Schizotaxia, schizotypy, schizophrenia. *American Psychologist, 17*, 827–838.

Meehl, P. E. (1964). *Manual for use with checklist of schizotypic signs. (No. PR-73-5)*. University of Minnesota Research Laboratories of the Department of Psychiatry.

Meehl, P. E. (1990). Toward an integrated theory of schizotaxia, schizotypy, and schizophrenia. *Journal of Personality Disorders, 4*, 1–99.

Menjivar Quijano, S. A., Ryczek, C. A., & Horne, M. R. (2022). The effect of schizotypy on spatial learning in an environment with a distinctive shape. *Frontiers in Psychology, 13*, 929653.

Mohr, C., & Claridge, G. (2015). Schizotypy--do not worry, it is not all worrisome. *Schizophrenia Bulletin, 41*(Suppl 2), S436–S443.

Morrison, S. C., Brown, L. A., & Cohen, A. S. (2013). A multidimensional assessment of social cognition in psychometrically defined schizotypy. *Psychiatry Research, 210*, 1014–1019.

Nelson, B., Yung, A., Markulev, C., & Nicoll, M. (2014). *The CAARMS: Assessing young people at ultra high risk of psychosis*. Orygen Youth Health Research Centre.

Peters, E. R., Joseph, S. A., & Garety, P. A. (1999). Measurement of delusional ideation in the normal population: Introducing the PDI (Peters et al. Delusions Inventory). *Schizophrenia Bulletin, 25*, 553–576.

Prévost, M., et al. (2010). Schizotypal traits and N400 in healthy subjects. *Psychophysiology, 47*, 1047–1056.

Rado, S. (1953). Dynamics and classification of disordered behaviour. *American Journal of Psychiatry, 110*, 406–416.

Raine, A. (1991). The SPQ: A scale for the assessment of schizotypal personality based on DSM-III-R criteria. *Schizophrenia Bulletin, 17*, 555–564.

Raine, A., & Benishay, D. (1995). The SPQ-B: A brief screening instrument for schizotypal personality disorder. *Journal of Personality Disorders, 9*, 346–355.

Raine, A., Reynolds, C., Lencz, T., Scerbo, A., Triphon, N., & Kim, D. (1994). Cognitive-perceptual, interpersonal and disorganized features of schizotypal personality. *Schizophrenia Bulletin, 20*, 191–201.

Raulin, M. L. (1986). Schizotypal Ambivalence Scale. Unpublished test (copies available from M.L. Raulin, Psychology Department, Youngstown State University, Youngstown, OH 44555; MikeRaulin.org).

Sahakyan, L., & Kwapil, T. R. (2016). Positive and negative schizotypy are associated with differential patterns of episodic memory impairment. *Schizophrenia Research Cognition, 5*, 35–40.

Sahakyan, L., Kwapil, T. R., Lo, Y., & Jiang, L. (2019). Examination of relational memory in multidimensional schizotypy. *Schizophrenia Research, 211*, 36–43.

Sahakyan, L. S., Meller, T., Evermann, U., Schmitt, S., Pfarr, J. K., Sommer, J., Kwapil, T. R., & Nenadić, I. (2021). Anterior vs. posterior hippocampal subfields in an extended psychosis phenotype of multidimensional schizotypy in a non-clinical sample. *Schizophrenia Bulletin, 47*, 207–218.

Sheinbaum, T., Bedoya, E., Ros-Morente, A., Kwapil, T. R., & Barrantes-Vidal, N. (2013). Association between attachment prototypes and schizotypy dimensions. *Psychiatry Research, 210*, 408–413.

Tallent, K. A., & Gooding, D. C. (1999). Working memory and Wisconsin card sorting test performance in schizotypic individuals: A replication and extension. *Psychiatry Research, 89*, 161–170.

Tandon, R., Nasrallah, H. A., & Keshavan, M. S. (2009). Schizophrenia, "just the facts" 4. Clinical features and conceptualization. *Schizophrenia Research, 110*, 1–23.

Thomas, E. H., et al. (2019). Do schizotypy dimensions reflect the symptoms of schizophrenia? *The Australian and New Zealand Journal of Psychiatry, 53*, 236–247.

Van Os, J., Linscott, R., Myin-Germeys, I., Delespaul, P., & Krabbendam, L. (2009). A systematic review and meta-analysis of the psychosis continuum. *Psychological Medicine, 39*, 179–195.

Vollema, M. G., & van den Bosch, R. J. (1995). The multidimensionality of schizotypy. *Schizophrenia Bulletin, 21*, 19–31.

Winterstein, B. P., Silvia, P. J., Kwapil, T. R., Kaufman, J. C., Reiter-Palmon, R., & Wigert, B. (2011). Brief assessment of schizotypy: Developing short forms of the Wisconsin Schizotypy Scales. *Personality and Individual Differences, 51*, 920–924.

Chapter 7
A (Cross-)Cultural Look at Schizotypy

Simone Cheli

A Cultural Premise

To define what a system is from within is an extremely difficult challenge. One of the most influential works of theoretical biology introduced the foundational idea that all living beings are embedded in their *Umwelt* (lit. German environment), that is, in their phenomenal world (von Uexküll, 1926). This *Umwelt* is distinctive from the surrounding so-called real world or, better, the world as experienced by the others (*Umgebung*). If we translate this perspective to the challenge of defining what culture is, we can appreciate how tricky and deceptive any answer can be.

Indeed, the construct of culture (and any attempt of mine to define schizotypy from a cultural point of view) is fully embedded in the Western society I have been born in. Several scholars have highlighted how the concept of culture is a Western construct that arose during the Enlightenment and implies a distinction between a meaning of culture as folk-spirit having a unique identity and culture as cultivation of waywardness or free individuality (Velkley, 2002). At the same time, modern anthropology and sociology suggest that culture would refer to a cumulative system of knowledge, beliefs, values, experiences, attitudes, and so on that are shared by a distinctive group of people. That said, this letter definition is again a Western one. It is embedded in the Western system of knowledge and beliefs that refers to a quite peculiar group of people that have developed across centuries a unique interest in features such as individualism, education, democracy, and many more (Henrich, 2020).

S. Cheli (✉)
Department of Psychology, St. John's University, Rome, Italy

Center for Psychology and Health, Tages Charity, Florence, Italy
e-mail: chelis@stjohns.edu

S. Cheli, P. H. Lysaker (eds.), *A Dimensional Approach to Schizotypy*,
https://doi.org/10.1007/978-3-031-41788-7_7

If we try to operationalize this information and question how to avoid cultural biases, we run the risk of entering into a spiraling paradox. The polymath Matteo Ricci (1552–1610) encountered a similar question and found a possible answer: that is, we cannot understand different cultures without changing who we are (somehow our *Umwelt*). He was a Jesuit asked to spread Christianity in China, a challenge that seemed (and maybe seems today) impossible. He subverted all the Jesuit rules and partly imbedded himself in Chinese culture: that is, he was not trying to better speak his own language, but rather changed his language, habits, clothes, and maybe beliefs. He never spread Christianity in China (and perhaps he was not really interested in that), but he was accepted at the court of the Ming Emperor, and he was shaped by Chinese culture (Fontana, 2011).

Thus, the idea of a cross-cultural perspective of schizotypy can be critical since it would imply that I am capable of comparing different cultures, and I do not think I am! In this chapter, instead, I will simply try to summarize a few cultural perspectives at the intersection between what we define in Western psychopathology as schizotypy and other aspects such as stigma, religiosity, and non-Western societies. My wish is that these pages invite the reader to maintain an inquisitive approach to what can be defined as culture and, therefore, schizotypy. In 1952 (Kroeber & Kluckhohn, 1952), there were 164 definitions of culture, and now this book aims to further extend the existing knowledge of a cross-cultural perspective of schizotypy. In order to avoid any dogmatic stance in exploring the cultural features of schizotypy, I propose to bear in mind two practical approaches. On one hand, the meaning beyond the Western construct of culture is better understood through a functional analysis of "the relation between a cultural performance and a human need" (Malinowski, 1960, p. 39). A people-specific system of knowledge and practices arises and perpetuates because it serves (or tries to serve) human scopes and needs. Consistent with an evolutionary perspective (Chap. 2), if a trait is maintained, it offers an advantage or is a sustainable cost associated with a greater advantage. A cultural inheritance system is a complex pattern that somehow extends and articulates well-known trajectories leading from genetic and epigenetic basis to ontogenetic processes (Boyd & Richerson, 1985). A cultural repertoire can be considered analogous to genotype and cultural transmission and learning to mating and nurturing from a biological point of view. On the other hand, as far as we acknowledge to be hyper-affiliative animals and that culture is by definition a social practice, we may embody what the Czech philosopher Jan Patočka (1947) defined as an ethical principle: that is, the Socratic I know that I know nothing. To the extent that we realize that we are embedded within relationships with others and that this implies that we do not have certainty in approaching our upcoming experiences because we cannot fully understand others; then we can be ethical in valuing this uncertainty. Any clinician who has approached phenomenologically the unique experience of a client has experienced this healthy doubt, and a diverse cultural background can be considered a clear reminder of the need for this ethical principle. As Wittgenstein once wrote, "Certainty is as it were a tone of voice in which one declares how things are, but one does not infer from the tone of voice that one is justified" (Wittgenstein, 1969, OC30).

Stigma and the West

> Rejection produces inferiority complexes.
> The difficulty of defending one's self-esteem devalorizes self-esteem.
> At the same time, susceptibility and hypersensitivity run high.
> – Frantz Fanon (In Gibson, 2014, p. 151)

In his works, Frantz Fanon (1925–1961) indicates a dramatic parallel between Western colonialism and the Western practice of psychiatry. Although Fanon's ideas can be compared and integrated with the ones of Ronald D. Laing (1960), Michel Foucault (1961), or Thomas Szasz (1961), his reflection goes far beyond that. Observing from the outside how the West has socially construed madness and psychiatry, he suggests that the same cultural function that underlies colonialism also underlies how Westerners deal with mental health. The function would be to control and sanction behaviors that deviate from a presumed normal standard that one is expected to adhere to as a matter of the *status quo*.

Fanon was the son of his times and experiences of being an Afro-Caribbean psychiatrist and Marxist philosopher who was born in a French colony. That said, his reflections can be delineated in modern times through two lines of research: (i) being a member of a minority would expose someone to a higher risk of severe mental disorders, with a possible contribution of some cultural precipitating factor; (ii) a normative and culturally insensitive approach to psychiatry would expose patients to a higher risk of stigmatization that, in turn, is associated with a higher distress.

First, large systematic reviews and meta-analyses support the idea that belonging to an ethnic minority group is associated with higher rates of being diagnosed with schizophrenia (Obert et al., 2018; Schwartz & Blankenship, 2014). For example, Black individuals are 2.4 times more likely to receive a diagnosis of schizophrenia than White individuals, and this finding was not affected by several contextual variables (e.g., time, healthcare setting, and diagnostic system). Consistently, young Black and Hispanic patients at risk for early psychosis have a higher probability of not receiving behavioral interventions and support compared to White patients (Heun-Johnson et al., 2021). These studies and those on minority stress (see, for sexual minority, Qi et al., 2020) do not offer any causal explanation of the phenomena, but rather raise several hypotheses. On one hand, clinicians may be seemingly affected by a bias so as to interpret divergent behaviors or beliefs as indicative of a diagnosis rather than consistent with a culture that is not their own. In the DSM-5 interview for personality disorders, for example, the item about having supernatural experiences should be explored with respect to one's religious background, rather than taking for granted it indicates a schizotypal trait. Just like nonprofessionals, clinicians can be affected by ingroup/outgroup biases that can become so rigid and pervasive that they become pathological (Bell & Dunbar, 2012). On the other hand, being a member of a minority group may also expose persons to chronic physical and mental health distress, disrupt well-being, and even cause premature mortality (Muscatell et al., 2022). Indeed, isolation, migration, changes in social status, and cultural transitions are associated with an increased risk for schizophrenia (Ku et al., 2021; Torrey et al., 1974).

Second, we need to make sense of two robust pieces of evidence about the role of stigma in mental health. Stigma is a complex construct that can be defined as a set of discriminatory or negative attitudes that others have about mental illness. In the field of psychiatry, it is also important to distinguish this broad issue from self- or internalized stigma (i.e., the internalized negative attitudes that persons diagnosed with mental disorders have about themselves) and institutional stigma (i.e., the set of intentional or unintentional negative attitudes that are generated and maintained by institutions). I have briefly summarized above how the prevalence of diagnosis and the access to services for those with schizophrenia or psychosis may be affected by clinicians' stigma (and possibly by the institutional stigma of their mental health systems). In this section, I would like to focus on the mechanisms affecting members of minority groups that are possibly diagnosed with one of the clinical manifestations of schizotypy. On one hand, it is well known how internalized stigma based on racial biases may affect the well-being of persons (David et al., 2019). Self-stigma distorts or restricts self-image by limiting and channeling the choices that a person makes, choices that will be closer to expectations consistent with internalized stigma than with real subjective needs. On the other hand, being diagnosed with schizophrenia, psychosis, or other common clinical manifestations of schizotypy is associated with an extremely high risk for reporting a self-stigma, and this, in turn, is associated with more severe symptoms, low self-confidence, poorer social functioning, and overall lower quality of life (Dubreucq et al., 2021; Vrbova et al., 2016). Therefore, those who are both members of a minority group and diagnosed with schizophrenia (or other clinical manifestations of schizotypy) are exposed to a double and extremely pernicious risk of experiencing greater suffering and not having access to the resources to cope with it.

Cultural Approaches to Schizophrenia and Psychosis

Cultural psychiatry is an emerging theoretical and applicative framework to explore the impact of culture on human behaviors and experiences. It has been suggested that this discipline has been shaped by three historical and successive "waves of development of the field from colonialist and comparative psychiatry to the mental health of ethnocultural communities and indigenous people in settler societies, and the post-colonial anthropology of psychiatry" (Kirmayer, 2018, p. 1). The rise of anti-colonialist movements and new eras of migration have fostered the development of a new perspective in psychiatry that aspires to be culturally sensitive. New theoretical tools have been proposed and new challenges have imposed change in overtly or covertly colonialist approaches to cultural psychiatry. Within this wider perspective, schizophrenia and schizotypy represent enlightening examples. The twentieth century saw the emergence of new cultural models in dealing with these clinical manifestations that made many of Falon's ideas their own (Woods, 2011).

Authors such as Thomas Szasz (1961), Ronald D. Laing (1960), and Gilles Deleuze (Deleuze & Guattari, 1974) have suggested how schizophrenia would represent emblematically how society imposes its norms over individuals and how these may manifest diverse forms of psychopathology as a way to defend themselves and hold together an inner world that is falling apart. On the contrary, they postulated how "the schizophrenic ceases to be schizophrenic when he meets someone by whom he feels understood. When this happens most of the bizarrerie which is taken as the 'signs' of the 'disease' simply evaporates" (Laing, 1961, p. 165).

More recently, these theoretical suggestions have been critically explored and tested in clinical work. This attempt to operationalize a cultural approach to schizophrenia has led to several important contributions. First, a social perspective to the emergence and persistence of psychosis and schizophrenia has been described (McKenzie & Shah, 2017). A culturally sensitive approach to prevention and research should include four interacting dimensions: (i) exposure to social factors at an individual level (e.g., social support); (ii) exposure to environmental factors at an ecological level (e.g., socio-economic status of the community); (iii) interaction between these previous factors (i and ii); and (iv) interactions between previous factors and time. This wider model aspires to support clinicians and researchers regardless of the cultural context of the setting and of the patient. For example, a deep conceptualization of schizotypal personality disorder (SPD) should integrate all these dimensions to better understand how diverse elements can be considered as maintaining or precipitating factors impeding treatment or fueling relapses, respectively. Second, commonly defined psychotic experiences such as hearing voices are increasingly understood through a cultural perspective (Luhrmann et al., 2015a, b). Indeed, different cultural contexts are associated with different experiences of hearing voices. Psychotic experiences are shaped by cultural context (social kindling hypothesis), and the more judgmental one's community is about this kind of experience, the more distress is reported by the hearer. Therefore, a better understanding of the cultural context of the client offers two major therapeutic advantages: (i) even the psychotic experience becomes meaningful and, therefore, manageable in session, and (ii) promoting a less judgmental and more compassionate stance in looking at one's self may be of great help for the patient. Therapeutic approaches such as compassion-focused therapy and evolutionary systems therapy are based on these very principles (see Chaps. 14 and 17). Third, even the apparently transcultural assumption of psychosis as personifying a fracture in the person's experience and as frequently associated with traumatic events may be another product of a Western monocultural perspective (Dhar, 2020). Diverse contexts are composed by diverse relationships, and the suggested framework to understand cultural diversity may be related to a broadly defined relational nature of our suffering: "People are constituted (in a very material way) by other people, lands, things, words, and intentions; and second, that intense affect like unfulfilled desire and acute suffering physically sticks to places and people across time and space" (Dhar, 2020, p. 126). Without contextualizing our conceptualization of presenting problems and the development of an intervention, we run the risk of not targeting the real problem. We have to be aware of how much psychotherapy and psychopharmacotherapy are embedded in our Western culture, and therefore, they may not be the most viable option for someone coming from another culture. For example, the Western way of thinking about efficacy and change has seemingly channelized the definition of therapeutic interventions. The philosopher François Julien (1997) has suggested several antitheses between West and China in this respect: We think in the West more in terms of immediate, agentic and dramatic action, whereas in China, they are more oriented toward a progressive and complex transformation based on a less is more perspective. These differences are consistent with studies showing how individuals in European and North American countries, when coping with stressors, are encouraged to focus on distinctiveness and act in accordance with their personal wishes, whereas in East Asian countries, individuals are encouraged to focus on their relationships and act in accordance with their communities (Lustig & Koester, 2017). The very idea of psychology as a scientific theory of mind is often indistinguishable from Western theory of mind and consequently at risk of several cultural biases (Bhatia & Priya, 2021). Therefore, it is difficult to think that there are interventions that are effective for everyone and every culture. This need for tailor-made interventions is even more important considering the very nature of schizotypal manifestations as primarily characterized by odd and bizarre experiences that by definition are divergent from a normative reference.

Creative, Religious, and Schizotypal Experiences

Schizotypy is a continuum of experiences ranging from subclinical or even healthy states to severe manifestations such as schizophrenia, psychosis, and SPD (see Chaps. 3 and 6). It has been suggested that the personality traits underlying this vulnerability are associated with high levels of healthy traits, such as openness to experience and introversion (Cheli, 2023). The most representative manifestation of schizotypy, that is SPD, would represent a failure in socialization to culminate in these healthy traits: that is, the curiosity in making experiences and proneness to change one's own beliefs (i.e., openness to experience) and the preference for focusing on inner thoughts and ideas, rather than what is happening externally (i.e., introversion). Evolutionarily speaking, persons with SPD would opt for risk-minimizing (i.e., social and emotional detachment) and unique-maximizing (i.e., psychoticism in the form of odd behaviors, emotions, cognitions) strategies when facing severe distress (Chap. 2).

Indeed, a growing body of evidence indicates a possible association between schizotypal traits and presumably divergent experiences, such as creative or religious ones. On one hand, large genetic studies on those diagnosed with schizophrenia and psychosis or on their healthy relatives have reported a relevant association between creative or artistic jobs and polygenic risk for schizophrenia (McCabe et al., 2018; Power et al., 2015). These findings cannot be interpreted as a causal link between schizotypal traits and creativity, but rather support a multi-trait perspective that schizotypy and creativity share a common background, consistent, in turn, with the association between openness to experience and schizotypy. Those with a greater proneness to intellectual curiosity when presenting a vulnerability for schizotypy may incur a higher risk for severe manifestations such as psychosis. On the other hand, anthropological or phenomenological studies suggest that cultural context may be a crucial protective factor against psychosis through religious and spiritual experiences (Cheli et al., 2021; Jackson, 1997; Luhrmann, 2020). To the extent that hearing a divine voice is experienced as an event that is consistent with both my system of values and the one of my community; the presumably psychotic experience is no longer experienced as such.

Ethnographic accounts suggest that religious practices, beliefs and experiences intrinsically interact with one another, even to the point of having experiences of relationships with supernatural agents (Luhrmann, 2020). Similar observations led the psychologist Mike Jackson (1997) to consider psychotic experiences within coherent religious experiences as a form of benign schizotypy. Similarly, Cheli et al. (2021) compared two groups of people hearing divine voices: one composed of persons diagnosed with psychosis, one composed of spiritual persons who were part of a religious community. The former group described the voices as mostly critical and causing distress and isolation, whereas the latter group reported a sense of compassionate connection with both the voice and their community. The case of religiosity has attracted the attention of researchers in psychology since Williams James (1902) and has seemingly played an important evolutionary role in our species, since we were hyper-affiliative animals spreading around all the globe. Robin Dunbar (2022) has postulated how religion served as an effective way to maintain social bonding despite the physical distance. Indeed, the relational dynamics and their association with specific traits can better explain the importance of these findings. It is reported that religious persons assuming either a leading/shamanic role or adept/follower role present very different personality profiles: The formers are higher in levels of openness to experiences and extroversion, whereas the latter of conscientiousness and agreeableness (Schnitker & Emmons, 2021). We can speculate how having a proneness to divergent ideas may have promoted and may promote within a certain context an evolutionary advantage.

Gathering together all these studies on creative, religious and schizotypal experiences, we can take a step further in respect to the previous studies on cultural psychiatry. The relational context and socializing strategies are seemingly the two most recurrent factors. Whenever the community, healthcare services, and mental health professionals are acting in an accepting, welcoming, and safe way, even bizarre and odd experiences might not lead to severe mental disorders. Whereas when the others are seemingly imposing a normative judgment about one's unique experience, the risk to transition to manifestations such as psychosis is seemingly high. Indeed, complex functions that therapists try to promote, such as "mentalization can be influenced by the social role one is in" (Liotti & Gilbert, 2011, p. 21). The more threatening this role is, the more difficult it will be for the person to mentalize.

A Possible Relational Synthesis

Emerging neurophysiological evidence supports a model of human experience that is profoundly relational, both at phylogenetic and ontogenetic level. The social brain theory explains the rise of the human complex neocortex as resulting from an increasingly qualitatively and quantitatively complex social environment (Dunbar, 2009). The neurocognitive demands of our social life were as massive; thus, we needed an extremely powerful device. The ability to mentalize others' minds increased exponentially in respect to other primates and mammals. Evolutionarily speaking, we traded greater complexity for greater risk in managing that complexity. It is reported that schizophrenia, as a failure of our newly evolved ability to mentalize, emerged with our species (Gregory et al., 2021). Similarly, our ontogenetic development is shaped by the relational experiences we are immersed in. As we develop, we begin forming ideas and a larger sense of the other before our self, and more ultimately, we form our identity and mentalize through our relationship with others (Faraji & Metz, 2023; Schore, 2021). The clinical manifestations of schizotypy, such as schizophrenia, psychosis, and SPD, are extensively associated with distorted early and adult intersubjective experiences, such as disorganized attachment, childhood maltreatment, bullying, social isolation, and so on (Bucci et al., 2017; Cheli, 2023; Gumley et al., 2014). Indeed, the perception of either an internal (e.g., self-criticism) or external (e.g., interpersonal criticism) threat may trigger a defensive response that, in turn, may hypo-activate areas involved in the mentalizing processes (e.g. prefrontal cortex) and indirectly activate areas involved in emotional hypervigilance (e.g., amygdala), leading to common psychological mechanisms or even psychotic symptoms (Heriot-Maitland et al., 2019; Petrocchi & Cheli, 2019).

This broad neuroscientific model might be applied to either schizotypy from a standard Western perspective or culturally sensitive experiences such as migrating or belonging to a minority. Moreover, it is not in contrast with a divergent perspective to severe manifestations of schizotypy, such as psychosis, either focusing on a non-Western society or a religious communitarian environment. From a more phenomenological point of view, if we suggest that we consider humans as hyper-affiliative animals, then this is consistent with a cross-cultural idea that we are made up of our relationships (see Dhar, 2020; Schore, 2021). The source of both psychopathology and healing is embedded in the relationships we have progressively constructed with persons, spaces, and environments. Therefore, a variety of experiences may lead either to mental health or emotional pain. In accordance with neuroscientific evidence of the multiplicity of our self (Klein & Gangi, 2010), I speculate about how we are not a unique self and in facing significant distress we do not need to recover an original unique self. Moreover, an experience of hearing voices or perceiving different persona or parts of self seems natural rather than odd. Any attempt to promote the well-being of someone hearing voices might work to the extent that it aims to welcome all the voices and connect them again with the persons, spaces, and environments where they arose (see Chaps. 14 and 17).

In conclusion, a culturally sensitive perspective to schizotypy is seemingly a fertile one. It may promote the integration of diverse fields of knowledge (such as cultural psychiatry, neuroscience, psychotherapy, religious studies, and anthropology) and inform the daily practice of any clinician. The sensitivity necessary to understand the uniqueness of a patient is the same that is useful to understand their cultural background. Finally, the complexity of schizotypal traits and their well-known association with divergent experiences such as creativity and religiosity represents an important area for further research.

> If you are a poet, you will see clearly that there is a cloud floating in this sheet of paper. Without a cloud, there will be no rain; without rain, the trees cannot grow; and without trees, we cannot make paper. The cloud is essential for the paper to exist. If the cloud is not here, the sheet of the paper cannot be here either. So we can say that the cloud and the paper inter-are. 'Interbeing' is a word that is not in the dictionary yet, but if we combine the prefix 'inter-' with the verb 'to be', we have a new verb, inter-be. Without a cloud, we cannot have paper, so we can say that the cloud and the sheet of paper inter-are.
> – Thich Nhat Hanh, 1998, p.3

References

Bell, C. C., & Dunbar, E. (2012). Racism and pathological bias a s a co-occurring problem in diagnosis and assessment. In T. A. Widiger (Ed.), *The Oxford handbook of personality disorders* (pp. 694–711). Oxford University Press.

Bhatia, S., & Priya, K. R. (2021). Coloniality and psychology: From silencing to re-centering marginalized voices in postcolonial times. *Review of General Psychology, 0*(0), 1–15. https://doi.org/10.1177/10892680211046507

Boyd, R., & Richerson, P. J. (1985). *Culture and the evolutionary process*. Chicago University Press.

Bucci, S., Emsley, R., & Berry, K. (2017). Attachment in psychosis: A latent profile analysis of attachment styles and association with symptoms in a large psychosis cohort. *Psychiatry research, 247*, 243–249. https://doi.org/10.1016/j.psychres.2016.11.036

Cheli, S. (2023). An evolutionary look at oddity and schizotypy: How the rise of social brain informs clinical practice. *New Ideas in Psychology, 68*. Advance online publication. https://doi.org/10.1016/j.newideapsych.2022.100993

Cheli, S., Petrocchi, N., & Cavalletti, V. (2021). Hearing divine voices: A qualitative enquiry about criticism, connectedness, and compassion. *Psychosis: Psychological, Social and Integrative Approaches*. https://doi.org/10.1080/17522439.2021.2011387

David, E. J. R., Schroeder, T. M., & Fernandez, J. (2019). Internalized racism: A systematic review of the psychological literature on racism's most insidious consequence. *Journal of Social Issues, 75*(4), 1057–1086. https://doi.org/10.1111/josi.12350

Deleuze, G., & Guettari, F. (1974). *L'Anti-Œdipe*. Minuit.

Dhar, A. (2020). *Madness and subjectivity: A cross-cultural examination of psychosis in the west and India*. Routledge.

Dubreucq, J., Plasse, J., & Franck, N. (2021). Self-stigma in serious mental illness: A systematic review of frequency, correlates, and consequences. *Schizophrenia Bulletin, 47*(5), 1261–1287. https://doi.org/10.1093/schbul/sbaa181

Dunbar, R. I. (2009). The social brain hypothesis and its implications for social evolution. *Annals of Human Biology, 36*(5), 562–572. https://doi.org/10.1080/03014460902960289

Dunbar, R. I. (2022). *How religion evolved: And why it endures*. Pelican Books.

Faraji, J., & Metz, G. A. S. (2023). Toward reframing brain-social dynamics: Current assumptions and future challenges. *Frontiers in Psychiatry, 14*, 1211442. https://doi.org/10.3389/fpsyt.2023.1211442

Fontana, M. (2011). *Matteo Ricci. A Jesuit at the Ming Court*. Rowaman & Littlefield Publishers.

Foucault, M. (1961). *Folie et déraison. Histoire de la folie à l'âge classique*. Plon.

Gibson, N. (2014). Decolonizing Madness. The Psychiatric Writings of Frantz fanon. New York: Palgrave Macmillan.

Gregory, M. D., Eisenberg, D. P., Hamborg, M., Kippenhan, J. S., Kohn, P., Kolachana, B., Dickinson, D., & Berman, K. F. (2021). Neanderthal-derived genetic variation in living humans relates to schizophrenia diagnosis, to psychotic symptom severity, and to dopamine synthesis. *American Journal of Medical Genetics. Part B, Neuropsychiatric Genetics: The Official Publication of the International Society of Psychiatric Genetics, 186*(5), 329–338. https://doi.org/10.1002/ajmg.b.32872

Gumley, A. I., Taylor, H. E., Schwannauer, M., & MacBeth, A. (2014). A systematic review of attachment and psychosis: measurement, construct validity and outcomes. *Acta psychiatrica Scandinavica, 129*(4), 257–274. https://doi.org/10.1111/acps.12172

Henrich, J. (2020). *The WEIRDest people in the world: : How the west became psychologically peculiar and particularly prosperous*. Farrar, Straus and Giroux.

Heriot-Maitland, C., McCarthy-Jones, S., Longden, E., & Gilbert, P. (2019). Compassion focused approaches to working with distressing voices. *Frontiers in Psychology, 10*, 152. https://doi.org/10.3389/fpsyg.2019.00152

Heun-Johnson, H., Menchine, M., Axeen, S., Lung, K., Claudius, I., Wright, T., & Seabury, S. A. (2021). Association between race/ethnicity and disparities in health care use before first-episode psychosis among privately insured young patients. *JAMA Psychiatry, 78*(3), 311–319. https://doi.org/10.1001/jamapsychiatry.2020.3995

Jackson, M. (1997). Benign schizotypy? The case of spiritual experience. In G. E. Claridge (Ed.), *Implications for illness and health*. Oxford University Press.

James, W. (1902). *The varieties of religious experience : A study in human nature*. Longmans.

Julien, F. (1997). *Traité de l'efficacité*. Grasset.

Kirmayer, L. J. (2018). Cultural psychiatry in historical perspective. In D. Bughra & K. Bhui (Eds.), *Textbook of cultural psychiatry* (2nd ed., pp. 1–17). Cambridge University Press.

Klein, S. B., & Gangi, C. E. (2010). The multiplicity of self: Neuropsychological evidence and its implications for the self as a construct in psychological research. *Annals of the New York Academy of Sciences, 1191*, 1–15. https://doi.org/10.1111/j.1749-6632.2010.05441.x

Kroeber, A. L., & Kluckhohn, C. (1952). Culture: A critical review of concepts and definitions. *Papers. Peabody Museum of Archaeology & Ethnology, Harvard University, 47*(1), viii, 223.

Ku, B. S., Compton, M. T., Walker, E. F., & Druss, B. G. (2021). Social fragmentation and Schizophrenia: A systematic review. *The Journal of Clinical Psychiatry, 83*(1), 21r13941. https://doi.org/10.4088/JCP.21r13941

Laing, R. D. (1960). *The divided self: An existential study in sanity and madness*. Harmondsworth: Penguin.

Liotti, G., & Gilbert, P. (2011). Mentalizing, motivation, and social mentalities: Theoretical considerations and implications for psychotherapy. *Psychology and Psychotherapy, 84*(1), 9–110. https://doi.org/10.1348/147608310X520094

Luhrmann, T. M. (2020). *How God becomes real: Kindling the presence of invisible others*. Princeton University Press.

Luhrmann, T. M., Padmavati, R., Tharoor, H., & Osei, A. (2015a). Differences in voice-hearing experiences of people with psychosis in the U.S.A., India and Ghana: Interview-based study. *The British Journal of Psychiatry : the Journal of Mental Science, 206*(1), 41–44. https://doi.org/10.1192/bjp.bp.113.139048

Luhrmann, T. M., Padmavati, R., Tharoor, H., & Osei, A. (2015b). Hearing voices in different cultures: A social kindling hypothesis. *Topics in Cognitive Science, 7*(4), 646–663. https://doi.org/10.1111/tops.12158

Lustig, M. W., & Koester, J. (2017). *Intercultural competence: interpersonal communication across cultures* (8th ed.). Allyn and Bacon.

MacCabe, J. H., Sariaslan, A., Almqvist, C., Lichtenstein, P., Larsson, H., & Kyaga, S. (2018). Artistic creativity and risk for schizophrenia, bipolar disorder and unipolar depression: A Swedish population-based case-control study and sib-pair analysis. *The British Journal of Psychiatry : the Journal of Mental Science, 212*(6), 370–376. https://doi.org/10.1192/bjp.2018.23

Malinowski, B. (1960). *A scientific theory of culture and other essays*. New York: Galaxy Book.

McKenzie, K., & Shah, J. (2017). Understanding the social etiology of psychosis. In L. J. Kirmayer, R. Lemelson, & C. A. Cummings (Eds.), *Re-visioning psychiatry cultural phenomenology, critical neuroscience, and global mental health* (pp. 317–342). Cambridge University Press.

Minkowski, B. (1960). *A scientific theory of culture and other essays*. Oxford University Press.

Muscatell, K. A., Alvarez, G. M., Bonar, A. S., Cardenas, M. N., Galvan, M. J., Merritt, C. C., & Starks, M. D. (2022). Brain-body pathways linking racism and health. *The American Psychologist, 77*(9), 1049–1060. https://doi.org/10.1037/amp0001084

Olbert, C. M., Nagendra, A., & Buck, B. (2018). Meta-analysis of Black vs. White racial disparity in schizophrenia diagnosis in the United States: Do structured assessments attenuate racial disparities? *Journal of Abnormal Psychology, 127*(1), 104–115. https://doi.org/10.1037/abn0000309

Patočka, J. (1947). *Sokarates*. Spolek posluchačů filosofie.

Petrocchi, N., & Cheli, S. (2019). The social brain and heart rate variability: Implications for psychotherapy. *Psychology and Psychotherapy, 92*(2), 208–223. https://doi.org/10.1111/papt.12224

Power, R. A., Steinberg, S., Bjornsdottir, G., Rietveld, C. A., Abdellaoui, A., Nivard, M. M., Johannesson, M., Galesloot, T. E., Hottenga, J. J., Willemsen, G., Cesarini, D., Benjamin, D. J., Magnusson, P. K., Ullén, F., Tiemeier, H., Hofman, A., van Rooij, F. J., Walters, G. B., Sigurdsson, E., Thorgeirsson, T. E., et al. (2015). Polygenic risk scores for schizophrenia and bipolar disorder predict creativity. *Nature Neuroscience, 18*(7), 953–955. https://doi.org/10.1038/nn.4040

Qi, R., Palmier-Claus, J., Simpson, J., Varese, F., & Bentall, R. (2020). Sexual minority status and symptoms of psychosis: The role of bullying, discrimination, social support, and drug use - findings from the Adult Psychiatric Morbidity Survey 2007. *Psychology and Psychotherapy, 93*(3), 503–519. https://doi.org/10.1111/papt.12242

Schnitker, S. A., & Emmons, R. A. (2021). Personality and religion. In O. P. John & R. W. Robins (Eds.), *Handbook of personality: Theory and research* (pp. 707–723). The Guilford Press.

Schore, A. N. (2021). The interpersonal neurobiology of intersubjectivity. *Frontiers in Psychology, 12*, 648616. https://doi.org/10.3389/fpsyg.2021.648616

Schwartz, R. C., & Blankenship, D. M. (2014). Racial disparities in psychotic disorder diagnosis: A review of empirical literature. *World Journal of Psychiatry, 4*(4), 133–140. https://doi.org/10.5498/wjp.v4.i4.133

Szasz, T. (1961). *The myth of mental illness: Foundations of a theory of personal conduct*. Harper & Row.

Thich Nhat Hanh. (1998). *The hearth of understanding. Commentaries to the Prajnaparamita Heart Sutra*. Berkeley: Parallax Press.

Torrey, E. F., Torrey, B. B., & Burton-Bradley, B. G. (1974). The epidemiology of schizophrenia in Papua New Guinea. *American Journal of Psychiatry, 131*, 567–573.

Velkley, R. L. (2002). *Being after Rousseau: Philosophy and culture in question*. University of Chicago Press.

von Uexküll, J. (1926). *Theoretical biology*. Harcourt, Brace & Co.

Vrbova, K., Prasko, J., Holubova, M., Kamaradova, D., Ociskova, M., Marackova, M., Latalova, K., Grambal, A., Slepecky, M., & Zatkova, M. (2016). Self-stigma and schizophrenia: A cross-sectional study. *Neuropsychiatric Disease and Treatment, 12*, 3011–3020. https://doi.org/10.2147/NDT.S120298

Wittgesntein, L. (1969). *On certainty*. Basil Blackwell.

Woods, A. (2011). *The sublime object of psychiatry: Schizophrenia in clinical and cultural theory*. Oxford University Press.

Part II
Transdiagnostic Mechanisms

Chapter 8
Understanding the Phenomenology of Schizotypy and Schizotypal Personality Disorder: An Application of the Integrative Model of Metacognition

Paul H. Lysaker and Courtney N. Wiesepape

Introduction

As discussed earlier in this volume, the term schizotypy is generally used to reflect an enduring set of personality traits that fall along a continuum that stretches from typical or healthy levels of psychosocial functioning to more impaired levels of psychosocial functioning. At relatively mild levels, schizotypy may reflect traits related to eccentricity that offer some social advantage as a marker of uniqueness and creativity. At more significant levels, it may represent forms of odd thought and detachment that significantly derail psychosocial functioning (Lenzenweger, 2006). When it reaches levels that could be deemed psychopathological, schizotypy has been suggested to fall at the mild end of the larger continuum of schizophrenia spectrum disorders (Nelson et al., 2013). When severe enough, schizotypy may manifest in maladaptive traits reflected in a diagnosis of schizotypal personality disorder (Verbeke et al., 2017). As originally conceptualized by Meehl (1962), these traits are present in approximately 10% of the general population and among those with schizotypy, 10% (approximately 1% of the total population) have impairments in functioning, which are severe enough to warrant a diagnosis of schizophrenia.

Like other features of schizophrenia spectrum disorders, it is unclear how to best characterize the psychological factors that underlie the emergence and persistence of schizotypy. Considerable literature exists examining potential biological processes that contribute to schizotypy including abnormalities in the neurobiology

P. H. Lysaker (✉)
Richard L Roudebush VA Medical Center, Department of Psychiatry, Indianapolis, IN, USA

Indiana University School of Medicine, Department of Psychiatry, Indianapolis, IN, USA
e-mail: plysaker@iupui.edu

C. N. Wiesepape
Indiana University School of Medicine, Department of Psychiatry, Indianapolis, IN, USA

S. Cheli, P. H. Lysaker (eds.), *A Dimensional Approach to Schizotypy*,
https://doi.org/10.1007/978-3-031-41788-7_8

that underlies optimal levels of arousal, executive functioning, and human attachment. However, at the level of phenomenology, what observable processes result in the development of the odd and detached behaviors which are described by schizotypy? As persons experience the world, what processes amplify those traits to levels where notable psychosocial dysfunction occurs? Answers to these questions are essential for developing psychosocial interventions which target more proximal causes of disorder.

To address these questions, this chapter will explore how the integrative model of metacognition may offer a framework for understanding different features of schizotypy. We will first describe the overlap between conceptual models of the features of schizotypy and schizophrenia disorders in general. We will next describe how the phenomenology of schizophrenia has been interpreted by one specific model—the integrative model of metacognition. Following this, we will explore how this model could be applied to understand the phenomenology observed in schizotypy as a personality organization and schizotypal personality disorder as a formal diagnostic category. Here we will propose that the behaviors that characterize schizotypy and schizotypal personality disorder may ultimately reflect metacognitive deficits or disturbances in persons' abilities to form integrative ideas of themselves and others in an ongoing and evolving manner that is responsive to dynamic changes in the world. Lastly, we will present supporting research and discuss limitations and future directions.

The Shared Phenomenology of Schizotypy and Schizophrenia Disorders

To date, the phenomenology of schizotypal personality disorder and schizotypy, as a general aspect of personality, includes a range of significantly different behaviors. One of the most common ways they have been organized is along multiple factors with varying solutions identifying separate positive, negative, and disorganized factors. In these models, positive expressions of schizotypy involve odd experiences and unusual modes of expressing oneself. Negative expressions of schizotypy, by contrast, involve a lack of social interest, anhedonia, and a lack of expression of emotions. Disorganized expressions reflect tangential and disorganized expressions of ideas or understandings of the world. Across models, these factors are conceptualized as dimensional with variation between persons ranging from subclinical levels where these experiences do not affect psychosocial function to more significant or clinical levels in which function is disrupted.

In parallel, the widely varying features of schizophrenia disorders have similarly been conceptualized as reflecting a number of factors (Bell et al., 1992). Important for the purposes of this chapter, a range of different approaches to studying schizophrenia include the same three factors as found in schizotypy: positive, negative, and disorganized (Fong et al., 2015). In schizophrenia spectrum disorders, in contrast to schizotypy, the factors tend to include clinical symptoms; however, the same themes pervade (Lim et al., 2021). Positive symptoms include odd experiences and beliefs such as hallucinations and delusions. Negative symptoms include a lack of internal experiences including lack of volition and interest in others and lack of expression of affect (e.g., blunted affect). Disorganized symptoms include conceptual disorganization and stereotyped and concrete thought processes.

The Integrated Model of Metacognition and the Phenomenology of Schizophrenia: A Brief Overview

In the integrated model, metacognition is conceptualized as a range of processes that support the formation of and reflection upon a sense of oneself, others, and one's action in the world. In this model, metacognition includes activities in which persons notice discrete experiences such as thoughts and feelings as well as interpret those in the context of a larger sense of oneself and others. Metacognition thus enables persons to notice errors and to be aware of one's preferred styles of thinking and learning. It also enables persons to recognize their own emotional state or habitual responses to the world. It facilitates the formation of ideas about what persons generally believe about themselves and others, and how they might best manage challenges as they emerge in life.

In short, all these forms of awareness are metacognitive because they are available for reflection. They are ideas and larger senses of things that persons can interpret or think about. They allow for reflection upon both what is happening at the moment and also the broader things that seem to be about oneself and others, including one's and others' purposes, possibilities, and place in the world (Lysaker et al., 2021). Metacognition thus allows persons to monitor and respond to experience not only at specific levels but at the level of the larger meanings which characterize a life. Importantly, metacognition is believed to involve several distinct foci including the self (self-reflectivity), others (awareness of the other), one's challenges and responses to those (mastery), and one's place in the larger community (decentration). These forms of awareness are further understood to be measurable independent of one another but also to interact. That interaction then is believed to be essential for human adaptation, allowing persons to form an evolving sense of themselves, others, and their communities, which is available to guide responses to a changing psychosocial environment (Davis et al., 2022).

In this evolving model, it has been suggested that metacognitive processes are supported by a broad range of social and biological processes. Accordingly, metacognition may fail to operate efficiently as a result of multiple factors (e.g., alterations in basic brain processes, trauma, and stigma) resulting in what could be described as metacognitive deficits. These metacognitive deficits then have been proposed to represent a transdiagnostic construct that might explain dysfunction across multiple conditions including bipolar disorder, borderline personality disorder, post-traumatic stress disorder, and substance use disorder (Lysaker et al., 2020b).

Perhaps, however, this model has received the most empirical attention as an application to schizophrenia. It is suggested that particularly severe decrements in metacognition function lead persons diagnosed with schizophrenia to have fragmented experiences of themselves, others, and their actions in the world (Lysaker et al., 2020c). Subjectively, this may appear as the experience of a self that lacks cohesion, and general confusion about the unique thoughts and feelings or others. With metacognitive deficits, persons may struggle to not only form coherent ideas about themselves but also find the challenges they are facing incomprehensible while having relatively little sense of being able to act in ways that might influence events. At this point, persons may experience themselves as having little to no sense of agency. They may feel that the trajectory of their lives has been altered if not in some sense obliterated, resulting in the sense of oneself as unconnected to the past or any potentially meaningful future.

To study this, researchers have assessed metacognitive capacity as persons diagnosed with schizophrenia spectrum disorders think about themselves, others, and their lives in semi-structured narrative interviews. In this research, the primary tool used to assess metacognitive capacity within narratives has been the Metacognitive Assessment Scale-Abbreviated, which generates separate scores for the capacity for self-reflectivity, awareness of others, understanding of one's actions (mastery), and awareness of one's place in their community (decentration). This work has to date found that adults with both first episode and in the later stages of schizophrenia produce more fragmented accounts of themselves, others, their actions, and place in their community (c.f. Lysaker et al., 2019). More specifically, persons with schizophrenia spectrum disorders have been found to have graver deficits in metacognitive capacity when compared to persons with less severe forms of mental illness, persons without serious mental illness who experience profound levels of social adversity from prolonged nonpsychiatric conditions and healthy controls (c.f. Lysaker et al., 2021).

In terms of general functioning, higher levels of metacognitive capacity have been linked with a range of healthier behaviors as disparate as levels of physical activity, coping style, ability to reject stigma, and self-compassion (c.f. Lysaker et al., 2020b). Regarding interpersonal functioning, greater metacognitive capacity has been similarly linked to a greater capacity for empathy, a heightened sense of social connection, more confidence in being able to rely on others, and more enduring social connections (c.f. Lysaker et al., 2021). At a more elemental level, research has suggested that with lower levels of metacognitive capacity, persons experience both increasingly lower levels of intrinsic motivation at the moment but also a heightened risk for lesser levels of intrinsic motivation in the future (Luther et al., 2016a). In one study (Luther et al., 2016b), lesser metacognitive capacity was linked to poorer social function in a path through lower levels of intrinsic motivation, after controlling for symptoms, neurocognition, and social cognition.

Turning to symptoms, most research to date has examined the relationship of metacognition with negative symptoms in schizophrenia spectrum disorders. Here, it has been proposed that with metacognitive deficits, persons may lose their sense of the larger purposes and possibilities they readily perceive in their lives leading to the loss of the intrinsic reasons and meanings, which previously supported goal-directed behavior and sharing of emotions with others. Research supporting this includes findings linking metacognition and negative symptoms in cross-sectional (Lysaker et al., 2020a; Trauelsen et al., 2016) and prospective studies (Austin et al., 2019; Faith et al., 2020; Hamm et al., 2012; Lysaker et al., 2015; McLeod et al., 2014). García-Mieres et al. (2020) have also reported that diminished emotional expression in schizophrenia spectrum disorders may occur as a result of an interaction between metacognitive deficits, alterations in higher-order language structures, and disorganized symptoms.

Metacognition has been proposed to influence the positive symptoms of schizophrenia in a less direct manner. Here, it has been proposed that metacognitive deficits limit persons' abilities to make sense of and manage emotional pain, which triggers positive symptoms. In other words, with relatively more intact metacognitive capacities, persons diagnosed with schizophrenia may be able to make sense of distressing states and not require delusional explanations for psychological challenges or descend into altered emotional states. Evidence supporting this includes findings that paranoia is more likely to be related to emotional distress among persons with less intact metacognitive capacity (Buck et al., 2020) and that metacognition moderates the relationship between positive symptoms and emotional distress (Faith et al., 2022).

Finally, a more complex relationship has been proposed to exist between disorganized symptoms and metacognition in schizophrenia spectrum disorders. Here, a feedback loop has been proposed in which disorganized thought contributes to deficits in metacognition and deficits in metacognition negatively impact the larger sense of meaning, which organizes experience resulting in verbal expressions that are less coherent. Research supporting this includes findings that deficits in metacognition are related to moderate levels of conceptual disorganization (Myers et al., 2023) and that disorganization may moderate the relationship of metacognition with neurocognition (Minor et al., 2015). In a particularly illustrative study, Hasson-Ohayon et al. (2018) performed a network analysis of multiple assessments of metacognition, social cognition, neurocognition, and symptoms including positive, negative, and disorganized symptoms. They found that the variables which played the most central role within this network, that is connected the most variables to one another, were disorganized symptoms and metacognition.

An Application of the Integrative Model of Metacognition to the Phenomenology Schizotypy

As noted above, parallels plainly exist between the phenomenology of schizotypy and schizophrenia spectrum disorders with both involving positive, negative, and disorganized features. It thus is intuitively appealing to consider whether psychological processes, such as metacognition, which affect these dimensions in schizophrenia and other disabling mental health conditions may offer insights into the experience of schizotypy.

Applied to schizotypy, it could be hypothesized that metacognitive deficits exist in various domains including awareness of the self, others, one's action, and one's larger community. Further, these disturbances may influence one another and significantly affect behavior. At a concrete level, this would suggest four potentially different kinds of disturbance in experience. First, persons with schizotypy might experience themselves in less integrated or coherent ways. They may be aware of different thoughts, emotions, or feelings that are occurring in their bodies but unsure how those relate to one another or unable to form a sense of how they may meaningfully change over time. They may, for example, realize they are thinking about someone who dislikes them and feel flushed in the face but be unaware that this is a reflection of being angry. Or, if they are aware that they are angry with the person who dislikes them, they may be unable to see that their anger is also a function of other things in their lives like a recent fight with a partner. They may not recognize that their thoughts and feelings change fluidly and as such are fallible or that experiences within one moment may be similar to experiences in other moments.

Second, persons with schizotypy may experience others in more fragmented and less integrated ways. In parallel with our last example, they may see that another person is talking loudly about an experience at work and that the face of the other seems flushed but not form the idea that the person is angry about something that happened at work. If they are aware the other is angry, they may struggle to see why the person is angry or to see the other as having other complex emotions that may be impacted by a range of internal and external experiences. They may also be unaware of what the other person is wanting of them at that moment and have difficulty understanding others' changing experiences overtime.

Third, with metacognitive deficits, persons with schizotypy may struggle to form coherent ideas of the challenges they are facing or to make sense of how they should respond to them in ways that uniquely consider their own thoughts, emotions, desires, and histories. With deficits in what is referred to as metacognitive mastery, they may be unsure how to characterize the challenges that are occurring and evolving naturally in their lives. For example, they may struggle to be able to describe how something has gone amiss in a romantic relationship or interpersonal struggles that are seeming to occur on the job. They may either fail to see these problems or form an incoherent or implausible explanation for them such as there being a conspiracy against them. Even if the person is able to see clearly a problem in a relationship or define another psychosocial challenge in their life, they may struggle to find a way to respond to it, at most feeling able to avoid things or rely on others for support. If they are able to think about taking effective actions such as deciding to talk to the partner or colleague at work, they may struggle to see in what ways this problem reflects unique struggles they or others around them have had in life. Thus, they may be unable to think about solutions that might be uniquely meaningful given who they or others are as unique beings.

Finally, in addition to difficulty forming integrated ideas about themselves, others, and their challenges and actions, persons with schizotypy may struggle to think about their place in their larger community. They may have difficulties seeing how others form their own valid perspective on events in the world which differs from their own. As a result, they may be unable to enrich their own understanding of the world by integrating different ideas and perspectives. They may struggle to see events that are not related to them as meaningful and be at a loss to think about the larger purposes and structure of the communities in which they live.

Importantly, these deficits in self-reflectivity, awareness of others, mastery, and decentration could readily be assumed to interact and have negative effects on behavior in complex and enduring ways. First, if we turn to the negative dimension of schizotypy, as has been suggested in schizophrenia disorders, persons may lose their sense of the larger purposes which have previously guided behavior and allowed certain activities to be perceived as more meaningful than others with metacognitive deficits. Whereas, for example, there was in the past a reason to make sacrifices for a partner or aspect of work, the reasons for making those sacrifices may no longer be apparent resulting in what seems like a failure to apply oneself to that relationship or the workplace. This certainly could be perceived as a lack of volition and motivation. Second, deficits in metacognition may limit persons' abilities to make sense of what is possible for them within interpersonal relationships culminating in a loss of coherent goal-directed behavior. They may see no meaningful gain from their actions in the wake of a loss of metacognitive mastery.

Just as a purpose for doing something might vanish with metacognitive deficits so might the potential end of doing something. For example, the achievement of greater intimacy or success in a work project may no longer appear possible and so again pursuit of that may diminish, appearing as avolition or abulia. Finally, greater metacognitive deficits may deprive persons of a sense of how they are connected to others, resulting in an absence of any potential for intersubjectivity and hence expression of emotion. With a limited sense of others and their needs and views, persons may fail to experience or anticipate pleasure in social relationships appearing increasingly anhedonic or morbidly introverted as characterizes negative schizotypy.

In terms of positive schizotypy, as in the case of schizophrenia, metacognitive deficits may leave persons struggling to make sense of the challenges they face and their aspirations in consensually valid ways. Following our last illustration, they may not be able to make sense of why a partner has left them for another person or why others are being given awards at work while fewer people talk to them. Still, with a need to explain these experiences, they may offer odd or unusual responses which may appear as magical or paranoid thinking. These difficulties in seeing how one belongs could make having an eccentric appearance a more appealing solution, as if to say, "it isn't that I don't fit in… I am just different in ways others do not appreciate." Finally, not being able to form an evolving sense of what others think and want could lead to a default sense that others might attack or seek harm, again appearing as paranoid or magical thinking.

Turning to disorganization symptoms, metacognitive deficits could interact with disorganized thought with the end result that both amplify one another. Persons with disorganized thoughts might be less likely to form integrated ideas about themselves, others, and their actions in the world. Conversely, with less coherent ideas about the self, others, and one's actions in the world, persons might communicate their experiences in less organized and more fragmented ways, that is, in ways that mirror their own experience. For example, if trying to talk about a difficult experience in a relationship or at work, with less coherent ideas about oneself and others, the report of those experiences might naturally appear more disorganized or tangential, appearing as a manifestation of the cognitive domain of schizotypy.

Metacognition and Schizotypy: Supporting Research

While there seems to be much appeal to the application of the integrated model of metacognition to schizotypy, research on this subject is still in the early stages. This has been promising, nevertheless. First, paralleling research on schizophrenia, several studies have suggested that higher levels of schizotypy are linked with metacognitive deficits. Chan et al. (2015) reported, for example, that a group of 22 individuals with high levels of schizotypy had significantly more maladaptive metacognitive beliefs relative to 20 individuals with relatively low levels of schizotypy. Debbané et al. (2012) also found a significant association between maladaptive beliefs and positive schizotypy among 179 adolescents. Consistent with relationships found between metacognition and negative symptoms in schizophrenia (Lysaker et al., 2020a), Rabin et al. (2014) found that more fragmented representations of the self were related to higher levels of negative schizotypy among 60 adults who did not have a diagnosis of a serious mental illness. Similarly, Davis et al. (2020) and Luther et al. (2023) found that lower levels of metacognitive mastery were related to higher levels of negative schizotypy in college samples.

Deficits in metacognition have also been found to predict greater challenges in psychosocial functioning among persons experiencing schizotypy. Springfield and Pinkham (2020), for example, found that high levels of schizotypy were linked to an underestimate of social competence among 137 undergraduate students. Webster et al. (2022) reported that having higher levels of maladaptive metacognitive beliefs mediated the relationship between levels of schizotypy with anxiety and depression in a large college sample of 344 participants. In parallel, lower levels of metacognition were associated with fewer experiences of social support among persons with higher degrees of schizotypy in the Davis et al. (2020) study while the negative effects of lower levels of metacognition upon social function were mediated by negative schizotypy in the Luther et al. (2023) study.

Concerning the presence and effects of metacognitive deficits in persons diagnosed with schizotypy-related disorders, several intensive case studies have reported that patients with these diagnoses experience significant decrements in the abilities to form integrated ideas about themselves, others, and their actions (Cheli et al., 2019; Dmitryeva et al., 2021). Cheli (2020) has also reported relatively low levels of metacognitive functioning in terms of self-reflectivity, awareness of others, decentration, and mastery among 12 adults diagnosed with schizotypal personality disorder. More recently, Cheli et al. (2023) confirmed the presence of relatively low levels of metacognitive function in baseline assessments of a randomized trial of a novel metacognitive-oriented intervention of 24 adults diagnosed with schizotypal personality disorder. Other less direct forms of evidence include studies of relatively larger samples of persons with different kinds of personality disorder, including schizotypal personality disorder, which have found the relatively ubiquitous presence of significant deficits in metacognition (Carcione et al., 2019; Semerari et al., 2014). Casework has also suggested metacognitive deficits in other personality disorders related to schizotypy including schizoid personality disorder (Cheli et al., 2022).

Finally, preliminary evidence also suggests that metacognitive deficits are not just present in schizotypy but that they also exert an influence upon functioning. In the casework noted above, psychotherapy that targeted metacognition was observed to result in patients forming more integrated sense of themselves (self-reflectivity), others (awareness of others), their actions (mastery), and place in their communities (decentration), leading to growth in those capacities, which was followed by improvements in psychosocial function and reductions in levels of schizotypal traits (Cheli et al., 2019; Dmitryeva et al., 2021). Similar findings were also reported in a more systematic way in the randomized trial conducted by Cheli et al. (2023). In this study, improvements in metacognitive capacity over time were significantly predictive of reductions in symptomatology.

Conclusions and Limitations

Recently, a model has been proposed suggesting that metacognitive deficits are a transdiagnostic construct that may underpin the phenomenology of multiple mental health disorders and contribute to psychosocial dysfunction. In this chapter, we have explored how that model has been applied to schizophrenia in particular and how that application could be adapted to explain the phenomenology of schizotypy, both as a personality organization and a form of personality disorder. Specifically, we have suggested that decrements in persons' abilities to form integrated senses of themselves, others, their actions, and place in their communities could play a role in the development of positive, negative, and disorganized dimensions of schizotypy. We have further reviewed initial evidence including findings of heightened levels of metacognitive deficits in persons with relatively high levels of schizotypy and significant schizotypal personality disorder traits and evidence that these metacognitive disturbances in both schizotypy and schizotypal personal disorder are closely linked to function.

Of note, there are limitations. Larger scale longitudinal studies are needed to track the potential complex relationships which exist between symptoms, function, and metacognition among persons with relatively high levels of schizotypy and significant schizotypal personality disorder traits. Studies are needed with simultaneously richer and broader assessments of different forms of metacognition (e.g., error monitoring, metacognitive beliefs, self-reflectivity, and mastery). Research is also needed comparing the metacognitive function of persons with relatively high levels of schizotypy, significant schizotypal personality disorder traits, and schizophrenia. It further remains unknown whether the metacognitive deficits potentially observed in these different groups have similar roots and courses over time.

With replication, there are important clinical implications from this work. For one, it offers a frame for understanding the complex and deeply subjective kinds of experiences persons with relatively high levels of schizotypy and significant schizotypal personality disorder traits face. As proposed by Cheli (2020), this may enable joint reflection and treatment plans that target the most proximal causes of dysfunction. If deficits in metacognition underlie the phenomenology and persistent dysfunction found in these groups, therapies that target metacognition may prove uniquely promising. Later in this volume, Wiesepape et al. (this volume) will offer a comprehensive presentation of one such approach that might address this.

References

Austin, S. F., Lysaker, P. H., Jansen, J. E., Trauelsen, A. M., Nielsen, H.-G. L., Pedersen, M. B., Haahr, U. H., & Simonsen, E. (2019). Metacognitive capacity and negative symptoms in first episode psychosis: Evidence of a prospective relationship over a 3-year follow-up. *Journal of Experimental Psychopathology, 10*(1). https://doi.org/10.1177/2043808718821572

Bell, M., Milstein, R., Beam-Goulet, J., Lysaker, P., & Cicchetti, D. (1992). The Positive and Negative Syndrome Scale and the Brief Psychiatric Rating Scale. Reliability, comparability, and predictive validity. *The Journal of Nervous and Mental Disease, 180*(11), 723–728. https://doi.org/10.1097/00005053-199211000-00007

Buck, B., Gagen, E. C., Luther, L., Kukla, M., & Lysaker, P. H. (2020). Dynamic relationships between emotional distress, persecutory ideation, and metacognition in schizophrenia. *Journal of Clinical Psychology, 76*(4), 716–724. https://doi.org/10.1002/jclp.22904

Carcione, A., Riccardi, I., Bilotta, E., Leone, L., Pedone, R., Conti, L., Colle, L., Fiore, D., Nicolò, G., Pellecchia, G., Procacci, M., & Semerari, A. (2019). Metacognition as a predictor of improvements in personality disorders. *Frontiers in Psychology, 10*, 170. https://doi.org/10.3389/fpsyg.2019.00170

Chan, C. C., Spencer, C. C., West, C., Viegas, C., & Bedwell, J. S. (2015). Metacognitive processes in psychometrically defined schizotypy. *Psychiatry Research, 230*(2), 279–286. https://doi.org/10.1016/j.psychres.2015.09.006

Cheli, S. (2020). Assessment and treatment planning for schizotypal personality disorder: A metacognitively oriented point of view. *Psychiatric Rehabilitation Journal, 43*(4), 335–343. https://doi.org/10.1037/prj0000429

Cheli, S., Lysaker, P. H., & Dimaggio, G. (2019). Metacognitively oriented psychotherapy for schizotypal personality disorder: A two-case series. *Personality and Mental Health, 13*(3), 155–167. https://doi.org/10.1002/pmh.1447

Cheli, S., Chiarello, F., & Cavalletti, V. (2022). A psychotherapy oriented by compassion and metacognition for schizoid personality disorder: A two cases series. *Journal of Contemporary Psychotherapy*, 1–10. https://doi.org/10.1007/s10879-022-09566-3

Cheli, S., Cavalletti, V., Lysaker, P. H., Dimaggio, G., Petrocchi, N., Chiarello, F., Enzo, C., Velicogna, F., Mancini, F., & Goldzweig, G. (2023). A pilot randomized controlled trial comparing a novel compassion and metacognition approach for schizotypal personality disorder with a combination of cognitive therapy and psychopharmacological treatment. *BMC Psychiatry, 23*(1), 113. https://doi.org/10.1186/s12888-023-04610-5

Davis, B. J., Firmin, R. L., Lysaker, P. H., Salyers, M. P., McGrew, J., & Minor, K. S. (2020). An investigation of metacognition in schizotypy: Evidence of linkage with negative traits. *Translational Issues in Psychological Science, 6*(1), 81–91. https://doi.org/10.1037/tps0000221

Davis, B. J., Bonfils, K. A., Zalzala, A., Lysaker, P. H., & Minor, K. S. (2022). Meaning-making processes across the lifespan: An investigation of the developmental course of metacognitive capacity. *Schizophrenia Research, 248*, 240–245. https://doi.org/10.1016/j.schres.2022.09.008

Debbané, M., Van der Linden, M., Balanzin, D., Billieux, J., & Eliez, S. (2012). Associations among metacognitive beliefs, anxiety and positive schizotypy during adolescence. *The Journal of Nervous and Mental Disease, 200*(7), 620–626. https://doi.org/10.1097/NMD.0b013e31825bfc1a

Dmitryeva, N., Chernov, N., Kostyuk, G., & Lysaker, P. H. (2021). Utilizing MERIT to promote recovery in schizotypal personality disorder: An illustrative case study. *Journal of Clinical Psychology, 77*(8), 1798–1806. https://doi.org/10.1002/jclp.23239

Faith, L. A., Lecomte, T., Corbière, M., Francoeur, A., Hache-Labelle, C., & Lysaker, P. H. (2020). Metacognition is uniquely related to concurrent and prospective assessments of negative symptoms independent of verbal memory in serious mental illness. *The Journal of Nervous and Mental Disease, 208*(11), 837–842. https://doi.org/10.1097/NMD.0000000000001219

Faith, L. A., Lecomte, T., Corbière, M., & Lysaker, P. H. (2022). Metacognitive mastery moderates the relationship between positive symptoms and distress in adults with serious mental illness. *Journal of Mental Health*, 1–8. https://doi.org/10.1080/09638237.2022.2091758

Fong, T. C., Ho, R. T., Wan, A. H., Siu, P. J., & Au-Yeung, F. S. (2015). Psychometric validation of the consensus five-factor model of the Positive and Negative Syndrome Scale. *Comprehensive Psychiatry, 62*, 204–208. https://doi.org/10.1016/j.comppsych.2015.07.015

García-Mieres, H., Lundin, N. B., Minor, K. S., Dimaggio, G., Popolo, R., Cheli, S., & Lysaker, P. H. (2020). A cognitive model of diminished expression in schizophrenia: The interface of metacognition, cognitive symptoms and language disturbances. *Journal of Psychiatric Research, 131*, 169–176. https://doi.org/10.1016/j.jpsychires.2020.09.008

Hamm, J. A., Renard, S. B., Fogley, R. L., Leonhardt, B. L., Dimaggio, G., Buck, K. D., & Lysaker, P. H. (2012). Metacognition and social cognition in schizophrenia: Stability and relationship to concurrent and prospective symptom assessments. *Journal of Clinical Psychology, 68*(12), 1303–1312. https://doi.org/10.1002/jclp.21906

Hasson-Ohayon, I., Goldzweig, G., Lavi-Rotenberg, A., Luther, L., & Lysaker, P. H. (2018). The centrality of cognitive symptoms and metacognition within the interacting network of symptoms, neurocognition, social cognition and metacognition in schizophrenia. *Schizophrenia Research, 202*, 260–266. https://doi.org/10.1016/j.schres.2018.07.007

Lenzenweger, M. F. (2006). Schizotypy: An organizing framework for schizophrenia research. *Current Directions in Psychological Science, 15*, 162–166.

Lim, K., Peh, O. H., Yang, Z., Rekhi, G., Rapisarda, A., See, Y. M., Rashid, N. A. A., Ang, M. S., Lee, S. A., Sim, K., Huang, H., Lencz, T., Lee, J., & Lam, M. (2021). Large-scale evaluation of the Positive and Negative Syndrome Scale (PANSS) symptom architecture in schizophrenia. *Asian Journal of Psychiatry, 62*, 102732. https://doi.org/10.1016/j.ajp.2021.102732

Luther, L., Firmin, R. L., Minor, K. S., Vohs, J. L., Buck, B., Buck, K. D., & Lysaker, P. H. (2016a). Metacognition deficits as a risk factor for prospective motivation deficits in schizophrenia spectrum disorders. *Psychiatry Research, 245*, 172–178. https://doi.org/10.1016/j.psychres.2016.08.032

Luther, L., Firmin, R. L., Vohs, J. L., Buck, K. D., Rand, K. L., & Lysaker, P. H. (2016b). Intrinsic motivation as a mediator between metacognition deficits and impaired functioning in psychosis. *The British Journal of Clinical Psychology, 55*(3), 332–347. https://doi.org/10.1111/bjc.12104

Luther, L., Hochheiser, J., Wiesepape, C., & Lysaker, P. H. (2023). Negative schizotypy mediates the relationship between metacognition and social functioning in a nonclinical sample. *The Journal of Nervous and Mental Disease, 211*(1), 74–78. https://doi.org/10.1097/NMD.0000000000001585

Lysaker, P. H., Kukla, M., Dubreucq, J., Gumley, A., McLeod, H., Vohs, J. L., Buck, K. D., Minor, K. S., Luther, L., Leonhardt, B. L., Belanger, E. A., Popolo, R., & Dimaggio, G. (2015). Metacognitive deficits predict future levels of negative symptoms in schizophrenia controlling for neurocognition, affect recognition, and self-expectation of goal attainment. *Schizophrenia Research, 168*(1–2), 267–272. https://doi.org/10.1016/j.schres.2015.06.015

Lysaker, P. H., Minor, K. S., Lysaker, J. T., Hasson-Ohayon, I., Bonfils, K., Hochheiser, J., & Vohs, J. L. (2019). Metacognitive function and fragmentation in schizophrenia: Relationship to cognition, self-experience and developing treatments. *Schizophrenia Research. Cognition, 19*, 100142. https://doi.org/10.1016/j.scog.2019.100142

Lysaker, P. H., Chernov, N., Moiseeva, T., Sozinova, M., Dmitryeva, N., Alyoshin, V., Faith, L. A., Karpenko, O., & Kostyuk, G. (2020a). Contrasting metacognitive profiles and their association with negative symptoms in groups with schizophrenia, early psychosis and depression in a Russian sample. *Psychiatry Research, 291*, 113177. https://doi.org/10.1016/j.psychres.2020.113177

Lysaker, P. H., Gagen, E., Klion, R., Zalzala, A., Vohs, J., Faith, L. A., Leonhardt, B., Hamm, J., & Hasson-Ohayon, I. (2020b). Metacognitive Reflection and Insight Therapy: A recovery-oriented treatment approach for psychosis. *Psychology Research and Behavior Management, 13*, 331–341. https://doi.org/10.2147/PRBM.S198628

Lysaker, P. H., Kukla, M., Leonhardt, B. L., Hamm, J. A., Schnakenberg Martin, A., Zalzala, A. B., Gagen, E. C., & Hasson-Ohayon, I. (2020c). Meaning, integration, and the self in serious mental illness: Implications of research in metacognition for psychiatric rehabilitation. *Psychiatric Rehabilitation Journal, 43*(4), 275–283. https://doi.org/10.1037/prj0000436

Lysaker, P. H., Cheli, S., Dimaggio, G., Buck, B., Bonfils, K. A., Huling, K., Wiesepape, C., & Lysaker, J. T. (2021). Metacognition, social cognition, and mentalizing in psychosis: Are these distinct constructs when it comes to subjective experience or are we just splitting hairs? *BMC Psychiatry, 21*(1), 329. https://doi.org/10.1186/s12888-021-03338-4

McLeod, H. J., Gumley, A. I., Macbeth, A., Schwannauer, M., & Lysaker, P. H. (2014). Metacognitive functioning predicts positive and negative symptoms over 12 months in first episode psychosis. *Journal of Psychiatric Research, 54*, 109–115. https://doi.org/10.1016/j.jpsychires.2014.03.018

Meehl, P. E. (1962). Schizotaxia, schizotypy, schizophrenia. *American Psychologist, 17*(12), 827–838. https://doi.org/10.1037/h0041029

Minor, K. S., Marggraf, M. P., Davis, B. J., Luther, L., Vohs, J. L., Buck, K. D., & Lysaker, P. H. (2015). Conceptual disorganization weakens links in cognitive pathways: Disentangling neurocognition, social cognition, and metacognition in schizophrenia. *Schizophrenia Research, 169*(1–3), 153–158.

Myers, E. J., Abel, D. B., Hardin, K. L., Bettis, R. J., Beard, A. M., Salyers, M. P., Lysaker, P. H., & Minor, K. S. (2023). Mild vs. moderate: How behavioral speech measures predict metacognitive capacity across different levels of formal thought disorder. *Journal of Psychiatric Research, 157*, 43–49. https://doi.org/10.1016/j.jpsychires.2022.11.013

Nelson, M. T., Seal, M. L., Pantelis, C., & Phillips, L. J. (2013). Evidence of a dimensional relationship between schizotypy and schizophrenia: A systematic review. *Neuroscience and Biobehavioral Reviews, 37*(3), 317–327. https://doi.org/10.1016/j.neubiorev.2013.01.004

Rabin, S. J., Hasson-Ohayon, I., Avidan, M., Rozencwaig, S., Shalev, H., & Kravetz, S. (2014). Metacognition in schizophrenia and schizotypy: Relation to symptoms of schizophrenia, traits of schizotypy and social quality of life. *The Israel Journal of Psychiatry and Related Sciences, 51*(1), 44–53.

Semerari, A., Colle, L., Pellecchia, G., Buccione, I., Carcione, A., Dimaggio, G., Nicolò, G., Procacci, M., & Pedone, R. (2014). Metacognitive dysfunctions in personality disorders: Correlations with disorder severity and personality styles. *Journal of Personality Disorders, 28*(6), 751–766. https://doi.org/10.1521/pedi_2014_28_137

Springfield, C. R., & Pinkham, A. E. (2020). Introspective accuracy for social competence in psychometric schizotypy. *Cognitive Neuropsychiatry, 25*(1), 57–70. https://doi.org/10.1080/13546805.2019.1683524

Trauelsen, A. M., Gumley, A., Jansen, J. E., Pedersen, M. B., Nielsen, H. L., Trier, C. H., Haahr, U. H., & Simonsen, E. (2016). Metacognition in first-episode psychosis and its association with positive and negative symptom profiles. *Psychiatry Research, 238*, 14–23. https://doi.org/10.1016/j.psychres.2016.02.003

Verbeke, L., De Clercq, B., Van der Heijden, P., Hutsebaut, J., & van Aken, M. A. (2017). The relevance of schizotypal traits for understanding interpersonal functioning in adolescents with psychiatric problems. *Personality Disorders, 8*(1), 54–63. https://doi.org/10.1037/per0000163

Webster, L., Norman, C., Jones, G., & Marriott, M. (2022). Mediating role for metacognitive processes in the relationship between schizotypy and anxiety and depression symptoms. *Cognitive Neuropsychiatry, 27*(6), 393–410. https://doi.org/10.1080/13546805.2022.2108388

Chapter 9
Linking Personality and Psychopathology: A Mentalization-Based Treatment Framework for the Understanding of Schizotypy-Related Psychopathology

George Salaminios and Martin Debbané

Introduction

Personality and psychopathology have been interconnected throughout history, particularly within the psychoanalytical and psychodynamic approaches devoted to the understanding and treatment of psychopathology (Luyten & Fonagy, 2022). Current empirical frameworks in the field of psychopathology research further attempt to link personality traits to psychopathology; for instance, the hierarchical taxonomy of psychopathology (HiTOP; Kotov et al., 2017) examines individual expression in symptoms, their relationships to psychopathological syndromes, and higher-order personality spectra of psychopathology within an overall hierarchical structure. However, the hierarchical approach remains disorder- rather than person-centered, which brings challenges to its application in everyday clinical work, particularly in the current era of personalized treatment. Other contemporary approaches to psychopathology choose to conceptualize associations and interactions between psychological processes and symptomatic manifestations through a network approach (Borsboom et al., 2013), thus offering a more dynamic view of symptom expression, in the absence of a disorder-syndromic approach. While the network approach

G. Salaminios
Research Department of Clinical, Educational and Health Psychology, University College London, London, UK

Research Department, British Association for Counselling and Psychotherapy, Lutterworth, Leicestershire, UK

M. Debbané (✉)
Research Department of Clinical, Educational and Health Psychology, University College London, London, UK

Developmental Clinical Psychology Research Unit, Faculty of Psychology and Educational Sciences, University of Geneva, Geneva, Switzerland
e-mail: martin.debbane@unige.ch

S. Cheli, P. H. Lysaker (eds.), *A Dimensional Approach to Schizotypy*,
https://doi.org/10.1007/978-3-031-41788-7_9

has sought to find applicability for personalized treatment (Mansueto et al., 2022), it is still very much based on data coming from large samples of individuals (Epskamp et al., 2018). As we will discuss below, when assessing the options for clinical and treatment strategies for schizotypy as a personality trait that entails liability to develop schizophrenia spectrum disorders (SSDs) (Lenzenweger, 2015), we find that contemporary psychodynamic approaches, such as mentalization-based therapy (MBT), may be well suited to formulate how psychological processes are connected to idiosyncratic psychopathological expression. In this chapter we offer the empirical and clinical rationale for adopting an MBT framework in the understanding and treatment of schizotypy-related psychopathology.

As is evident from previous chapters, the historical conceptualization of schizotypy was originally construed within a disorder-centered approach by the theorist Paul H. Meehl, who was a practicing psychoanalyst at the time he developed the concept of schizotypy (Meehl, 1962). Within this framework adopted from another psychoanalyst, Sandor Rado, who first coined the term "schizotypy," one can find both a strong taxonomic, disorder-centered view of schizotypy and a developmentally sensitive understanding of how individual liability to schizophrenia spectrum psychopathology unfolds within the development of each individual's unique personal history and social context. Indeed, in his model, Meehl specifies how environmental potentiators are necessary to understand the unfolding of schizophrenic psychopathology (Debbané & Barrantes-Vidal, 2014), beyond the putatively causal neural defect (schizotaxia), which he hypothesized as the necessary condition for developing SSDs. Those who have criticized Meehl's taxonic model as placing increased emphasis on schizotypy as a pathological personality organization have put forward a fully dimensional proposition of schizotypy. According to this view, schizotypy does not reflect a neural defect present only among a relatively small number of genetically liable individuals, but rather a *neural type,* which is dimensionally distributed across the general population. Indeed, Gordon Claridge emphasized the psychological processes that would underlie such a neural type and that these processes were not inherently psychopathological (Claridge, 1997). Yet the fully dimensional view proposed by Claridge did not specify the environmental interactions that would sustain a "happy," as opposed to a psychopathological outcome to the unfolding of the personality trait through development. We could characterize the fully dimensional view of schizotypy as a personality-centered alternative to the disorder-centered concept proposed by Meehl. However, we also argue that neither of these models lend themselves easily to a personalized treatment approach for schizotypy-related psychopathology. Indeed, it may well be that schizotypy interacts with both specific psychopathological factors (e.g., depression and anxiety) and general psychopathology factors present across different forms of psychopathology (Sun et al., 2022; Badcock et al., 2016). Recent longitudinal studies have shed some light into the complex associations linking personality to psychopathology. For instance, research to date suggests that schizotypy and a general psychopathology factor common across all psychopathological manifestations (i.e., p-factor, see Caspi et al., 2014) constitute independent constructs, which can longitudinally interact through psychological processes critically involving representations of self and others (such as rumination; see Sun et al., 2022). Importantly, these psychological processes involved in the formation of mental representations appear to be transdiagnostic and implicated across traditional diagnostic categories (Fonagy & Bateman, 2016). In order to think clearly about the treatment of psychopathology linked to schizotypy (we will refer to SSDs mainly in this chapter—but specific forms of internalizing and externalizing disorders and suicidality should be kept in mind too), we would argue that the disorder-centered or personality-centered approaches can benefit from the integration of a psychodynamic person–centered perspective. Specifically with regard to clinical and treatment issues related to schizotypy, such a perspective offers itself to personalized psychological treatment as it seeks to explore how each individual's specific personality organization and interpersonal experiences may interact across development to uniquely shape how they make sense of themselves and others around them.

In this chapter, we emphasize the mentalization-based therapy framework (MBT) for SSDs that we and others have developed to illustrate our argument (Debbané et al., 2016a, b; Brent & Fonagy, 2014). Mentalizing refers to the set of psychological processes dedicated to thinking about mental states, both in oneself and others, to make sense of behavior; ultimately mentalizing sustains social cognition, communication, and collaboration (Fonagy et al., 2002). The main argument for focusing on mentalizing in the context of clinical treatment is that it lies at the interface of the individual's relationship to oneself and to others (Fonagy et al., 2002). As such mentalizing is one of the key processes that contributes to sustaining both self-continuity and continuity in meaningful relationships (Debbané et al., 2022), both of which are critical in terms of sustaining mental health (Fonagy & Bateman, 2016). Because schizotypy and SSDs involve profound alterations in one's self-experience (Raballo & Parnas, 2011), as well in the experience of other people (Cohen et al., 2015), mentalizing as a psychological process necessarily comes into play, not as a causal factor, but rather as we have suggested elsewhere, as a protective factor against the psychotic pathogenesis potentially associated with the interaction between schizotypy and environmental risk factors (Debbané et al., 2016b).

In order to achieve an integration between disorder- or personality-centered approaches and our person-centered psychodynamic approach, we propose that conceptualizing treatment along the continuum spanning from benign schizotypy to SSDs requires: (1) a developmental perspective; (2) within this perspective, a clear assessment of the schizotypy facets that augment risk for severe psychopathology; and (3) a developmental understanding of within- and between-person psychological processes that increase or mitigate the risk for the unfolding of SSDs and in particular the mentalizing dimensions that can influence the development of psychopathology. In the following section, we outline how schizotypy and mentalizing facets have been studied in relation to the risk for SSDs. In section "Evidence Linking Mentalizing and Schizotypy Along the Developmental Continuum of Psychosis Expression", we review empirical findings elucidating the links between mentalizing and schizotypy along its continuum of psychopathological expression. In the final section, we outline how a clinical conceptualization of psychotic manifestations as prementalizing modes of thinking can be informative to individual patients and assist in treatment formulation within a personalized treatment approach.

Schizotypy and Mentalizing Throughout Development

In this section, we attempt to provide an overview of the developmental trajectories that occur with regard to schizotypy and mentalizing. Schizotypy is commonly studied through an investigation of three connected, yet autonomous phenotypic dimensions: the positive, negative, and disorganization dimensions. Other dimension denominations have also been proposed by the personality-centered approach. For instance, using the O-Life questionnaire, studies have suggested a four-factor structure composed by unusual experiences, cognitive disorganization, introvertive anhedonia, and impulsive nonconformity (Mason & Claridge, 2006). Broadly speaking, our interest is to clinically distinguish between positive/unusual perceptual phenomena (ranging from perceptual distortions to hallucinations and from eccentric beliefs to delusional ideation), negative/anhedonic phenomena (encompassing diminished feelings of emotion, pleasure, and motivational drive that seem to relate to experiences of social anxiety and aversion and can progress to strongly avoidant behavior as that seen in clinical social isolation), and disorganization phenomena (which range from verbal, cognitive, and behavioral eccentricity; cognitive disorganization; thought disturbances; language oddities; and bizarre behaviors). Longitudinal studies examining the early manifestations of schizotypy first focused on the positive dimension. Notably, data from the original prospective study on the Dunedin cohort showed that individuals reporting early positive manifestations at age 11 had an increased propensity for developing the equivalent of SSDs at age 26 (Poulton et al., 2000). Later studies on this same sample, however, moderated the initial enthusiasm showing that employing positive symptoms alone as the signal of risk for SSDs in fact carried very poor sensitivity and specificity indices (Fisher et al., 2013). Other studies taking into account the ensemble of schizotypy dimensions consistently found the negative and disorganized dimensions of schizotypy to be the most predictive dimensions for an increased risk for SSDs (Debbané et al., 2014a). Furthermore, the continuity of positive schizotypy expression during adolescent development appears to be dependent on the negative and disorganized dimension expressions (Dominguez et al., 2010; Debbané et al., 2013). In general population and in prodromal or high-risk samples, the negative dimension appears to be the only predictive dimension (Flückiger et al., 2016). In family-risk and personality-disorder samples, the transition rate to clinically significant SSDs is approximately 12%, and the negative and disorganization dimensions appear to carry a predictive value to conversion (Johnstone et al., 2005). It thus appears that the negative dimension of schizotypy is the most inclined to signal risk for future SSDs. Interestingly, the negative dimension is also linked to atypical brain morphology maturation during adolescence, as suggested by recent longitudinal evidence (Derome et al., 2020).

In parallel, mentalizing abilities appear to develop throughout childhood (Fonagy et al., 2002) and specialize during adolescence and early adulthood (Choudhury et al., 2006; Dumontheil et al., 2010; Vetter et al., 2013). It is probable that mentalizing specializes across the life span, in response to evolving contextual complexities (i.e., personal, familial, and group relationships) that characterize any individual's social ecosystem (Fonagy et al., 2002). Mentalizing is commonly assessed as an individual's capacity to attend (mostly automatically and unconsciously) to mental state information that can concern other minds as well as one's own mind. Research protocols commonly distinguish between emotion (feelings, affects, etc.) and cognitions (beliefs, desire, etc.) as these systems are separately studied in cognitive neuroscience (Fonagy & Luyten, 2009). This framework gives four interlinked mental state information processing systems that can be experimentally and clinically evaluated: self, other, cognitive, and affective mentalizing. For example, theory of mind (ToM) tasks typically investigate the cognitive-other systems of mentalizing: "*What is Sally thinking*?", while mindfulness tasks typically capture self-oriented processing (both cognitive and affective): "*Take the time to describe what you are feeling at the present moment*".

It is important to note that mentalizing develops within the early attachment relationships to caregivers. A number of studies have shown that secure attachment confers an advantage in terms of mentalizing during childhood (Fonagy et al., 1997; Steele et al., 2008; Sharp & Fonagy, 2008). For instance, Fonagy et al. (1997) reported that the level of attachment security, measured by a separation anxiety test (Klagsburn and Bowlby, 1976), was positively correlated with ToM performance among a sample of children aged between 3 and 6 years. Steele et al. (2008) tested basic facial emotion recognition capacities in a sample of 6-year-old children (n = 63) that had previously undergone an assessment of mother–infant attachment (Strange Situation Procedure, Ainsworth et al., 2015) at 1 year of age. The authors reported that 6-year-old children who were classified as having an insecure attachment to their mother at 1 year of age were significantly less accurate in their emotion recognition judgments compared with children that were classified as securely attached.

While early attachment relationships during infancy and childhood are considered critical for the establishment of basic mentalizing capacities (Fonagy & Target, 1996), increasing evidence suggests that adolescence represents a key developmental period for the maturation and elaboration of mentalizing processes (Fonagy et al., 2002). For instance, data suggest that significant structural and functional brain changes occur in key neural networks implicated in mentalizing during adolescence (Blakemore, 2008; Choudhury et al., 2006), and these have been shown to significantly contribute to the cerebral specialization of mentalizing processes (Badoud et al., 2016). Simultaneously, within the interpersonal and social domains, young people's decreasing dependence on family systems and the initiation of new interpersonal relationships (e.g., peer and romantic) contribute to the elaboration of mentalizing processes as a means to navigate a social world of increasing complexity (Fonagy et al., 2002). Indeed, a growing number of behavioral data suggest that mentalizing performance continues to improve throughout adolescence and into young adulthood (Choudhury et al., 2006; Dumontheil et al., 2010; Vetter et al., 2013). Therefore, the capacity to form representations of one's own and other people's mental states appears to be shaped both through adolescent brain development and through the social learning opportunities that typically arise in adolescence (Fonagy et al., 2002; Poznyak et al., 2019).

Studies simultaneously investigating schizotypy and mentalizing report significant associations between the two in adolescent and young adult samples who exhibit subclinical to clinical forms of risk for psychosis (Debbané et al., 2016b). We have previously suggested that such developmental associations are underpinned by at least five key neurobiological pathways through which early trauma and attachment adversity may partly account for developmental transactions between personality, the individual's relational and social context, and psychosis risk. To outline a schematic overview, attachment adversity during critical periods of neurodevelopment has been linked to hyperactivation of the hypothalamic–pituitary–adrenal (HPA) stress-response system (Heim et al., 2008); increased dopamine synthesis and release in response to increased stress (Howes & Kapur, 2009; Strathearn, 2011); reduced oxytocin levels (Brent & Fonagy, 2014); chronic neuroinflammation (Kirkpatrick & Miller, 2013); and oxidative stress damage (Do et al., 2009). Critically, each of these pathways appears to impact on the neurodevelopmental function of cortical brain regions that normally sustain the regulation of self-referential processing, from basic cognitive processes involved in assigning salience to stimuli and differentiating self from non-self-cues, to more complex reflective abilities pertaining to one's own thoughts, beliefs, and feelings (Debbané et al., 2016b). In the next section, we review the empirical evidence linking mentalizing dimensions to schizotypy during development.

Evidence Linking Mentalizing and Schizotypy Along the Developmental Continuum of Psychosis Expression

Contemporary research has identified two putative risk stages for psychosis, the premorbid and the clinical (prodromal) high-risk stages, where the level of pathophysiology developmentally augments from subtle premorbid personality manifestations to prodromal psychotic states, respectively (Debbané et al., 2014a, 2016b). These are understood to precede the first episode of psychosis (FEP), which marks the conversion point at which symptomatic expression will for the first time reach the severity, duration, and functional impairment thresholds needed for a formal diagnosis of SSDs.

First, the premorbid risk stage is characterized by schizotypal personality manifestations (Meehl, 1962; Claridge, 1997; Kwapil & Barrantes-Vidal, 2015), which represent the phenotypic expression of an underlying liability for psychosis and encompass a wide range of nonclinical and relatively stable *trait* abnormalities manifesting primarily within the perceptual, interpersonal, and neurocognitive domains. These typically emerge during preadolescent and early adolescent development, are subjectively experienced as common aspects of one's personality functioning, and confer a distal risk for clinical psychosis (Kwapil & Barrantes-Vidal, 2015). Second, following the premorbid period, the prodromal stage most proximally linked to clinical psychosis during late adolescence and young adulthood is best defined by the clinical high risk (CHR) approach (Fusar-Poli et al., 2013), which captures newly emergent transient psychotic states that are subjectively experienced as marked deviations from one's common functioning and signal imminent risk for transition to clinical illness.

Overall, it appears that the trajectory of psychosis risk overlaps developmentally with the progression from childhood and adolescence to young adulthood. Most interestingly, perhaps, empirical data suggest that the process of emerging psychotic pathogenesis across the premorbid, prodromal, and clinical stages spanning from adolescence to young adulthood can correlate with increasing levels of mentalizing dysfunction (Armando et al., 2019). In this section, we briefly review empirical evidence suggesting that dysfunctions in the capacity to accurately infer and recognize mental states in oneself and others, commonly observed among adults suffering with SSDs and young adults meeting the CHR criteria, are preceded by more subtle difficulties in these domains during childhood and adolescence, and these relate to schizotypal trait manifestations.

As introduced above, mentalizing represents a complex psychological construct that has been operationalized as organized along different but interrelated dimensions (Fonagy & Luyten, 2009). Indeed, at any given moment, the focus of mentalizing activity may center on oneself or other people (self/other dimension). In a similar vein, the content of mentalizing activity of both the self and others may focus on cognitive (e.g., thoughts and intentions) or affective (e.g., emotions) material at varying degrees (cognitive/affective dimension). Within this framework, different forms of mental state understanding reflect different facets of the wider mentalizing construct (Choi-Kain & Gunderson, 2008). For instance, inferences about other people's thoughts or intentions would overlap with the cognitive, other-oriented facet of mentalizing, while attributions about others' emotional states capture the affect, other-oriented dimensions of mentalizing. Similarly, self-oriented "metacognitive" processes involving the ability to recognize, monitor, and reflect on one's own thoughts, experiences, and beliefs would overlap with the cognitive/self-oriented aspect of mentalizing (Debbané et al., 2016a, b).

Empirical data suggest that adults suffering with SSDs exhibit difficulties in the capacity to accurately infer the mental states of others (Brüne, 2005), and these have been shown to relate to the level of negative (Corcoran and Frith, 2003; Corcoran et al., 1995; Weijers et al., 2018), positive (Sarfati et al., 1997; Frith & Corcoran, 1996), and disorganization symptoms (Sarfati et al., 1999; Mazza et al., 2001). In line with the findings from samples suffering with SSDs, data suggest that young adults who report prodromal CHR manifestations (i.e., attenuated and intermittent psychotic symptoms) also display difficulties in understanding the mental states of others (Chung et al., 2008), and these are prospectively linked with transition to SSDs (Kim et al., 2011; Boldrini et al., 2020).

Further evidence in support of the links between mentalizing and early signs of psychosis risk comes from studies in nonclinical adults, children, and young people who score high on measures of schizotypy. Cross-sectional studies in adults have reported associations between high scores on positive schizotypy and reduced ToM scores (Langdon & Coltheart, 1999; Pickup, 2006; Fyfe et al., 2008). In line with the findings from adult samples, research has also shown that expressions of positive schizotypy are associated with reduced ToM scores among community adolescents (Barragan et al., 2011) and with a hypermentalizing pattern in nonclinical children (Clemmensen et al., 2014, 2016). Overall, data indicate that difficulties in inferring mental states in others are linked to early trait signs of emerging psychosis.

Critically, however, evidence also suggests that difficulties extending beyond the other-oriented dimension of mentalizing relate to psychotic phenomena across the premorbid, prodromal, and clinical levels of expression from adolescence to young adulthood. Functional neuroimaging studies among patients suffering with SSDs, as well as nonclinical adults and adolescents who report high schizotypy have identified atypical neural activation patterns in cortical brain regions that normally sustain self-referential processing and the differentiation between self- and non-self-cues (Murphy et al., 2010; Shad et al., 2011; Debbané et al., 2012, 2014b). In line with neuroscientific evidence, experimental paradigms have consistently shown that adults suffering with SSDs and young adults who meet the CHR criteria can struggle to monitor the source of self-generated mental events and tend to misattribute these as externally perceived and real (Keefe et al., 1999; Docherty, 2012; Franck et al., 2000; Johns et al., 2010; Gaweda et al., 2018; Bentall et al., 1991; Brébion et al., 2000). Similarly, research using narrative methodologies suggests that individuals suffering with SSDs exhibit difficulties in synthesizing information about their inner states (i.e., thoughts, beliefs, and emotions) and personal experiences to form coherent representations of themselves and their relation to others (Lysaker et al., 2021; Rabin et al., 2014).

Importantly, difficulties in self-oriented mentalizing appear to already be present, albeit at an attenuated degree, among nonclinical samples who score high on measures of schizotypy, suggesting an early developmental pathway that may be linked to risk progression. For instance, experimental studies have shown that nonclinical adults reporting positive schizotypy tend to experience difficulties in differentiating self-generated thoughts and actions from externally perceived stimuli (Peters et al., 2007; Humpston et al., 2017; Versmissen et al., 2007). In addition, studies using narrative assessment methods suggest that dysfunctions in more complex self-reflective abilities correlate with measures of negative schizotypy in nonclinical samples (Rabin et al., 2014).

A small amount of empirical research has also explored the links between schizotypy and self-oriented mentalizing processes during adolescence. Experimental studies in samples of young people have shown that impairments in the capacity to monitor the source of self-generated mental events are associated with both positive (Debbané et al., 2008, 2009) and negative schizotypy (Salaminios et al., 2020). In line with these findings, self-reported schizotypy in adolescence has been shown to correlate with atypical neural activation patterns in the prefrontal cortex during self-monitoring evaluations (Lagioia et al., 2011; Debbané et al., 2014b; Dahoun et al., 2013). Furthermore, findings from a community adolescent sample using a self-report measure of mentalizing that primarily included items referring to mental state inferences about the self showed that schizotypal trait features of social anxiety and odd speech were associated with increased uncertainty in understanding mental states (Salaminios et al., 2021). Thus, emerging evidence appears to support the early links between schizotypal manifestations and impairments in self-oriented mentalizing processes.

Interestingly, studies among both nonclinical and SSD samples show correlated task performance and shared neural activation patterns in the prefrontal cortex during self- and other-oriented mentalizing evaluations (Fisher et al., 2008; Murphy et al., 2010; Shad et al., 2011). The overlap between dysfunctions in self-understanding and understanding of others in SSDs suggests that these may be indicative of a more fundamental disturbance of the self (Murphy et al., 2010). Indeed, contemporary clinical models suggest that early dysfunctions in self-oriented mentalizing processes, particularly in the context of schizotypal trait expression, may contribute to the aberrant explanations of social experiences observed during the prodromal and clinical stages of SSDs (Brent & Fonagy, 2014; Salaminios & Debbané, 2021). In line with phenomenologically oriented approaches (Sass & Parnas, 2003), these models highlight the critical role of disturbed self-awareness in SSDs, while at the same time offering a developmental account on how this may emerge through associations across the personality, interpersonal, and psychological domains.

While the precise nature of the associations between schizotypy and mentalizing dysfunction remains unclear, we have previously proposed that the two may dynamically impact on each other across childhood and adolescence to undermine the development of the self and augment vulnerability for SSDs (Debbané et al., 2016b; Salaminios & Debbané, 2021). Specifically, among genetically predisposed individuals and in the context of early attachment difficulties, the phenotypic expression of schizotypy during childhood and early adolescence (e.g., suspiciousness and social withdrawal) may negatively impact on the close interpersonal relationships and social learning opportunities that normally sustain the capacity to monitor, reflect on, and regulate one's own mental states. Concurrently and in the context of adolescent-specific biopsychosocial challenges, failures to reflect on and regulate one's own mental states (including the subtle perceptual aberrations of schizotypy) may facilitate the progression of the underlying schizotypal "seed," leading to anomalous self-experiences, as captured by the basic symptoms approach (Schultze-Lutter et al., 2007), prodromal impairments in social understanding (e.g., delusional ideation), and ultimately the transition to clinically diagnosable SSDs. Here, we want to highlight that in the context of an undermined ability to form mental representations of one's self-experiences, dysfunctions of social understanding and associated difficulties in social functioning during the prodromal and clinical stages of psychosis expression do not represent "deficits," but rather dynamic compensatory attempts of adaptation (by diminishing uncertainty) in a social world of increasing complexity. Problematically, however, the dysfunction of self and other mentalizing processes will impede the type of emotion regulation so critical to developing safe, trustworthy, and continuous relationships with significant others (Luyten et al., 2020). Given the centrality of mentalizing in affect regulation within the interpersonal domain, as well as within the relationship one maintains to oneself during adolescence and early adulthood, a robust capacity to think about mental states may represent a protective factor against the anxieties that early signs of schizotypy tend to exacerbate (Benerjee & Henderson, 2001). Conversely, impairments or developmental delays in mentalizing in the context of schizotypy may promote avoidant coping strategies that can exacerbate into clinically relevant social withdrawal and paranoid ideation (Michail & Birchwood, 2009). Therefore, affect regulation provided by accurate mentalizing, when impaired, may contribute to give way to risk for SSDs in the context of schizotypy expression. From our perspective, any therapeutic approach designed to address clinical risk should sensitively take into account the affective developmental dynamics in the emergence of SSDs during adolescence and early adulthood.

In the conclusion of this chapter, we develop a clinical perspective of psychotic phenomena across the continuum of their expression, from schizotypal trait manifestations to clinical symptoms, through the identification of exaggerated forms of "prereflective" modes of thinking about mental states, which serve to regulate cognitive and affective disturbances, and aim at maintaining a minimal sense of self-coherence in the face of increasing emotional and interpersonal complexity. Against this background, we suggest that the critical value of mentalizing in emerging psychosis is to sustain self-continuity and afford resilience against the psychopathological effects of an underlying trait liability for the illness. On this basis, the clinical framework offered by MBT can assist clinicians in case formulation and clinical intervention with a focus on increasing mentalizing skills in the face of challenging subjective states and interpersonal difficulties. As further developed in another Chap. 18, MBT can increase resilience in the face of emerging SSDs.

Conclusion: Toward a Person-Centered Integration of the Schizotypy Framework for Clinical Intervention

In the context of MBT, the clinical translation of key empirical findings reviewed above follows a set of simple principles that can legitimately relate to the patient's subjective experience, thereby sustaining alliance for the initiation of therapeutic intervention. We propose a stepwise rationale that can be individually adapted and integrated to each patient's formulation prior to beginning treatment: (1) Schizotypy can stimulate psychological distress, in response to which the individual may resort to idiosyncratic "prementalistic" thinking patterns in order to regulate distress and threats to self-coherence; (2) these patterns represent attempts to regulate cognitive and emotional disturbances through explanations that maintain a minimal sense of self-coherence in the face of perceived threat triggering schizotypy distressing expression; (3) these patterns will affect how the individual holds oneself and others in mind and may therefore affect interpersonal communication; (4) while providing temporary solutions to idiosyncratic triggers, if these thinking patterns become dominant on a regular basis, they can significantly impede thought flexibility, emotion regulation, and behavioral control; and (5) when crystalized, these patterns increasingly isolate the individual in their own way of perceiving reality and underminine trust in meaningful interpersonal relations that normally sustain resilience against clinical psychopathology. As such, individuals become impervious to and can increasingly feel threatened by the mentalizing of others' minds, which reinforces prementalistic explanations of self in relation to others.

The main objective of MBT along the continuum of SSDs is to sustain and help develop mentalizing skills to strengthen thought flexibility about mental states, to enable a better understanding of self and others, and to promote a more robust regulation of emotions encountered in the social domain through calibrated mentalizing. Because the identification of prementalistic thinking patterns is essential to MBT treatment along the continuum of SSDs (Bateman et al., 2023; Debbané & Bateman, 2019), it may be useful to describe how in order to regulate their experience of themselves and others, individuals with impaired mentalizing may turn to "prementalistic" forms of thinking (the teleological, psychic equivalence and pretend modes). These modes of thinking find their source in early self-development during infancy and early childhood, preceding the emergence of mentalizing and the establishment of a coherent self (Fonagy et al., 2002). They have been described as playing a role in other forms of psychopathology affecting emotion regulation and coherence of self, as in borderline personality disorder (Fonagy & Luyten, 2009). Experiences of intense affective arousal and interpersonal complexity can lead to the temporary dominance of the prementalizing modes of thinking for any individual, which naturally requires other minds to help reestablish a balance (decreased uncertainty and increased predictability) in the relationship to oneself and others. Below we illustrate how these modes manifest in the expression of schizotypal traits and in the phenomenology of psychotic symptoms.

The *teleological mode* (Fonagy & Bateman, 2006) refers to the most basic form of self-organization, in which internal states in the self and others are mainly inferred on the basis of behaviors and actions. When this mode of thinking dominates, the individual becomes extremely vulnerable to overdetermining intentions on the basis of everyday actions, and therefore, physical actions in the interpersonal context can be experienced as overwhelmingly hostile. For instance, experiences of suspiciousness based solely on others' physical actions may indicate teleological mode functioning (e.g., "she looked at me when she was talking to her friend so she must have said something bad about me"). In clinical psychosis, teleological mode functioning can adopt a more overtly delusional quality (e.g., she looked at me when she was talking to her friend because she knows all my secrets and now they are planning on exposing me to everyone). Differentiation between the mind of oneself and others is absent when the teleological mode dominates interpretations of reality, and mentalistic activity attempts to make sense of the individual's experience based solely on sensory evidence.

The *psychic equivalence mode* (Fonagy & Target, 1996) refers to a type of thinking pattern in which one's thoughts and feelings are taken as unequivocally real. When this mode dominates thinking activity, the capacity to consider alternative perspectives of one's own internal experience is severely compromised. Beliefs in mind-reading often signify psychic equivalence functioning as one assumes they know what is in the other's mind. Similarly, ideas of reference also entail psychic equivalence thinking as the opacity of other people's mental states is refuted (i.e., a belief that people on the TV are directly addressing oneself). In clinical psychosis, paranoid delusional ideation represents a prototypical example of psychic equivalence functioning because beliefs about others' intentions are held with absolute conviction (i.e., they do not constitute possibilities but certainties). As in teleological mode, boundaries between minds are blurred through nondifferentiation (*what I think you think is what you think*), and mentalistic activity attempts to ground the individual's experience solely on the basis of cognitive evidence.

Finally, in the *pretend mode* thinking pattern (Fonagy & Target, 1996), mentalizing activity objectifies the self and its experience as a subject of rational thought, decoupled from the lived, affective dimension of experience. When this mode dominates thinking activity, hyper-reflexivity tends to overdetermine the individual's understanding of reality. Boundaries between different minds are subject to extremes, experienced as greatly distanced or fused with one another. Consequently, the capacity to genuinely reflect on and communicate inner states, particularly within interpersonal relationships, is disrupted. Risk for dissociative symptoms is exacerbated when pretend mode dominates. For instance, individuals may engage in hyper-reflexive descriptions of their experience, which however remain devoid of affective content and tone. In clinical psychosis, the exacerbation of pretend mode thinking further contributes to affective blunting and anhedonia, which can lead to severe forms of dissociation, such as experiencing parts of oneself as split-off from one another.

We underline that the prementalizing modes of thinking are not psychopathological in themselves; rather, they characterize states where an individual is attempting to regulate disturbances in cognition, affect, and, most significantly, self-coherence. Indeed, adopting such modes of thinking does often afford significant regulation. A common and most often benign example of prementalizing modes of thinking can be found in conspiracy theories: They are held with certainty, usually overdetermine others' intentions on the basis of little evidence, and can themselves be a base for further expanding on malevolent motives. While these may help individuals make sense of complex issues that stir significant cognitive and affective disturbances in one's relation to the world, they become problematic when they are rigidly held, as well as when they lead the individual to despair, to lose trust in others and mentally isolate, or to feel that violence is the only way out of such difficult circumstances. Similarly, the expression of schizotypy is usually benign and can be compensated by adaptive mechanisms, such as mentalizing, which can support individuals maintain flexibility and emotional regulation in the face of potentially disturbing experiences. In the context of impaired mentalizing, however, the individual is more vulnerable to the pathogenic effects of schizotypy expression, which may exacerbate into clinically relevant psychopathology characterized by rigid delusional thinking patterns and social isolation.

We have argued that a mentalization-informed perspective on psychological treatment along the continuum of schizotypy trait expression is justified, both empirically and clinically. A number of clinical studies provide preliminary evidence in the case of clinical high-risk symptoms (Armando et al., 2019; Debbané et al., 2016a) and for patients with nonaffective SSDs (Weijers et al., 2020). Although as discussed above the prementalizing modes of functioning represent early thinking about mental states, they appear to significantly disrupt the establishment of a more integrated sense of self and impede meaningful relatedness with others. Within this context, we have previously suggested that among individuals faced with a trait risk for psychosis the critical value of mentalizing may be to confer resilience by sustaining emotion regulation through a better understanding of one's own and others' mental states, affording greater self-continuity and attenuating experiences of confusion within interpersonal relationships (Debbané et al., 2016b; Salaminios & Debbané, 2021). In turn, treatment that focuses on strengthening mentalizing may help individuals on the schizophrenia spectrum to engage and sustain increased trust in meaningful relationships. These resources are key to mental health and to fostering safe and meaningful relationships to oneself and others.

References

Ainsworth, M. D. S., Blehar, M. C., Waters, E., & Wall, S. N. (2015). *Patterns of attachment: A psychological study of the strange situation*. Psychology Press.

Armando, M., Hutsebaut, J., & Debbané, M. (2019). A mentalization-informed staging approach to clinical high risk for psychosis. *Frontiers in Psychiatry, 10*, 385.

Badcock, J. C., Barkus, E., Cohen, A. S., Bucks, R., & Badcock, D. R. (2016). Loneliness and schizotypy are distinct constructs, separate from general psychopathology. *Frontiers in Psychology, 7*, 1018.

Badoud, D., Speranza, M., & Debbané, M. (2016). Vers un modèle du développement des dimensions de la mentalisation a l'adolescence. *Revue québécoise de psychologie, 37*(3), 49–68.

Banerjee, R., & Henderson, L. (2001). Social-cognitive factors in childhood social anxiety: A preliminary investigation. *Social Development, 10*(4), 558–572.

Barragan, M., Laurens, K. R., Navarro, J. B., & Obiols, J. E. (2011). 'Theory of Mind', psychotic-like experiences and psychometric schizotypy in adolescents from the general population. *Psychiatry Research, 186*(2), 225–231.

Bateman, A., Fonagy, P., Campbell, C., Luyten, P., & Debbané, M. (2023). *Cambridge Guide to Mentalization-Based Treatment (MBT)* (Cambridge Guides to the Psychological Therapies). Cambridge University Press.

Bentall, R. P., Baker, G. A., & Havers, S. (1991). Reality monitoring and psychotic hallucinations. *British Journal of Clinical Psychology, 30*(3), 213–222.

Blakemore, S. J. (2008). The social brain in adolescence. *Nature Reviews Neuroscience, 9*(4), 267–277.

Boldrini, T., Pontillo, M., Tanzilli, A., Giovanardi, G., Di Cicilia, G., Salcuni, S., et al. (2020). An attachment perspective on the risk for psychosis: Clinical correlates and the predictive value of attachment patterns and mentalization. *Schizophrenia Research, 222*, 209–217.

Borsboom, D., & Cramer, A. O. (2013). Network analysis: An integrative approach to the structure of psychopathology. *Annual Review of Clinical Psychology, 9*, 91–121.

Brébion, G., Amador, X., David, A., Malaspina, D., Sharif, Z., & Gorman, J. M. (2000). Positive symptomatology and source-monitoring failure in schizophrenia—An analysis of symptom-specific effects. *Psychiatry Research, 95*(2), 119–131.

Brent, B. K., & Fonagy, P. (2014). A mentalization-based treatment approach to disturbances of social understanding in schizophrenia. In P. H. Lysaker, G. Dimaggio, & M. Brune (Eds.), *Social cognition and metacognition in schizophrenia: Psychopathology and treatment approaches* (pp. 245–259). Elsevier Science and Technology.

Brüne, M. (2005). "Theory of mind" in schizophrenia: A review of the literature. *Schizophrenia Bulletin, 31*(1), 21–42.

Caspi, A., Houts, R. M., Belsky, D. W., Goldman-Mellor, S. J., Harrington, H., Israel, S., et al. (2014). The p factor: One general psychopathology factor in the structure of psychiatric disorders? *Clinical Psychological Science, 2*(2), 119–137.

Choi-Kain, L. W., & Gunderson, J. G. (2008). Mentalization: Ontogeny, assessment, and application in the treatment of borderline personality disorder. *American Journal of Psychiatry, 165*(9), 1127–1135.

Choudhury, S., Blakemore, S.-J., & Charman, T. (2006). Social cognitive development during adolescence. *Social Cognitive and Affective Neuroscience, 1*(3), 165–174.

Chung, Y. S., Kang, D. H., Shin, N. Y., Yoo, S. Y., & Kwon, J. S. (2008). Deficit of theory of mind in individuals at ultra-high-risk for schizophrenia. *Schizophrenia Research, 99*(1–3), 111–118.

Claridge, G. E. (1997). *Schizotypy: Implications for illness and health*. Oxford University Press.

Clemmensen, L., van Os, J., Skovgaard, A. M., Væver, M., Blijd-Hoogewys, E. M., Bartels-Velthuis, A. A., & Jeppesen, P. (2014). Hyper-theory-of-mind in children with psychotic experiences. *PLoS One, 9*(11), e113082.

Clemmensen, L., Van Os, J., Drukker, M., Munkholm, A., Rimvall, M. K., Vaever, M., et al. (2016). Psychotic experiences and hyper-theory-of-mind in preadolescence—A birth cohort study. *Psychological Medicine, 46*(1), 87–101.

Cohen, A. S., Mohr, C., Ettinger, U., Chan, R. C., & Park, S. (2015). Schizotypy as an organizing framework for social and affective sciences. *Schizophrenia Bulletin, 41*(suppl_2), S427–S435.

Corcoran, R., & Frith, C. (2003). Autobiographical memory and theory of mind: Evidence of a relationship in schizophrenia. *Psychological Medicine, 33*(5), 897.

Corcoran, R., Mercer, G., & Frith, C. D. (1995). Schizophrenia, symptomatology and social inference: Investigating "theory of mind" in people with schizophrenia. *Schizophrenia Research, 17*(1), 5–13.

Dahoun, T., Eliez, S., Chen, F., Badoud, D., Schneider, M., Larøi, F., & Debbane, M. (2013). Action simulation in hallucination-prone adolescents. *Frontiers in Human Neuroscience, 7*, 329.

Debbané, M., & Barrantes-Vidal, N. (2014). Schizotypy from a developmental perspective. *Schizophrenia Bulletin, 41*(suppl_2), S386–S395.

Debbané, M., & Bateman, A. W. (2019). Psychosis. In A. W. Bateman & P. E. Fonagy (Eds.), *Handbook of mentalizing in mental health practice*. American Psychiatric Publishing.

Debbané, M., Van der Linden, M., Glaser, B., & Eliez, S. (2008). Source monitoring for actions in adolescents with 22q11. 2 deletion syndrome (22q11DS). *Psychological Medicine, 38*(6), 811–820.

Debbané, M., Van der Linden, M., Gex-Fabry, M., & Eliez, S. (2009). Cognitive and emotional associations to positive schizotypy during adolescence. *Journal of Child Psychology and Psychiatry, 50*(3), 326–334.

Debbané, M., Lazouret, M., Lagioia, A., Schneider, M., Van De Ville, D., & Eliez, S. (2012). Resting-state networks in adolescents with 22q11. 2 deletion syndrome: Associations with prodromal symptoms and executive functions. *Schizophrenia Research, 139*(1–3), 33–39.

Debbané, M., Badoud, D., Balanzin, D., & Eliez, S. (2013). Broadly defined risk mental states during adolescence: Disorganization mediates positive schizotypal expression. *Schizophrenia Research, 147*(1), 153–156.

Debbané, M., Eliez, S., Badoud, D., Conus, P., Flückiger, R., & Schultze-Lutter, F. (2014a). Developing psychosis and its risk states through the lens of schizotypy. *Schizophrenia Bulletin, 41*(suppl_2), S396–S407.

Debbané, M., Vrtička, P., Lazouret, M., Badoud, D., Sander, D., & Eliez, S. (2014b). Self-reflection and positive schizotypy in the adolescent brain. *Schizophrenia Research, 152*(1), 65–72.

Debbané, M., Benmiloud, J., Salaminios, G., Solida-Tozzi, A., Armando, M., Fonagy, P., & Bateman, A. (2016a). Mentalization-based treatment in clinical high-risk for psychosis: A rationale and clinical illustration. *Journal of Contemporary Psychotherapy, 46*(4), 217–225.

Debbané, M., Salaminios, G., Luyten, P., Badoud, D., Armando, M., Tozzi, A. S., Fonagy, P., & Brent, B. K. (2016b). Attachment, neurobiology, and mentalizing along the psychosis continuum. *Frontiers in Human Neuroscience, 10*, 406.

Debbané, M., Prada, P., Bouteloup, M., Speranza, M., & Perroud, N. (2022). *Mentaliser: la clédes interactions humaines: Concepts et applications*. De Boeck Supérieur.

Derome, M., Zöller, D., Modinos, G., Schaer, M., Eliez, S., & Debbané, M. (2020). Developmental trajectories of subcortical structures in relation to dimensional schizotypy expression along adolescence. *Schizophrenia Research, 218*, 76–84.

Do, K. Q., Cabungcal, J. H., Frank, A., Steullet, P., & Cuenod, M. (2009). Redox dysregulation, neurodevelopment, and schizophrenia. *Current Opinion in Neurobiology, 19*(2), 220–230.

Docherty, N. M. (2012). Missing referents, psychotic symptoms, and discriminating the internal from the externalized. *Journal of Abnormal Psychology, 121*(2), 416.

Dominguez, M. D. G., Saka, M. C., Lieb, R., Wittchen, H. U., & van Os, J. (2010). Early expression of negative/disorganized symptoms predicting psychotic experiences and 265 subsequent clinical psychosis: A 10-year study. *American Journal of Psychiatry, 167*(9), 1075–1082.

Dumontheil, I., Apperly, I. A., & Blakemore, S. J. (2010). Online usage of theory of mind continues to develop in late adolescence. *Developmental Science, 13*(2), 331–338.

Epskamp, S., Borsboom, D., & Fried, E. I. (2018). Estimating psychological networks and their accuracy: A tutorial paper. *Behavior Research Methods, 50*, 195–212.

Fisher, M., McCoy, K., Poole, J. H., & Vinogradov, S. (2008). Self and other in schizophrenia: A cognitive neuroscience perspective. *American Journal of Psychiatry, 165*(11), 1465–1472.

Fisher, H. L., Caspi, A., Poulton, R., Meier, M. H., Houts, R., Harrington, H., et al. (2013). Specificity of childhood psychotic symptoms for predicting schizophrenia by 38 years of age: A birth cohort study. *Psychological Medicine, 43*(10), 2077–2086.

Flückiger, R., Ruhrmann, S., Debbané, M., Michel, C., Hubl, D., Schimmelmann, B. G., et al. (2016). Psychosis-predictive value of self-reported schizotypy in a clinical high-risk sample. *Journal of Abnormal Psychology, 125*(7), 923.

Fonagy, P., & Bateman, A. W. (2006). Mechanisms of change in mentalization-based treatment of BPD. *Journal of Clinical Psychology, 62*(4), 411–430.

Fonagy, P., & Bateman, A. W. (2016). Adversity, attachment, and mentalizing. *Comprehensive Psychiatry, 64*, 59–66.

Fonagy, P., & Luyten, P. (2009). A developmental, mentalization-based approach to the understanding and treatment of borderline personality disorder. *Development and Psychopathology, 21*(4), 1355–1381.

Fonagy, P., & Target, M. (1996). Playing with reality I. *The International Journal of Psychoanalysis, 77*(2), 217.

Fonagy, P., Redfern, S., & Charman, T. (1997). The relationship between belief-desire reasoning and a projective measure of attachment security (SAT). *British Journal of Developmental Psychology, 15*(1), 51–61.

Fonagy, P., Gergely, G., Jurist, E. L., & Target, M. (2002). *Affect regulation, mentalization and the development of the self.* Routledge.

Franck, N., Rouby, P., Daprati, E., Daléry, J., Marie-Cardine, M., & Georgieff, N. (2000). Confusion between silent and overt reading in schizophrenia. *Schizophrenia Research, 41*(2), 357–364.

Frith, C. D., & Corcoran, R. (1996). Exploring 'theory of mind'in people with schizophrenia. *Psychological Medicine, 26*(3), 521–530.

Fusar-Poli, P., Borgwardt, S., Bechdolf, A., Addington, J., Riecher-Rössler, A., Schultze-Lutter, F., et al. (2013). The psychosis high-risk state: A comprehensive state-of-the-art review. *JAMA Psychiatry, 70*(1), 107–120.

Fyfe, S., Williams, C., Mason, O. J., & Pickup, G. J. (2008). Apophenia, theory of mind and schizotypy: Perceiving meaning and intentionality in randomness. *Cortex, 44*(10), 1316–1325.

Gawęda, Ł., Li, E., Lavoie, S., Whitford, T. J., Moritz, S., & Nelson, B. (2018). Impaired action self-monitoring and cognitive confidence among ultra-high risk for psychosis and first-episode psychosis patients. *European Psychiatry, 47*, 67–75.

Heim, C., Newport, D. J., Mletzko, T., Miller, A. H., & Nemeroff, C. B. (2008). The link between childhood trauma and depression: Insights from HPA axis studies in humans. *Psychoneuroendocrinology, 33*(6), 693–710.

Howes, O. D., & Kapur, S. (2009). The dopamine hypothesis of schizophrenia: Version III—The final common pathway. *Schizophrenia Bulletin, 35*(3), 549–562.

Humpston, C. S., Linden, D. E., & Evans, L. H. (2017). Deficits in reality and internal source monitoring of actions are associated with the positive dimension of schizotypy. *Psychiatry Research, 250*, 44–49.

Johns, L., Allen, P., Valli, I., Winton-Brown, T., Broome, M., Woolley, J., Tabraham, P., Day, F., Howes, O., & Wykes, T. (2010). Impaired verbal self-monitoring in individuals at high risk of psychosis. *Psychological Medicine, 40*(9), 1433–1442.

Johnstone, E. C., Ebmeier, K. P., Miller, P., Owens, D. G., & Lawrie, S. M. (2005). Predicting schizophrenia: Findings from the Edinburgh high-risk study. *The British Journal of Psychiatry, 186*(1), 18–25.

Keefe, R. S., Arnold, M., Bayen, U., & Harvey, P. (1999). Source monitoring deficits in patients with schizophrenia; a multinomial modelling analysis. *Psychological Medicine, 29*(4), 903–914.

Kirkpatrick, B., & Miller, B. J. (2013). Inflammation and schizophrenia. *Schizophrenia Bulletin, 39*(6), 1174–1179.

Klagsbrun, M., & Bowlby, J. (1976). Responses to separation from parents: A clinical test for young children. *British Journal of Projective Psychology & Personality Study*.

Kotov, R., Krueger, R. F., Watson, D., Achenbach, T. M., Althoff, R. R., Bagby, R. M., et al. (2017). The Hierarchical Taxonomy of Psychopathology (HiTOP): A dimensional alternative to traditional nosologies. *Journal of Abnormal Psychology, 126*(4), 454.

Kwapil, T. R., & Barrantes-Vidal, N. (2015). Schizotypy: Looking back and moving forward. *Schizophrenia Bulletin, 41*(suppl_2), S366–S373.

Lagioia, A., Eliez, S., Schneider, M., Simons, J. S., Van der Linden, M., & Debbané, M. (2011). Neural correlates of reality monitoring during adolescence. *NeuroImage, 55*(3), 1393–1400.

Langdon, R., & Coltheart, M. (1999). Mentalising, schizotypy, and schizophrenia. *Cognition, 71*(1), 43–71.

Lenzenweger, M. F. (2015). Thinking clearly about schizotypy: Hewing to the schizophrenia liability core, considering interesting tangents, and avoiding conceptual quicksand. *Schizophrenia Bulletin, 41*(suppl_2), S483–S491.

Luyten, P., & Fonagy, P. (2022). Integrating and differentiating personality and psychopathology: A psychodynamic perspective. *Journal of Personality, 90*(1), 75–88.

Luyten, P., Campbell, C., Allison, E., & Fonagy, P. (2020). The mentalizing approach to psychopathology: State of the art and future directions. *Annual Review of Clinical Psychology, 16*, 297–325.

Lysaker, P. H., Cheli, S., Dimaggio, G., Buck, B., Bonfils, K. A., Huling, K., et al. (2021). Metacognition, social cognition, and mentalizing in psychosis: Are these distinct constructs when it comes to subjective experience or are we just splitting hairs? *BMC Psychiatry, 21*(1), 1–14.

Mansueto, A. C., Wiers, R. W., van Weert, J., Schouten, B. C., & Epskamp, S. (2022). Investigating the feasibility of idiographic network models. *Psychological Methods*.

Mason, O., & Claridge, G. (2006). The Oxford-Liverpool Inventory of Feelings and Experiences (O-LIFE): Further description and extended norms. *Schizophrenia Research, 82*(2–3), 203–211.

Mazza, M., De Risio, A., Surian, L., Roncone, R., & Casacchia, M. (2001). Selective impairments of theory of mind in people with schizophrenia. *Schizophrenia Research, 47*(2–3), 299–308.

Meehl, P. E. (1962). Schizotaxia, schizotypy, schizophrenia. *American Psychologist, 17*(12), 827.

Michail, M., & Birchwood, M. (2009). Social anxiety disorder in first-episode psychosis: Incidence, phenomenology and relationship with paranoia. *The British Journal of Psychiatry, 195*(3), 234–241.

Murphy, E. R., Brent, B. K., Benton, M., Pruitt, P., Diwadkar, V., Rajarethinam, R. P., & Keshavan, M. S. (2010). Differential processing of metacognitive evaluation and the neural circuitry of the self and others in schizophrenia: A pilot study. *Schizophrenia Research, 116*(2–3), 252–258.

Peters, M. J., Smeets, T., Giesbrecht, T., Jelicic, M., & Merckelbach, H. (2007). Confusing action and imagination: Action source monitoring in individuals with schizotypal traits. *The Journal of Nervous and Mental Disease, 195*(9), 752–757.

Pickup, G. (2006). Theory of mind and its relation to schizotypy. *Cognitive Neuropsychiatry, 11*(2), 117–192.

Poulton, R., Caspi, A., Moffitt, T. E., Cannon, M., Murray, R., & Harrington, H. (2000). Children's self-reported psychotic symptoms and adult schizophreniform disorder: A 15-year longitudinal study. *Archives of General Psychiatry, 57*(11), 1053–1058.

Poznyak, E., Morosan, L., Perroud, N., Speranza, M., Badoud, D., & Debbané, M. (2019). Roles of age, gender and psychological difficulties in adolescent mentalizing. *Journal of Adolescence, 74*, 120–129.

Raballo, A., & Parnas, J. (2011). The silent side of the spectrum: Schizotypy and the schizotaxic self. *Schizophrenia Bulletin, 37*(5), 1017–1026.

Rabin, S. J., Avidan, M., Rozencwaig, S., & Shalev, H. (2014). Metacognition in schizophrenia and schizotypy: Relation to symptoms of schizophrenia, traits of schizotypy and Social Quality of Life. *Israel Journal of Psychiatry, 51*(1), 44.

Salaminios, G., & Debbané, M. (2021). A Mentalization-based treatment framework to support the recovery of the self in emerging psychosis during adolescence. In *The recovery of the self in psychosis* (pp. 12–35). Routledge.

Salaminios, G., Morosan, L., Toffel, E., Tanzer, M., Eliez, S., & Debbané, M. (2020). Self-monitoring for speech and its links to age, cognitive effort, schizotypal trait expression and impulsivity during adolescence. *Cognitive Neuropsychiatry, 25*(3), 215–230.

Salaminios, G., Morosan, L., Toffel, E., Tanzer, M., Eliez, S., Badoud, D., et al. (2021). Associations between schizotypal personality features, mentalizing difficulties and thought problems in a sample of community adolescents. *Early Intervention in Psychiatry, 15*(3), 705–715.

Sarfati, Y., Hardy-Baylé, M. C., Besche, C., & Widlöcher, D. (1997). Attribution of intentions to others in people with schizophrenia: A non-verbal exploration with comic strips. *Schizophrenia Research, 25*(3), 199–209.

Sarfati, Y., Hardy-Baylé, M. C., Brunet, E., & Widlöcher, D. (1999). Investigating theory of mind in schizophrenia: Influence of verbalization in disorganized and non disorganized patients. *Schizophrenia Research, 37*(2), 183–190.

Sass, L. A., & Parnas, J. (2003). Schizophrenia, consciousness, and the self. *Schizophrenia Bulletin, 29*(3), 427–444.

Schultze-Lutter, F., Klosterkötter, J., Picker, H., Steinmeyer, E. M., & Ruhrmann, S. (2007). Predicting first-episode psychosis by basic symptom criteria. *Clinical Neuropsychiatry, 4*(1), 11–22.

Shad, M. U., Brent, B. K., & Keshavan, M. S. (2011). Neurobiology of self-awareness deficits in schizophrenia: A hypothetical model. *Asian Journal of Psychiatry, 4*(4), 248–254.

Sharp, C., & Fonagy, P. (2008). The parent's capacity to treat the child as a psychological agent: Constructs, measures and implications for developmental psychopathology. *Social Development, 17*(3), 737–754.

Steele, H., Steele, M., & Croft, C. (2008). Early attachment predicts emotion recognition at 6 and 11 years old. *Attachment & Human Development, 10*(4), 379–393.

Strathearn, L. (2011). Maternal neglect: Oxytocin, dopamine and the neurobiology of attachment. *Journal of Neuroendocrinology, 23*(11), 1054–1065.

Sun, X., So, S. H., Chung, L. K., Chiu, C. D., Chan, R. C., & Leung, P. W. (2022). Longitudinal bifactor modelling of anxiety, depression and schizotypy-The role of rumination as a shared mechanism. *Schizophrenia Research, 240*, 153–161.

Versmissen, D., Myin-Germeys, I., Janssen, I., Franck, N., Georgieff, N., Campo, J., et al. (2007). Impairment of self-monitoring: Part of the endophenotypic risk for psychosis. *The British Journal of Psychiatry, 191*(S51), s58–s62.

Vetter, N. C., Altgassen, M., Phillips, L., Mahy, C. E., & Kliegel, M. (2013). Development of affective theory of mind across adolescence: Disentangling the role of executive functions. *Developmental Neuropsychology, 38*(2), 114–125.

Weijers, J., Fonagy, P., Eurelings-Bontekoe, E., Termorshuizen, F., Viechtbauer, W., & Selten, J. (2018). Mentalizing impairment as a mediator between reported childhood abuse and outcome in nonaffective psychotic disorder. *Psychiatry Research, 259*, 463–469.

Weijers, J., Ten Kate, C., Viechtbauer, W., Rampaart, L. J. A., Eurelings, E. H. M., & Selten, J. P. (2020). Mentalization-based treatment for psychotic disorder: A rater-blinded, multi-center, randomized controlled trial. *Psychological Medicine*, 1–10.

Chapter 10
The Role of Attachment Processes in the Psychosis Spectrum

Katherine Berry, Anvita Vikram, and Claire Muller

Attachment Theory

According to Bowlby, the founder of attachment theory, the attachment system developed due to an evolutionary need for safety and security (Bowlby, 1969). From an evolutionary perspective, the attachment system promotes closeness to the caregiver and so ensures protection for the vulnerable infant and a felt sense of security. However, attachment theory is a life span developmental theory. The theory argues that relationships with significant others in the early years have a significant bearing on a person's way of relating to others throughout their life (Bowlby, 1969). This is because early experiences lead to the formation of "internal working models" that are essentially mental representations of the self, others, and relationships with those others. These working models influence how the individual interprets later life experiences and guides the way in which they interact with, and behave toward, others. In support of the theory, there is empirical evidence that childhood experiences and attachments influence attachments to others in adult life and that adult attachment style predicts social functioning, interpersonal difficulties, and mental health problems (Bartholomew & Horowitz, 1991; Berry et al., 2006; Platts et al., 2002).

Individual differences in attachment styles have been described in both the child and adult literatures. In adulthood, a "secure" attachment style is associated with a

---

K. Berry (✉)
University of Manchester, Manchester, UK

Greater Manchester Mental Health NHS Foundation Trust, Manchester, UK
e-mail: Katherine.Berry@manchester.ac.uk

A. Vikram
Pennine Care NHS Foundation Trust, Manchester, UK

C. Muller
Greater Manchester Mental Health NHS Foundation Trust, Manchester, UK

S. Cheli, P. H. Lysaker (eds.), *A Dimensional Approach to Schizotypy*,
https://doi.org/10.1007/978-3-031-41788-7_10

positive view of the self, distress tolerance, and a value of close relationships (Mikulincer & Shaver, 2012). Adult insecure attachment styles are suggested to encompass three main types: anxious, avoidant, and fearful and/or disorganized (Bartholomew & Horowitz, 1991; Main & Solomon, 1990). An anxious attachment style, also known as "preoccupied" or "anxious-ambivalent," is characterized by a negative view of the self, worry in relation to the availability of others, and an increased negative affect. Avoidant attachment, also known as "dismissing," is characterized by a negative view of others, a relatively positive view of self, social withdrawal and the suppression of negative affect. A fearful attachment reflects a combination of negative beliefs about the self and others. This is largely associated with a desire for close relationships and a simultaneous fear, and consequent avoidance, of others (Bartholomew & Horowitz, 1991). Fearful attachment as assessed on adult attachment measures has been argued to have a conceptual overlap with the disorganized concept of attachment in infancy, with some suggesting that fearful attachment in adulthood is the equivalent of the disorganized attachment in childhood (Bartholomew & Horowitz, 1991). Disorganized attachment has been linked to experiences of parental maltreatment and interpersonal trauma (Lyons-Ruth & Jacobvitz, 1999) and is understood to be the product of the child experiencing an attachment figure (who is meant to provide protection and a sense of security) as frightening and/or unpredictable. Disorganized attachment in adulthood has been associated with dissociative experiences in response to trauma (Liotti, 2004), and there is a growing interest in the relevance of this concept to understanding psychotic experiences (Harder, 2014). However, disorganized attachment is rarely assessed in psychosis research as it is not well captured using self-report measures of attachment, which are the primary method of assessing attachment in research (Berry et al., 2017). For example, studies often use the fearful attachment subscales to assess disorganized attachment, but this approach has been criticized for failing to capture the dissociative responses that are one of the key features of the disorganized attachment (Pollard et al., 2020, 2023).

Given the role of attachment in potentially explaining the development of interpersonal functioning and mental health problems, a number of researchers have argued that attachment theory can help extend existing models and conceptualizations of psychosis (Berry et al., 2007, 2017; Korver-Nieberg et al., 2015; Read & Gumley, 2010; Berry & Bucci, 2016). The link between childhood adversity and psychosis is well established (Varese et al., 2012), and attachment difficulties have been identified as a key potential mediating factor in this relationship (Williams et al., 2018).

The empirical evidence for the role of attachment difficulties in psychosis has lagged behind theoretical developments. However, over the past decade, there has been a significant increase in research measuring attachment styles or patterns in psychosis (Carr et al., 2018). Studies have identified an association between insecure attachment and psychotic experiences primarily in people diagnosed with schizophrenia (Carr et al., 2018). However, there is also a related body of research investigating attachment and its association with psychotic phenomena in nonclinical samples (Korver-Nieberg et al., 2013; Carr et al., 2018). These nonclinical studies are useful in psychosis research, as psychotic experiences are hypothesized to lie on a continuum with normal experiences (Berry et al., 2006). The predominance of studies in nonclinical samples investigates associations between attachment and schizotypal personality traits. Below we summarize the studies investigating attachment and schizotypy. In line with the single-symptom approach to psychosis (Bentall et al., 2014), we also consider the role of attachment experiences in relation to the individual constructs of paranoia, hallucinatory phenomena, and negative symptoms.

An Overview of Attachment Styles and Schizotypy

Carr et al. (2018) carried out a meta-analysis of studies investigating the prevalence of insecure attachment across the psychosis spectrum and the association with types and severity of psychosis spectrum experiences. Nonclinical samples in this review mainly comprised healthy adult volunteers ($k = 10$), and a small number were exclusively involved student populations ($k = 4$). Studies used a range of different measures to assess subclinical psychosis and schizotypy. These included the revised Launay–Slade Hallucination Scale (rLSHS; Morrison et al., 2000), a self-report measure of hallucinatory experiences in nonclinical populations; the Green et al.'s Paranoid Thoughts Scale (GPTS; Green et al., 2008) and the Persecution and Deservedness Scale (PaDS; Melo et al., 2009), measures of paranoia commonly used in other nonclinical studies of paranoia; and the Community Assessment of Psychic Experience (CAPE; Stefanis et al., 2002), which is a commonly used self-reported psychotic-like experiences in the general population. Across the psychosis continuum, Carr et al. (2018) reported a small but significant relationship between positive symptom severity and insecure attachment and a significant relationship between negative symptom severity and insecure attachment in the nonclinical analysis, which was not found in the clinical group. The authors explain these discrepant findings between the clinical and nonclinical groups in terms of the increased use of schizotypy measures within nonclinical studies. They argue that while high scores on measures of negative schizotypy are indicative of subclinical negative psychotic-like experiences, the constructs that are assessed (e.g., social anhedonia—which is defined as an increased disinterest in all aspects of interpersonal relationships and a lack of pleasure in social situations) could have a more significant overlap with the construct of avoidant attachment. The authors also argue that the absence of associations between avoidant attachment and negative symptoms in clinical samples may be due to lower rates of symptom reporting by clinical participants with avoidant coping styles or their poor engagement in mental health services and research, meaning that they are not represented by clinical research samples.

Attachment Styles and Paranoia

Nonclinical studies published after the Carr et al. (2018)'s review have replicated associations between insecure attachment and paranoia (Ascone et al., 2020; Martinez et al., 2021; Mertens et al., 2021). Martinez et al. (2021) and Mertens et al. (2021) reported associations between both anxious and avoidant attachment and paranoia. However the study by Ascone et al. (2020) found only associations between anxious attachment but not avoidant attachment in their nonclinical control sample. The slightly more robust relationship between anxious attachment and paranoia compared to that between avoidant attachment and paranoia was also evident from a systematic review of clinical studies assessing associations between insecure attachment and paranoia (Lavin et al., 2020).

Anxious attachment style may be related to paranoia as this attachment style is characterized by preoccupation/worry, increased negative affect, and increased interpersonal sensitivity (Mikulincer & Shaver, 2012), which may predispose an individual toward a hypervigilance for threat in the social world (Lavin et al., 2020). For example, Freeman et al.'s (2002) threat anticipation model of paranoia argues that affective processes, such as anxiety and worry, along with interpersonal sensitivity, are important casual factors in paranoia. Negative affect and interpersonal sensitivity make a negative interpretation of others' behaviors more likely, which can drive paranoid ideation (Freeman & Garety, 2014). A negative self-self perception that is also a characteristic of attachment anxiety may also lead individuals to perceive themselves as vulnerable and thus increase a sense of threat and harm from others (Freeman & Garety, 2014).

However, this is not to say that attachment avoidance does not also play a role. Attachment avoidance is characterized by a negative view of others, minimization of affect, and social withdrawal (Mikulincer & Shaver, 2012). Individuals with attachment avoidance downregulate their affect through avoidance strategies and can have a positive view of self but a negative view of others (Bartholomew & Horowitz, 1991). Both social withdrawal and negative beliefs about others are also implicated in models of paranoia (Freeman et al., 2002), suggesting that this attachment style may increase vulnerability to the development and maintenance of paranoia.

In order to develop and test theoretical models explaining associations between attachment and paranoia, researchers have carried out studies exploring the potential role of mediators through statistical analysis or through experimental designs. Given the dominance of cognitive models of psychosis, it is not surprising that the majority of studies have investigated the role of cognitive factors as potential mediators in the relationship between insecure attachment and paranoia. For example, a cross-sectional survey by Pickering et al. (2008) involving 350 undergraduate students found that associations between insecure attachment and paranoia were partially mediated by measures such as self-esteem, anticipation of threat, and the perception of others as powerful. These findings in relation to self-esteem were replicated in a similar survey by the same research group (Wickham et al., 2014). A large and a more recent study by Martinez et al. (2021) from the same research group involving 1121 participants recruited using stratified sampling also explored the mediating role of self-esteem as well as the role of mistrust. The authors argued that mistrust was an independent construct from self-esteem and a particularly important explanatory factor in the context of subclinical paranoia as it is a subcomponent of the paranoia spectrum often present in subclinical populations. In support of their hypotheses, the authors found that both mistrust and negative self-esteem mediated the association between attachment anxiety and paranoia, but only mistrust mediated the association between attachment avoidance and paranoia. The authors argued that these findings are explained by the fact that attachment avoidance reflects a negative view of others, whereas attachment anxiety reflects a negative view of oneself as well as others.

Although there is good evidence from cross-sectional surveys that insecure attachment and paranoia are associated and negative self-beliefs and related constructs mediate the relationship between insecure attachment and paranoia, the majority of research relies on measured (rather than manipulated) variables that preclude causal inferences. A series of recent studies have used attachment priming that involves the manipulation of attachment to demonstrate more convincingly that attachment styles cause changes in paranoia and explore potential mediators including beliefs about self and others and cognitive fusion. Cognitive fusion describes the extent to which people are able to "decenter" (Teasdale et al., 2002) or distance themselves (Gillanders et al., 2014) from internal experience. The inability to step back from thoughts, feelings, and urges and recognize these as transient states of the mind (rather than accurate reflections of reality) is associated with mental distress across a range of different mental health conditions.

Sood et al. (2021) recruited 303 adults with high nonclinical paranoia online who were asked to engage in an imagery task designed to elicit secure, anxious, or avoidant attachment. As expected, the authors found that paranoia, anxiety, and cognitive fusion decreased from pre- to post-imagery in the secure condition and increased over time in the anxious and avoidant conditions. The authors then conducted parallel mediation to test whether cognitive fusion and negative beliefs about self and others mediate the association between attachment imagery and paranoia. In support of a cross-sectional research and study hypotheses, the authors found that cognitive fusion and negative beliefs about self and others mediated the association between attachment imagery (anxious/avoidant vs. secure) and paranoia. Relative to the secure group, the anxious and avoidant imagery groups were more fused with their negative cognitions, held more negative beliefs about self and others and, therefore, felt more paranoid and anxious. These findings replicated an earlier, smaller less sophisticated study by the same authors comparing just secure and insecure attachment primes (Sood & Newman-Taylor, 2020) and another study during which the primes were repeated over time (Newman-Taylor et al., 2021).

Another recent study by Lawrence et al. (2022) used a novel experience sampling methodology to capitalize on the idea that attachment is a fluctuating concept and to investigate the causal role of shifts in attachment behaviors in paranoia. The authors recruited 60 nonclinical participants who completed 3423 assessments of state stress, proximity seeking (a proxy measure of attachment), and paranoia over a 6-day period in response to random alerts. Participants also completed measures at attachment style at the start of the study. Although changes in proximity seeking were not associated with momentary reports of paranoia, for individuals with an avoidant attachment style, greater shifts in proximity seeking resulted in greater subsequent reports of paranoia. The authors conclude that for those with an avoidant attachment style, an active attachment system may increase paranoid thoughts due to a coming online of attachment-related beliefs, such as one should be fearful of unavailable others and instead rely oneself to down-regulate affect.

Attachment Styles and Hallucinatory Phenomena

The aforementioned review by Carr et al. exploring associations between attachment and psychotic symptoms across the psychosis spectrum included a review of studies exploring associations between insecure attachment and subclinical hallucinatory experiences (Carr et al., 2018). These studies primarily adopted a single-symptom approach to explore the independent role of insecure attachment in both paranoia and subclinical hallucinatory experiences (e.g., Pickering et al., 2008; Wickham et al., 2014). For example, in a sample of 350 university students, Pickering et al. (2008) used statistical methods to control for comorbidity between paranoia and hallucinations and found that insecure attachment predicted paranoia, but not hallucinations. The authors therefore conclude that attachment processes play a role in paranoia, but not hallucinatory experiences. They argue that childhood abuse plays a more important role in the development of hallucinations due to robust associations with childhood abuse when studied in terms of clinical hallucinations and hallucination proneness (Bentall & Sitko, 2019).

Research examining specific mechanisms underlying psychotic symptoms is complicated by the fact that many people experience both paranoia and distressing voices, which is the rationale given for statistically controlling for different symptoms when testing theories of paranoia or hallucinatory experiences. However, the traumatic events themselves that are hypothesized to drive symptoms cannot be so easily disentangled. For example, the experience of childhood abuse, particularly if the perpetrator is a caregiver or if the caregiver fails to protect/appropriately support the victim, is also likely to influence the individual's attachment system given that the functioning of the attachment system is so closely determined by relationships with the early caregivers. Some authors have argued that previous research has failed to find robust associations between attachment and hallucinatory experiences because studies have not assessed the form of attachment difficulties that are most likely to play a role in the development of hallucinations. These authors argue that disorganized attachment may play a more important role in explaining hallucinatory experiences. Although studies have often included measures of the related concept of fearful attachment, this is not the same construct as disorganized attachment, which is characterized by dissociative processes and trauma histories (Pollard et al., 2023).

Studies published since the Carr et al.'s review have examined the role of attachment, trauma, and subclinical voice-hearing phenomenon, which mirror studies of people with psychosis (Pearce et al., 2017; Pilton et al., 2016). These studies also typically include a measure of dissociation (although notably not disorganized attachment as until very recently there has not been an adequate self-report measure of this construct). Dissociation is defined as the disruption in the 'normal integration of consciousness, memory, identity, emotion, perception, body representation, motor control, and behaviour' (American Psychiatric Association, 2013, p. 291). It is hypothesized to develop as a response to traumatic life experiences and is recognized as an adaptive response to such experiences (Liotti & Gumley, 2008). It has also been theoretically linked to the concept of disorganization attachment (Berry et al., 2017). For example, Berry et al. have developed the cognitive attachment model of voices (CAV), which proposes that experiences of trauma in childhood increase vulnerability to voice-hearing experiences by leading to the disruption of the attachment system and the development of subsequent dissociative states in response to stress (see Berry & Bucci, 2016; Berry et al., 2017). Although the model was developed to account for voice-hearing experiences in psychosis, the continuum model of psychosis would suggest that the concepts would extend to subclinical hallucinatory experiences.

In support of the CAV and its application to subclinical psychotic phenomena, Berry et al. (2018) investigated the relative contribution of childhood adversity, dissociation, and adult attachment in explaining hallucination proneness in a sample of 123 participants. The authors found that insecure attachment, childhood trauma, and dissociative symptoms were all associated with hallucination proneness. The authors controlled for confounds such as negative affect and age, but, unlike the earlier studies, they did not, however, control for paranoia. Whether associations are upheld when controlling for paranoia is a question for future research, but one which presents challenges to statistical modeling given the almost inevitable impact of earlier life traumas on attachment processes.

Attachment Styles and Negative Symptoms

As indicated previously, the review by Carr et al. (2018) reported a significant association negative symptom severity and insecure attachment in the nonclinical analysis, which was not found in the clinical group. Associations between insecure attachment and negative schizotypy traits reflect associations between avoidant attachment and social anhedonia or apathy. For example, in a sample of 323 university students, Berry et al. (2006) found that correlation between avoidance and social anhedonia was significantly greater than the correlation between anxiety and social anhedonia. These findings were replicated in later undergraduate sample study by Berry et al. (2007), investigating the related concept of introverted anhedonia assessed using the Oxford-Liverpool Inventory of Feelings and Experiences Scale (Mason & Claridge, 2006). The relationship between avoidant attachment and negative symptomatology is unsurprising given that negative symptoms are interpersonal in nature and are associated with social isolation and constricted displays of affect (Tiliopoulos & Goodall, 2009).

Another similar study by Sheinbaum et al. (2013) involving a large combined sample of student and general population of nonclinical samples in the United States and Spain looked at unique associations between four types of attachment (secure, preoccupied, dismissing, and fearful) and positive and negative schizotypy as measured by the Wisconsin Schizotypy Scales (Eckblad et al., 1982). The authors found that dismissing attachment significantly correlated with negative schizotypy, preoccupied attachment with positive schizotypy, and fearful attachment (which they compared to disorganized attachment) with both schizotypy dimensions. The authors argue that fearful attachment, which is characterized by an oscillation between hyperactivating and deactivating tendencies and thus lacks a coherent strategy of affect regulation (Simpson & Rholes, 2002; Shaver & Mikulincer, 2007), would be expected to relate to both schizotypy dimensions. Sheinbaum et al. (2014) reported the results from the undergraduate sample ($n = 546$) that formed part of the dataset from the 2013 study in a separate paper and showed that fearful attachment mediated the relationship between physical/emotional trauma and both positive and negative schizotypy (Sheinbaum et al., 2014). The authors suggest that individuals with fearful attachment have negative working models of both the self and others and develop opposing approach and avoidance strategies, which ultimately contribute to emotional and cognitive disorganization (Sheinbaum et al., 2014). Interestingly, research with clinical samples with psychosis has also suggested that disorganized attachment and dissociative experiences may mediate the association between childhood trauma and negative symptoms (Degnan et al., 2022).

Others authors have highlighted the important role of mentalization in explaining the association between insecure attachment and negative schizotypy. Mentalization is a social cognitive process, by which the individual uses knowledge of the mental states of the self and others to understand social relationships and interactions (Fonagy et al., 2000). In support of this theory, there is a growing evidence of the role of early trauma and attachment on higher-order cognitive processes such as mentalization (Debbané et al., 2016).

Limitations and Future Research

There is relatively strong evidence that insecure attachment patterns are associated with positive and negative schizotypal symptoms in nonclinical samples, although the role that specific types of attachment play in the development and maintenance of different symptoms requires further research. It is especially important that researchers include more specific measures of disorganized attachment, given the potentially important role of this construct in explaining psychotic experiences across the continuum. In this regard, Pollard et al. (2020) have recently adapted the Psychosis Attachment Measure to include a disorganized attachment scale. Besides this development, it is important to note that the majority of research in this field has been based on nonclinical samples (which are often undergraduate students or comprising a significant proportion of undergraduate students). While the recruitment of such samples facilitates data collection enabling large sample sizes, the generalizability of these findings to those experiencing schizotypal symptoms with greater impairments in functioning or higher levels of distress is called into question.

Relatedly, there has been a debate about whether schizotypy measures are assessing sub-clinical symptom experiences or instead assessing trait characteristics. However, a recent review argued that existing measures of schizotypy are robust at assessing both subclinical psychotic-like experiences and characterological traits (Mason, 2015), suggesting that these measurements are appropriate for assessing the symptoms of psychosis across the continuum.

However, perhaps the most significant limitation in the existing literature pertains to the predominance of cross-sectional research. Even studies that claim to test mediation effects have done so through statistical modeling as opposed to through longitudinal designs or experimental manipulation. There are nonetheless promising developments in this area particularly in relation to paranoia where researchers have manipulated attachment states of mind or assessed momentary fluctuations in attachment behaviors. Future research should develop these paradigms to explore more fully causal relationships and the role of mediators and moderators in the association between attachment and different types of schizotypal symptoms.

Clinical Implications

Associations between insecure attachment and schizotypy symptoms suggest that interventions aimed at helping people understand the role that attachment difficulties may play in relationship difficulties may be helpful. For example, during psychological therapies for schizotypy, therapists may help clients understand attachment theory and formulate the role earlier relationship experiences played in the development of their own attachment patterns and the implications of these later relationships. Interventions aimed at increasing attachment security may also be beneficial in terms of reducing distress and difficulties in functioning associated with schizotypy. There is evidence that psychological therapies have the potential to lead people with insecure attachment patterns to develop more secure attachment patterns (Taylor et al., 2014). Although identifying which therapeutic mechanisms or techniques lead to change requires further empirical investigation, attachment theories would argue that the therapeutic relationship itself (in the form of a reliable, consistent, and sensitive therapist) has the potential to provide a corrective emotional experience (Bowlby, 1988), which is used as a platform to help clients try out alternative ways of relating to others outside of the therapy room. However, perhaps the most important clinical implication that we can take from associations between insecure attachment and schizotypy is the importance of early intervention in the form of parenting programs and other social enrichment programs during the early years. Indeed, there is promising evidence from longitudinal research that such programs can reduce the risk of developing schizotypal symptoms in young adulthood (Raine et al., 2003).

References

American Psychiatric Association. (2013). *Diagnostic and statistical manual of mental disorders* (5th ed.). American Psychiatric Association. https://doi.org/10.1176/appi.books.9780890425596

Ascone, L., Schlier, B., Sundag, J., & Lincoln, T. M. (2020). Pathways from insecure attachment dimensions to paranoia: The mediating role of hyperactivating emotion regulation versus blaming others. *Psychology and Psychotherapy: Theory, Research and Practice, 93*(1), 72–87. https://doi.org/10.1111/papt.12208

Bartholomew, K., & Horowitz, L. M. (1991). Attachment styles among young adults: A test of a four-category model. *Journal of Personality and Social Psychology, 61*(2), 226. https://doi.org/10.1037//0022-3514.61.2.226

Bentall, R. P., & Sitko, K. (2019). The specific role of insecure attachment in paranoid delusions. In *Attachment theory and psychosis* (pp. 23–42). Routledge.

Bentall, R. P., de Sousa, P., Varese, F., Wickham, S., Sitko, K., Haarmans, M., & Read, J. (2014). From adversity to psychosis: Pathways and mechanisms from specific adversities to specific symptoms. *Social Psychiatry and Psychiatric Epidemiology, 49*, 1011–1022. https://doi.org/10.1007/s00127-014-0914-0

Berry, K., & Bucci, S. (2016). What does attachment theory tell us about working with distressing voices? *Psychosis, 8*(1), 60–71. https://doi.org/10.1080/17522439.2015.1070370

Berry, K., Wearden, A., Barrowclough, C., & Liversidge, T. (2006). Attachment styles, interpersonal relationships and psychotic phenomena in a non-clinical student sample. *Personality and Individual Differences, 41*(4), 707–718. https://doi.org/10.1016/j.paid.2006.03.009

Berry, K., Barrowclough, C., & Wearden, A. (2007). A review of the role of adult attachment style in psychosis: Unexplored issues and questions for further research. *Clinical Psychology Review, 27*(4), 458–475. https://doi.org/10.1016/j.cpr.2006.09.006

Berry, K., Varese, F., & Bucci, S. (2017). Cognitive attachment model of voices: Evidence base and future implications. *Frontiers in Psychiatry, 8*, 111. https://doi.org/10.3389/fpsyt.2017.00111

Berry, K., Fleming, P., Wong, S., & Bucci, S. (2018). Associations between trauma, dissociation, adult attachment and proneness to hallucinations. *Behavioural and Cognitive Psychotherapy, 46*(3), 292–301. https://doi.org/10.1017/S1352465817000716

Bowlby, J. (1969). *Attachment. Attachment and loss: Vol. 1. Loss*. Basic Books.

Bowlby, J. (1988). *A secure base: Parent-child attachment and healthy human development*. Basic Books.

Carr, S. C., Hardy, A., & Fornells-Ambrojo, M. (2018). Relationship between attachment style and symptom severity across the psychosis spectrum: A meta-analysis. *Clinical Psychology Review, 59*, 145–158. https://doi.org/10.1016/j.cpr.2017.12.001

Debbané, M., Salaminios, G., Luyten, P., Badoud, D., Armando, M., Solida Tozzi, A., et al. (2016). Attachment, neurobiology, and mentalizing along the psychosis continuum. *Frontiers in Human Neuroscience, 10*, 406. https://doi.org/10.3389/fnhum.2016.00406

Degnan, A., Berry, K., Humphrey, C., & Bucci, S. (2022). The role of attachment and dissociation in the relationship between childhood interpersonal trauma and negative symptoms in psychosis. *Clinical Psychology & Psychotherapy, 29*(5), 1692–1706. https://doi.org/10.1002/cpp.2731

Eckblad, M. L., Chapman, L. J., Chapman, J. P., & Mishlove, M. (1982). *The revised social anhedonia scale: Unpublished test*. University of Wisconsin at Madison.

Fonagy, P., Target, M., & Gergely, G. (2000). Attachment and borderline personality disorder: A theory and some evidence. *Psychiatric Clinics of North America, 23*, 103–122. https://doi.org/10.1016/S0193-953X(05)70146-5

Freeman, D., & Garety, P. (2014). Advances in understanding and treating persecutory delusions: A review. *Social Psychiatry and Psychiatric Epidemiology, 49*, 1179–1189. https://doi.org/10.1007/s00127-014-0928-7

Freeman, D., Garety, P. A., Kuipers, E., Fowler, D., & Bebbington, P. E. (2002). A cognitive model of persecutory delusions. *British Journal of Clinical Psychology, 41*(4), 331–347. https://doi.org/10.1348/014466502760387461

Gillanders, D. T., Bolderston, H., Bond, F. W., Dempster, M., Flaxman, P. E., Campbell, L., et al. (2014). The development and initial validation of the cognitive fusion questionnaire. *Behavior Therapy, 45*(1), 83–101. https://doi.org/10.1016/j.beth.2013.09.001

Green, C. E. L., Freeman, D., Kuipers, E., Bebbington, P., Fowler, D., Dunn, G., & Garety, P. A. (2008). Measuring ideas of persecution and social reference: The Green et al. Paranoid Thought Scales (GPTS). *Psychological Medicine, 38*(1), 101–111. https://doi.org/10.1017/S0033291707001638

Harder, S. (2014). Attachment in schizophrenia--implications for research, prevention, and treatment. *Schizophrenia Bulletin, 40*(6), 1189–1193. https://doi.org/10.1093/schbul/sbu133.

Korver-Nieberg, N., Fett, A. K. J., Meijer, C. J., Koeter, M. W., Shergill, S. S., de Haan, L., & Krabbendam, L. (2013). Theory of mind, insecure attachment and paranoia in adolescents with early psychosis and healthy controls. *The Australian and New Zealand Journal of Psychiatry, 47*(8), 737–745. https://doi.org/10.1177/0004867413484370

Korver-Nieberg, N., Berry, K., Meijer, C., de Haan, L., & Ponizovsky, A. M. (2015). Associations between attachment and psychopathology dimensions in a large sample of patients with psychosis. *Psychiatry Research, 228*(1), 83–88. https://doi.org/10.1016/j.psychres.2015.04.018

Lavin, R., Bucci, S., Varese, F., & Berry, K. (2020). The relationship between insecure attachment and paranoia in psychosis: A systematic literature review. *British Journal of Clinical Psychology, 59*(1), 39–65. https://doi.org/10.1111/bjc.12231

Lawrence, K., Bucci, S., Berry, K., Carter, L. A., & Taylor, P. (2022). Fluctuations in proximity seeking and paranoia. *British Journal of Clinical Psychology, 61*(4), 1019–1037. https://doi.org/10.1111/bjc.12372

Liotti, G. (2004). Trauma, dissociation, and disorganized attachment: Three strands of a single braid. *Psychotherapy: Theory, Research, Practice, Training, 41*(4), 472. https://doi.org/10.1037/0033-3204.41.4.472

Liotti, G., & Gumley, A. (2008). An attachment perspective on schizophrenia: The role of disorganized attachment, dissociation and mentalization. *Psychosis, Trauma and Dissociation: Emerging Perspectives on Severe Psychopathology, 14*, 117–133. https://doi.org/10.1002/9780470699652.ch9

Lyons-Ruth, K., & Jacobvitz, D. (1999). Attachment disorganization: Unresolved loss, relational violence, and lapses in behavioral and attentional strategies. In J. Cassidy & P. R. Shaver (Eds.), *Handbook of attachment: Theory, research, and clinical applications* (pp. 520–554). The Guilford Press.

Main, M., & Solomon, J. (1990). Procedures for identifying infants as disorganized/disoriented during the Ainsworth strange situation. *Attachment in the Preschool Years: Theory, Research, and Intervention, 1*, 121–160.

Martinez, A. P., Agostini, M., Al-Suhibani, A., & Bentall, R. P. (2021). Mistrust and negative self-esteem: Two paths from attachment styles to paranoia. *Psychology and Psychotherapy: Theory, Research and Practice, 94*(3), 391–406. https://doi.org/10.1111/papt.12314

Mason, O. J. (2015). The assessment of schizotypy and its clinical relevance. *Schizophrenia Bulletin, 41*(suppl_2), S374–S385. https://doi.org/10.1093/schbul/sbu194

Mason, O., & Claridge, G. (2006). The Oxford-Liverpool Inventory of Feelings and Experiences (O-LIFE): Further description and extended norms. *Schizophrenia Research, 82*(2–3), 203–211. https://doi.org/10.1016/j.schres.2005.12.845

Melo, S., Corcoran, R., Shryane, N., & Bentall, R. P. (2009). The persecution and deservedness scale. *Psychology and Psychotherapy: Theory, Research and Practice, 82*(3), 247–260. https://doi.org/10.1348/147608308X398337

Mertens, Y. L., Racioppi, A., Sheinbaum, T., Kwapil, T., & Barrantes-Vidal, N. (2021). Dissociation and insecure attachment as mediators of the relation between childhood emotional abuse and nonclinical paranoid traits. *European Journal of Psychotraumatology, 12*(1), 1888539. https://doi.org/10.1080/20008198.2021.1888539

Mikulincer, M., & Shaver, P. R. (2012). An attachment perspective on psychopathology. *World Psychiatry, 11*(1), 11–15. https://doi.org/10.1016/j.wpsyc.2012.01.003

Morrison, A. P., Wells, A., & Nothard, S. (2000). Cognitive factors in predisposition to auditory and visual hallucinations. *British Journal of Clinical Psychology, 39*(1), 67–78. https://doi.org/10.1348/014466500163112

Newman-Taylor, K., Sood, M., Rowe, A. C., & Carnelley, K. B. (2021). The impact of repeated attachment priming on paranoia, mood and help-seeking intentions in an analogue sample. *Brain Sciences, 11*(10), 1257. https://doi.org/10.3390/brainsci11101257

Pearce, J., Simpson, J., Berry, K., Bucci, S., Moskowitz, A., & Varese, F. (2017). Attachment and dissociation as mediators of the link between childhood trauma and psychotic experiences. *Clinical Psychology & Psychotherapy, 24*(6), 1304–1312. https://doi.org/10.1002/cpp.2100

Pickering, L., Simpson, J., & Bentall, R. P. (2008). Insecure attachment predicts proneness to paranoia but not hallucinations. *Personality and Individual Differences, 44*(5), 1212–1224. https://doi.org/10.1016/j.paid.2007.11.016

Pilton, M., Bucci, S., McManus, J., Hayward, M., Emsley, R., & Berry, K. (2016). Does insecure attachment mediate the relationship between trauma and voice-hearing in psychosis? *Psychiatry Research, 246*, 776–782. https://doi.org/10.1016/j.psychres.2016.10.050

Platts, H., Tyson, M., & Mason, O. (2002). Adult attachment style and core beliefs: Are they linked? *Clinical Psychology & Psychotherapy, 9*(5), 332–348. https://doi.org/10.1002/cpp.345

Pollard, C., Bucci, S., MacBeth, A., & Berry, K. (2020). The revised psychosis attachment measure: Measuring disorganized attachment. *British Journal of Clinical Psychology, 59*(3), 335–353. https://doi.org/10.1111/bjc.12249

Pollard, C., Bucci, S., & Berry, K. (2023). A systematic review of measures of adult disorganized attachment. *British Journal of Clinical Psychology*. https://doi.org/10.1111/bjc.12411

Raine, A., Mellingen, K., Liu, J., Venables, P., & Mednick, S. A. (2003). Effects of environmental enrichment at ages 3–5 years on schizotypal personality and antisocial behavior at ages 17 and 23 years. *American Journal of Psychiatry, 160*(9), 1627–1635. https://doi.org/10.1176/appi.ajp.160.9.1627

Read, J., & Gumley, A. (2010). Can attachment theory help explain the relationship between childhood adversity and psychosis? In S. Benamer (Ed.), *Telling stories? Attachment-based approaches to the treatment of psychosis* (pp. 51–94). Karnac Books.

Shaver, P. R., & Mikulincer, M. (2007). Adult attachment strategies and the regulation of emotion. In *Handbook of emotion regulation* (pp. 446–465). The Guilford Press.

Sheinbaum, T., Bedoya, E., Ros-Morente, A., Kwapil, T. R., & Barrantes-Vidal, N. (2013). Association between attachment prototypes and schizotypy dimensions in two independent non-clinical samples of Spanish and American young adults. *Psychiatry Research, 210*(2), 408–413. https://doi.org/10.1016/j.psychres.2013.07.020

Sheinbaum, T., Kwapil, T. R., & Barrantes-Vidal, N. (2014). Fearful attachment mediates the association of childhood trauma with schizotypy and psychotic-like experiences. *Psychiatry Research, 220*(1–2), 691–693. https://doi.org/10.1016/j.psychres.2014.07.030

Simpson, J. A., & Rholes, W. S. (2002). Fearful-avoidance, disorganization, and multiple working models: Some directions for future theory and research. *Attachment & Human Development, 4*(2), 223–229. https://doi.org/10.1080/14616730210154207

Sood, M., & Newman-Taylor, K. (2020). Cognitive fusion mediates the impact of attachment imagery on paranoia and anxiety. *Cognitive Therapy and Research, 44*, 1150–1161. https://doi.org/10.1007/s10608-020-10127-y

Sood, M., Carnelley, K., & Newman-Taylor, K. (2021). How does attachment imagery for paranoia work? Cognitive fusion and beliefs about self and others mediate the impact on paranoia and anxiety. *Psychology and Psychotherapy: Theory, Research and Practice, 94*(4), 973–993. https://doi.org/10.1111/papt.12354

Stefanis, N. C., Hanssen, M., Smirnis, N. K., Avramopoulos, D. A., Evdokimidis, I. K., Stefanis, C. N., et al. (2002). Evidence that three dimensions of psychosis have a distribution in the general population. *Psychological Medicine, 32*(2), 347–358. https://doi.org/10.1017/S0033291701005141

Taylor, G. J., Bagby, R. M., Kushner, S. C., Benoit, D., & Atkinson, L. (2014). Alexithymia and adult attachment representations: Associations with the five-factor model of personality and perceived relationship adjustment. *Comprehensive Psychiatry, 55*(5), 1258–1268. https://doi.org/10.1016/j.comppsych.2014.03.015

Teasdale, J. D., Moore, R. G., Hayhurst, H., Pope, M., Williams, S., & Segal, Z. V. (2002). Metacognitive awareness and prevention of relapse in depression: Empirical evidence. *Journal of Consulting and Clinical Psychology, 70*(2), 275. https://doi.org/10.1037/0022-006X.70.2.275

Tiliopoulos, N., & Goodall, K. (2009). The neglected link between adult attachment and schizotypal personality traits. *Personality and Individual Differences, 47*(4), 299–304. https://doi.org/10.1016/j.paid.2009.03.017

Varese, F., Smeets, F., Drukker, M., Lieverse, R., Lataster, T., Viechtbauer, W., et al. (2012). Childhood adversities increase the risk of psychosis: A meta-analysis of patient-control, prospective-and cross-sectional cohort studies. *Schizophrenia Bulletin, 38*(4), 661–671. https://doi.org/10.1093/schbul/sbs050

Wickham, S., Sitko, K., & Bentall, R. P. (2014). Insecure attachment is associated with paranoia but not hallucinations in psychotic patients: The mediating role of negative self-esteem. *Psychological Medicine, 45*(7), 1495–1507. https://doi.org/10.1017/S0033291714002633

Williams, B., Jalilianhasanpour, R., Matin, N., Fricchione, G. L., Sepulcre, J., Keshavan, M. S., et al. (2018). Individual differences in corticolimbic structural profiles linked to insecure attachment and coping styles in motor functional neurological disorders. *Journal of Psychiatric Research, 102*, 230–237. https://doi.org/10.1016/j.jpsychires.2018.04.006

Chapter 11
Compassion-Focused Therapy and Schizotypy: An Exploration of an Evolution-Informed Biopsychosocial Approach

Paul Gilbert

The Basic Science of CFT

Although psychotherapy research has been very keen on outcome studies, CFT has always taken the view that therapies must be developed from understanding processes, informed by the biopsychosocial sciences (Gilbert, 1989, 1992, 1995, 2019, 2022a). CFT is an evolution-informed, biopsychosocial approach that maps onto the four evolved functions of mind: motives; emotions, competencies, and behaviors (Davey, 2018; Gilbert, 2014, 2022a); their facilitators and inhibitors; and their biological, psychological, and social regulators (Gilbert, 1989, 2005, 2020a; Gilbert & Mascaro, 2017; Keltner et al., 2014; Petrocchi et al., 2022; Seppälä et al., 2017; Stevens & Woodruff, 2018; Vrtička et al., 2017). Exploring these functions enables understanding of how they support compassion but also how each of these functions can be compromised in schizotypy and why CFT may be helpful. These are outlined in Fig. 11.1 and are described below. This chapter then focuses primarily on self-to-self relating, and therapeutic compassion focused interventions.

Evolved functions have adaptive and maladaptive ranges (Buss, 2019; Cheli, 2023; Gilbert, 1998). For example, diarrhea and vomiting are good for removing toxic substances, but if they are poorly regulated, they can kill us through dehydration. Our autoimmune systems defend against viruses, but if they turn against us, we end up with unpleasant diseases. For the "depressions," the ability to regulate positive affect and explorative behavior in different contexts of safeness or dangerousness is highly adaptive, but this variation does not mean that depressions, as complex syndromes, are adaptive (Gilbert, 2006). Indeed, recent adaptations over the last few million years that enable insight, complex metacognition, objective self-awareness,

P. Gilbert (✉)
Centre for Compassion Research and Training, College of Health, Psychology and Social Care, University of Derby, Derby, UK
e-mail: P.Gilbert@derby.ac.uk

S. Cheli, P. H. Lysaker (eds.), *A Dimensional Approach to Schizotypy*,
https://doi.org/10.1007/978-3-031-41788-7_11

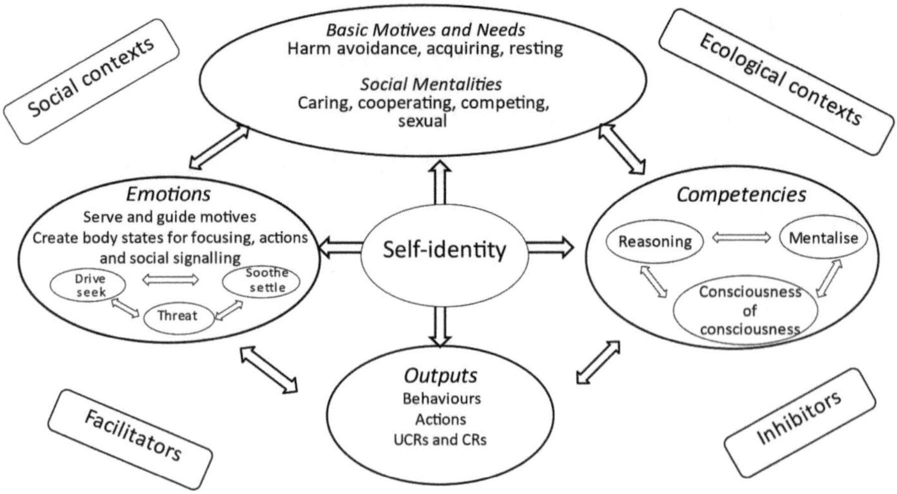

Fig. 11.1 Mapping the functions of the mind. (Adapted from Gilbert, 2020a © Paul Gilbert)

and self-evaluation, and also social cultures that promote high competitiveness, can now drive mental health problems. Understanding the evolved mechanisms of processes does not imply that they function helpfully in all contexts. This raises the question of what evolved functions, in what contexts, and in what forms underpin mental health difficulties.

Exploring the Basic Functions of Mind

There are different ways in which psychology distinguishes between different functions of mind, but a reasonably standard distinction of functions is between motives, emotions, competencies, and specific behavioral output systems. These are depicted in Fig. 11.1 and are discussed below.

Motives Motives evolve because they solve survival and reproductive challenges (Buss, 2019; Workman et al., 2020). The three life challenges, tasks, and major motives for most living things are: (1) identifying and defending against threat and harms—that is, harm avoidance motives; (2) acquiring the resources necessary for survival and reproduction, such as food, shelter, and mating partners; and (3) being able to rest and digest when not under threat or needing to seek resources. All three motivational systems can be compromised in people with schizotypy. First, people with this mental health problem have elevated sensitivity to potential harm and are prone to high anxiety. Horton et al. (2014) found that "Paranoia had a strong association with positive schizotypy, a moderate association with social anxiety, and a minimal association with negative schizotypy. The results are consistent with paranoia being part of a multidimensional model of schizotypy and schizophrenia" (p. 1). Second, these people have reduced capacities for positive emotions, linked to poor social engagement and social anhedonia (Barkus & Badcock, 2019; Brown et al., 2008). Third, people with this condition can struggle to feel safe, content and at peace, and instead often have a constant sense of threat (White et al., 2013).

These three evolved motives, with their unique feature detectors, responses and physiological infrastructures, coregulate each other. Motivational conflicts can be (Gilbert, 2020a, b) central to mental health difficulties, can present as ambivalence (Gilbert, 2000a; Huang & Bargh, 2014), and can produce dissociative states (Dell & O'Neil, 2009). Over 100 years ago, for example, motivational conflict was understood to be seen as important for people with schizotypy (Ellenberger, 1970), especially whether to approach or avoid social situations. For example, people with schizotypy find it difficult to resolve emotional conflict and can become disorientated in emotional conflict paradigms such as the Stroop test (Jia et al., 2023).

Social Motives as Social Mentalities Social species are motivated to interact with conspecifics in specific ways. They may form groups as a form of protection, engage in conflict with each other to establish hierarchies and access to resources, and engage in mating behavior and care for offspring. Social motives are called *social mentalities* because they differ from other basic nonsocial motives in that they require specific information-processing systems to decode social communication (Camilleri et al., 2023; Gilbert, 1989, 2005, 2017, 2020a, b, 2022c).

At a basic level is the need to distinguish between signals of friendliness versus hostility and between sexual interest and disinterest. Social mentalities have to coevolve via interactions. For example, in any species infants could not evolve care-seeking behavior if, at the same time, parents were not evolving competencies to be attentive to such behavior and provide care. Sexual motives are the same in that, for the different sexes, each needs to be able to identify appropriate sexual signals from the other. One implication of this is that social mentalities are evolved to be triggered by social stimuli. For example, the infant's care-seeking motivational system cannot grow and mature until s/he *receives* care signals from another. In essence, the motive is waiting for a signal. Like spoken language, if, for any reason, social mentalities do not have access to key social inputs that the motivational system needs, or if the system cannot recognize or respond to those social inputs/signals, then that motivational system will struggle to mature. Children with autism, for example, can struggle to recognize and respond to signals of caring (affectionate eye gaze, voice tones, and stroking) from others and thus to build affiliative interactions (Baron-Cohen, 2011).

In species that compete with each other, one key cognitive task is to work out if an individual is stronger or weaker than the self. That in turn is linked to both the functions and forms of social behavior and resource-seeking behavior, such that if an individual evaluates itself to be the stronger, then it may assert dominance and reap the rewards (pleasures) of access to resources. In contrast, if an animal evaluates itself to be weaker, and the other is threatening and potentially harmful, this can trigger the psychophysiological defenses for submissive responding such as running away, withdrawing, suppressing resource-seeking behavior, and/or expressing submissive postures (Gilbert, 1992, 2000b). Submissive signals usually trigger a de-escalation of conflict. This reciprocal dynamic pattern of interacting clearly has to coevolve, and without it, conflicts would commonly end in injury or death. To put this another way, animals have the potential to threaten others to acquire dominance and also the potential to take a submissive defense. This is part of that mentality, but as we will consider below, attack and defend interactions can become unhelpfully stimulated within forms of self-criticism (Gilbert & Irons, 2005). In this situation, people can generate hostile, attacking signals to themselves and then respond to them with submissive, anxious, and depressive reactions.

Emotions Emotions are linked to the three fundamental motives and life tasks (Gilbert, 2015, 2022c). Harm avoidance and threat emotions tend to be connected with emotions such as anger, anxiety, disgust, and longer-term brain states of shutdown. Emotions associated with resource acquisition tend to be ones of activation served by psychophysiological processes for exploration, the pleasure from achieving, acquiring, and consuming (Depue & Morrone-Strupinsky, 2005). These emotions vary as to whether they are social rewards or material rewards (Keltner et al., 2018). In contrast, emotions associated with rest and digest (not protecting or striving) tend to be lower arousal states associated with contentment and calmness (Depue & Morrone-Strupinsky, 2005). These are shown in Fig. 11.2. This figure also indicates that the threat system has different possible responses for short-term versus long-term threats. In addition, when a threat has occurred that resulted in a loss, the consequent process is sadness and grief (Harris & Ho, 2023).

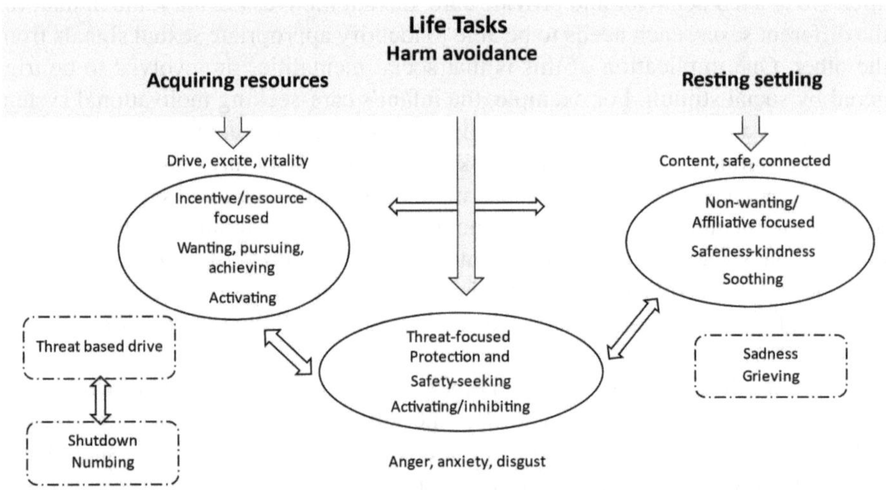

Fig. 11.2 Three functions of emotions. (Adapted from Gilbert, 2010 © Paul Gilbert)

As part of the affect or felt component of an emotion, there are other processes, such as cognition about meaning and implication, metacognition, behavioral impulses, and memories. Hence, cognitive and behavioral manifestations of an emotional reaction to an event can vary greatly (Keltner et al., 2018). Control over a defensive behavior is also important because, while some forms of anxiety involve the response of running away, if escape routes are blocked or running would involve greater risk (attract a predator), a demobilization response might be part of the defense-threat response (Beck et al., 1985). In addition, studies of learned helplessness suggest that when individuals cannot control or escape a threat or harm (e.g., electric shock), they show a demobilization response, which can underpin shutdown states (Seligman, 1975), and anhedonia (Gilbert et al., 2002). Gilbert (1992, 2001a, b; Gilbert & Allan, 1998) suggested that in addition to the perception of control, focus can be on the way some defensive responses are blocked or arrested and constitute forms of entrapment. Measuring both the strength of the flight motivation and also the degree to which the actual behavior was arrested, Gilbert and Allan (1998) revealed entrapments to be highly associated with depression, anhedonia (Gilbert et al., 2002) and some forms of self-harm (Clarke et al., 2016). Indeed, many studies have now indicated that entrapment and defeat are powerfully linked to numerous mental health problems (Taylor et al., 2011). They are also highly linked to people with schizotypy, and a sense of defeat may well explain elements of social anhedonia. Grant et al. (1998) found lower D_2 dopamine receptors among subordinate monkeys, hypothesizing that the stress of subordination produced a downregulation of D_2 dopamine receptors in monkeys. Watt et al. (2014) showed that social defeats in adolescent rats produced hypofunction of the prefrontal cortex D_2 receptor. Defeats are associated with animals *losing interest* in their environments and in resource acquisition (Willner, 1993). This may be adaptive in that a "loss of interest" means that animals are not motivated to pursue resources in a social environment where to do so might elicit injurious downrank attacks. Voruganti and Awad (2006) have shown that alpha-methyl-para-tyrosine (AMPT)-induced dopamine depletion leads to blunted pleasure responsivity, clouded thinking, loss of motivation, and lowered vigilance in humans. This is a profile of changes that overlaps with the phenomenology of negative symptoms found in schizotypal problems.

These three emotion systems coregulate each other and often form blends. For example, excitement can involve both drive and threat; play can involve both drive and safeness. It is the motivations that prime the emotions. For example, in the case of trauma, individuals have elevated motives to detect threat quickly and respond quickly. Hence, this has an impact on priming threat detection and processing. Since part of threat processing is to reach conclusions quickly, "better safe than sorry," people can often jump to conclusions about threats.

One of the major problems related to schizotypy, and its spectrum of disorders, is alexithymia. There are different elements to alexithymia. Yang et al. (2020) found a strong relationship between alexithymia, reduced empathy, and social and physical anhedonia. Difficulty describing and verbalizing emotions seems particularly associated with schizotypal difficulties (Larøi et al., 2008).

Competencies Humans have evolved (at least) three types of complex cognitive competencies: The first includes competencies for reasoning, meta-cognition, insight into complexity (Baron-Cohen, 2020; Byrne, 2016), and thinking in time (Suddendorf, 2018). The second are competencies for insight into the minds of self and others via empathy and mentalization (Luyten et al., 2020). The third are competencies for consciousness of consciousness, which gives rise to forms of mindfulness and knowing awareness, including self-awareness (Brown et al., 2015; Sears et al., 2011). There are many models of emotion that distinguish between the rapidly activated behavioral programs for an emotion and these types of newly evolved cognitive processing competencies that are important for giving meaning and feeling (see Epstein, 2003; Ledoux, 2020, 2022). People with schizotypy can be compromised in all three types of cognitive competency and functioning. Difficulties in reading the intentions of others can link to tendencies for paranoia (Langdon et al., 1997). Török and Kéri (2022) showed that mentalization problems were independent of working memory and mindfulness skills. Nonetheless, mindfulness is another competency that is compromised in people with schizotypy and linked to alexithymia (Bronchain & Chabrol, 2020). Dickey et al. (2011) found that people with schizotypal difficulties "face two hurdles in terms of daily social interactions. They have problems both in correctly interpreting others' facial expressions and in generating socially attractive and unambiguous facial expressions" (p. 242). These issues can also be seen as part of the problems connected with alexithymia, which impacts people's mentalization competencies (Yang et al., 2020). In general, then, people with schizotypy have problems with the recently evolved cognitive competencies that seem to be poorly integrated with earlier evolved behavioral emotion programs for emotion and motivation (Cheli, 2023).

Self-Evaluation and Self-Attacking

As noted in the introduction, this chapter focuses on self-to-self relating, self-attacking, and self-reassurance/compassion. The above three competencies enable self-evaluation and self-judgement in relationship to internalized ideals and to others (Gilbert, 1989, 1992, 2022a, b). This enables individuals to work out how they should relate to others in order to elicit advantageous interactions and avoid harmful ones. However, as noted above, humans have different social mentalities that link to the creation of interactional processes and social roles. Social mentality theory suggests that we can relate to ourselves using the same biopsychosocial systems as we relate to others. For example, when we are self-critical, that stimulates brain systems that evolved to respond to being criticized by others, and when we are self-reassuring and compassionate, that stimulates brain systems that evolved to respond to receiving compassion from others. Hence, the important aspects of self-to-self relating is that they play off and through evolved brain systems that were designed for social relating (Gilbert, 1989, 2005, Gilbert, 2020a, b, 2022a, b).

One of the greatest social relating challenges for all species is how they interact with their conspecifics, particularly when it comes to mating and conflict over resource acquisition (Buss, 2019; Gilbert, 1992, 2000b). Individuals have to work out their ability to secure and challenge for resources, including the probability of stimulating conflict that may be harmful to them. In other words, in any competitive encounter, for many species, internal evaluative systems assess the relative probabilities of success and danger in challenging or resource-seeking where others may want to stop you from securing those resources. Basically, this means that in various social encounters we try to work out whether the people we engage with will be supportive, neutral, or potentially critical and rejecting. When we perceive others to be potentially harmful, social defenses can activated. These can be some form of counter-defense or attack or a submissive and/or social withdrawal defense (Gilbert, 2000b). The degree of social anxiety and threat sensitivity will be linked to processes such as social trust and sense of social safeness (Armstrong et al., 2020) and confidence in oneself.

Social mentality theory notes that just as we can relate to others in different roles and styles so we can relate to ourselves. This means that we can be friendly to ourselves and supportive to ourselves or become disappointed, critical, and hostile. The style of our relationships with ourselves has implications for what brain systems we are stimulating within ourselves. When we generate a signal of hostile criticism within ourselves, this will stimulate defenses too. Then we can literally end up feeling defeated and submissive to our own self-attacks. Indeed, some of the forms of self-criticism are extremely hostile, for example, people may think and say to themselves *you're fat and ugly*; *you are inadequate, a stupid/bad person* [shame labelling], and *nobody will like you or want to be with you*; *people will hate you if they know about you* [threat prediction]. Because these inner dialogues can come with intense hostile emotion, they maintain threat processing. Such self-derogations are common in people who hear hostile voices (Birchwood et al., 2000; Legg & Gilbert, 2006). In fact, there is now good evidence that certain forms of self-criticism stimulate brain systems involved with threat processing (Kim et al., 2020; Longe et al., 2010).

Forms of self-criticism that relate to an awareness that one has made errors or could improve are helpful especially if the motivation is one of helpfulness and caring. However, harmful self-criticism is a multi-textured, complex process of hostility to the self (Gilbert, 1992, 2022b; Gilbert et al., 2004). Hence, the core dimension of self-criticism in relationship to mental health has to do with to its *punitive and hostile forms*; indeed, early discussions of self-criticism and mental health have, until recently, always highlighted the inherent hostility to the self (Carver & Ganellen, 1983). Whelton and Greenberg (2005) found clear evidence that the content of criticism was far less pathogenic than its emotional tone and motivational intent of it. Indeed, when conducting functional analysis of problematic self-criticism, these commonly have a hostile intent-motive, that is, to create distress in the self, to express anger, and to punish or shame the self for failure (see Gilbert, 2022b for worked examples). In fact, one of the measures on Gilbert et al.'s (2004) self-criticism scales is self-persecution, with items of "wanting to take revenge on oneself, to destroy part of oneself, to harm part of oneself, to punish self, to get at things one hates" (p. 38). Gilbert et al. (2010) found that in a mixed clinical population of day and in-patients, self-persecution was highly linked to self-harm, and self-hating was highly associated with depression. These differ from criticizing oneself to stop oneself from making mistakes or to keep oneself in check. This is one of the reasons that scales measuring self-criticism need to distinguish between forms and functions (Gilbert et al., 2004; Gilbert, 2022b). Interestingly, in nonclinical populations, measures of "hating the self" are low and therefore rarely emerge as a separate factor (Halamová et al., 2018), but in clinical populations, hating the self is highly predictive of problems (Castilho et al., 2015; Werner et al., 2019).

In the area of psychosis spectrum disorders and schizotypy, self-condemning, contemptuous, shaming, hostile, and persecutory self-critical messages are less identified as coming from the self and more from external agencies in the form of voices. These are linked to both positive and negative symptoms (Hickey et al., 2022). Birchwood et al. (2000) showed that people who feel inferior and dominated by their voices can also feel like this in relationship to other people in general. Gilbert et al. (2001) found that individuals who felt threatened by their hostile voices also felt dominated by them and subordinate to them. In comparing voice-hearers with those with depression and self-criticism, both felt trapped and defeated by the, emotional tone and content of their 'voices' (see Heriot-Maitland & Murphy, Chap. 14, this volume).

Different theories have different explanations for why self-criticism can become so vicious. One idea is that the attack impulse is actually generated because of rage toward another, but it is inhibited out of fear. Freud's (1917) original exploration of self-criticism in melancholia borrowed Nietzsche's dictum that "no one blames themselves without a secret wish for vengeance" (Ellenberger, 1970). He saw the self-derogations of melancholic patients as diverted anger: They were actually angry with people they depended on. They were frightened to express their anger for fear of retaliation from them. The submissive-appeasing, "anger suppression," and "fight inhibition" styles can be common in religious groups, especially when individuals perceive their gods as powerful and potentially punitive. The Aztecs, for example, sacrificed many individuals to their sun god in order to try to secure the harvests and avoid droughts. When the sacrifices did not work, they did not show anger toward the gods for "cheating on the deal," but made assumptions that they had done something wrong (self-blame) and increased their sacrifices. Bowlby (1980) highlighted similar issues that he called *defensive exclusion*. This is where children have unconsciously learnt to screen out information or avoid the conclusion that indicates their parent is "bad" when the parent shames or attacks them in some way.

Ferster (1973) offered a classical conditioning explanation for these problems of the inhibition of anger and the adoption of self-blame as a defense blaming others and expressing anger. When children are blamed and criticized in the context of hostile emotion from the parent (e.g., being shouted at) and/or if the parent is punitive toward the child's assertiveness, then anxiety becomes associated and conditioned to inner cues of anger. In other words, "anger-fight" impulses are under inhibitory control from threat contingencies, as they are when a person is under attack for more powerful dominant attackers. Ferster's classical conditioning view is adopted within CFT and can be explained to clients in detail (Gilbert, 1992). In addition, in contrast to expressing defiance or anger, anger inhibition, self-blame, and apology provide the potential to settle, or at least tone down, the hostility in the parent or dominant others. For example, imagine a child has knocked over a drink and the parent flies into a temper, calling the child stupid and clumsy. The child can't fight back and is more likely to cry and apologize ("I am so sorry, please don't hurt me"), trying to placate the aggression in the parent. In addition, as many therapies point out, the child internalizes the judgement of the parent. Crucially, it sensitizes the child's social mentality for how they view themselves as existing in the minds of others (e.g., as flawed and vulnerable to attack) and primes their submissive defensive strategy (e.g., taking the blame and anger-fight suppression). This is important because when working with self-criticism, the therapist must establish the origins of the critical process as best s/he can. CFT makes a distinction between a critical process that has become fused with the self and a critical process that is an echo of another's criticism (e.g., a bully). There is now good evidence that harsh and hostile forms of self-criticism are linked to forms of trauma and neglect (Carvalho et al., 2019; Cox et al., 2004; Lee, 2022). However, the link between trauma, self-criticism, and posttraumatic stress disorder (PTSD) is complex. Kline et al. (2021) found that in sexual assault survivors, self-blame and criticism predicted severity of PTSD at Time 1 of the study but not subsequently. At later time points, the direction was reversed such that the severity of PTSD predicted self-blame. This makes sense from a social mentality point of view, in that the severity of PTSD symptoms indicates the degree of internalized fear/threat. The more one lives with a sense of threat from hostile others, the more automatic the submissive defensive strategies are.

There is also experimental evidence for this process of self-criticizing and self-blaming in the context of frightening power. Gilbert and Irons (2005) reviewed a number of studies exploring how individuals engage in submissive and self-blaming behavior in contexts where dominant authorities could be harmful to them if they didn't do so. Trower et al. (1998) conducted an experimental study where socially anxious students were invited to have a conversation with a lecturer. The research was suggested to be an observation of conversation, but the lecturer (part of the study) regularly broke conversational rules by butting in when a student was speaking or by changing the subject. We found that nonsocially anxious students blamed the lecturer for these interruptions as simply being rude and inappropriate. In contrast, socially anxious students blamed themselves for being boring or for having some other defect.

In a different paradigm, psychodynamic therapist Abbass (2015) has also shown that individuals with somatic problems often carry fears of anger and unprocessed anger. These can be held in the body in striatal and smooth muscle, giving rise to somatic problems. He highlights a different mechanism of *guilt* whereby the child experiences hostile feelings toward the parent but then feels guilt and is fearful of harming the parent. Again, they see themselves as bad rather than the parent as bad.

Psychotherapy is partly aimed at helping clients process these feared and avoided feelings. Linked to this can be issues where clients begin to acknowledge unprocessed anger toward somebody they wanted to be cared or loved by. However starting to acknowledge and feel anger, and "fight impulses" stimulates the fear of becoming "a bad, ungrateful, unlovable, and shamed self." It can also create feelings of disloyalty and betrayal and thereby the risk of losing the sense of connectedness to others (Gilbert & Irons, 2005). Another fear can arise of being highly vulnerable to a powerful counter-attack. Clients may not be able to consciously articulate these experiences and fears in this way, but instead have *body* experiences of fear, indicating the importance of classical conditioning. The therapist helps the client begin to develop body and mind awareness for what can be an undifferentiated fear, or even terror, as the client begins to engage and access hostility and rage impulses. Similar problems can arise in people who escape cults where they have been under the control of powerful, charismatic, dominant individuals. Working with these processes can mark a stage of tension in the therapy and the risk of therapeutic rupture because clients often want to avoid this journey into experiencing the unloved or unlovable self. One of my clients could not distinguish feelings of anger from feelings of violence. When trying to work on anger, the only thing that would come up for her was violence, which was frightening. As her awareness of her anger to past trauma increased, it also linked to feeling more "undesirable" and increased her desire to self-harm. Helping people deal with repressed anger is important because without being able to process anger, people can't move to mature, helpful assertiveness, and without helpful assertiveness, individuals can feel defenseless and fearful.

Another area where self-criticism is problematic, and linked to competitiveness, is perfectionism. These are individuals who are fearful of making mistakes and demand high standards of themselves, but also think other people demand high standards of them. They create inner models of their ideal self, and when the actual self doesn't match up to it, this generates a threat response of frustration-linked (narcissistic) anger (see Gilbert, 2022b for examples). Dunkley et al. (2003) suggest that self-critical perfectionists experience chronic dysphoria "because they experience minor hassles in catastrophic terms and perceive others as condemning, unwilling, or unavailable to help them in times of stress" (p. 235). Although not always consciously available, they can have underlying fears of rejection and social disconnection.

People also differ in their attributions for sources of their setbacks. Attribution theorists have made distinctions between: stable and unstable, global and specific, and internal and external. When a trauma or some undesired event happens, people attribute the cause of it to something. Those who attribute causes of misfortune to stable, internal, and global reasons (e.g., being inadequate) have more difficulties coping. Hence, there are distinctions between behavioral self-blame and characterological self-blame. Breitenbecher (2006) looked at individuals who had suffered sexual assaults in relationship to perpetrator blame, characterological self-blame, situational factors and/or chance blame, behavioral self-blame, and societal blame. They found that "characterological self-blame, but not behavioral self-blame, was associated with negative outcomes, including increased psychological distress and increased frequency of past victimization." Hence, the type of attribution plays a role in the impact of self-criticism. However, such attributions may be generated through fast processing systems and conditioning of the subordinate defense system.

Another dimension of attacking self-criticism is that of self disliking. Some individuals simply do not like themselves, and others experience self-hating. Self-disliking is different to criticizing oneself for particular failures or setbacks. Gilbert et al. (2004) found some evidence that some individuals were self-critical because they were trying to self-improve; they did not dislike themselves and felt that they were capable of being better and being good. In contrast, some individuals feel that they can't trust themselves to make good decisions or to be in emotional control. Some individuals feel they have come to dislike themselves after trauma, but not before, or they dislike what the trauma has done to them. One client acknowledged that it was after her sexual assault, and how it was handled, that she had come to distrust people and carried a lot of anger—"I used to be a happy-go-lucky sort of soul, but now I hate what I've become *as a result* of my trauma; I really don't like being me" (not an exact quote). All of these textures require awareness within the therapeutic process.

In regard to studies of the psychophysiological effects of self-criticism, few studies have used clinical populations. In student and nonclinical populations, self-hating and self-persecution tend to be low and are rarely part of the assessment. Nonetheless, both Longe et al. (2010) and Kim et al. (2020), who used nonclinical populations, showed that self-criticism to setback events stimulates the amygdala and other areas of the brain linked to threat processing, whereas self-reassurance to the same imagined scenarios creates different patterns of brain activation linked to empathy and compassion.

Overview The above indicates that difficulties for people with schizotype problems are found in *all main domains* of functioning linked to motives, emotions, cognitive competencies, and (social) behavior. Therefore, psychotherapy for complex conditions like schizotypy has to be biopsychosocial and multidimensional. One of the crucial overarching domains of CFT (and social mentality approaches) is that individuals with various mental health problems can experience the outside world as hostile and rejecting and also their internal world as hostile and rejecting. This scenario is highly disorganizing of psychophysiological systems because, as discussed below, the human brain evolved to require social helpful relationships. These stimulate physiological systems that underpin safeness and the maturation of key frontal cortical mechanisms that support emotion regulation, confidence, and prosocial behavior (Cassidy & Shaver, 2016; Seppälä et al., 2017). Hence, the concern is how people process their interactions with external others and also their relationships with themselves given that we are a species different to others that can self-monitor, self-evaluate, self-reflect, self-judge, and self-attack or self-reassure (Gilbert, 1992; Gilbert et al., 2004, 2022a) Hence, what is called for is to stimulate care motivational systems because motives are major organizing processes. They arrange a range of psychophysiology processes with multiple psychological functions such as attention, thinking, empathy, self-judgement, and so forth. To indicate how compassion can have multiple effects, the chapter now turns to the evolution of compassion and the psychophysiological processes involved with care and compassion.

The Evolution and Therapeutic Use of Compassion

The evolution of compassion has a number of different pathways. One is via rescuing behavior (Kessler, 2020; Spikins, 2015); a second is via attachment and caring for the young (Cassidy & Shaver, 2016); and a third is via developing a reputation for altruism and helpfulness to others (Barkow, 1989) and building reciprocating friendships (Camilleri et al., 2023; Dunbar, 2022). As compassion is rooted in and emerges from the evolution of care motivation, then like all motives, it is underpinned by the stimulus response *if* A *then* do B algorithm, where "A" is dependent on evolved feature detectors that trigger "B" action responses. Whether it is protecting from threats, seeking food, or enabling sexual encounters, understanding the algorithms of a motive is essential to exploring its biopsychosocial manifestations. Harm avoidance motives need feature detectors for threat, feeding needs feature detectors to identify edible foods and how to find them, and sexual motives need feature detectors for sexual opportunities that stimulate bodily processes for courting and mating behavior. The evolution of feature detectors means that the brain is able to monitor for the presence or absence of stimuli that convey information about particular motive needs and opportunities.

Over hundreds of millions of years, caring algorithms have been evolving around the basic processes of [A] evolved feature detectors (enabling attention sensitivity) for stimuli and signals of suffering/need that then [B] trigger appropriate actions to alleviate suffering. Hence, we can define compassion as derived from its basic algorithm, which is [A] *sensitivity to suffering in self and others with* [B] *a commitment to try to alleviate and prevent it* (Gilbert, 2014, 2020a). With small variations, most secular and Buddhist approaches to compassion define it something like this (Mascaro et al., 2020). It is important to see the processes underpinning engagement and action separately, with different effects and competencies (Di Bello et al., 2021; Gilbert & Choden, 2013).

In the last 20 years, substantial research has been conducted on the psychophysiological mechanisms underpinning compassion (for reviews see Gilbert & Simos, 2022; Seppälä et al., 2017; Stevens & Woodruff, 2018). Compassion is linked to the organization of the autonomic nervous system (Keltner et al., 2014), especially the vagus nerve (Porges, 2017, 2021), certain neurocircuits (Kim et al., 2020; Singer & Engert, 2019; Vrtička et al., 2017), and hormones like oxytocin (Kucerova et al., 2023). The essence of CFT is to seek to trigger these processes in the context of working with the source of mental health difficulty. More specifically, CFT identifies core competencies for the ability to engage with and move toward suffering rather than away from it. This includes basic motivation, with forms of mindfulness, distress tolerance, empathic understanding about the causes of distress, and the ability to be relatively accepting rather than self-critical or condemning. The second function of compassion is action, with specific interventions that help people develop compassionate actions linked to forms of attention, the use of imagery and visualisation on what might be helpful, metacognition, acting in the mindset of their compassionate self, chairwork, planned behavior, body regulation via breathing patterns, and other practices (see Gilbert & Simos, 2022 for major overviews). These guide clients through a series of practices designed to stimulate key psychophysiological systems such as the vagus nerve and neural circuits that regulate threat and enable change and growth and a move towards supportive forms of social relating. As a biopsychosocial approach, CFT seeks to produce changes in biological, psychological, and social domains of functioning. By bringing compassion into people's internal world and to the ways they relate to others, CFT seeks to reduce over-sensitivity to threat and create the psychophysiological textures for feeling socially safe(r), which in turn facilitates improved integrated executive functions.

To date, there have been no specific studies on CFT for schizotype, but there have been for people with problems such as psychosis (Braehler et al., 2013; Brown et al., 2020; Laithwaite et al., 2009; Mayhew & Gilbert, 2008; Waite et al., 2015; and see Herriot-Maitland et al., 2019; Heriot-Maitland & Longden, 2022; Heriot-Maitland & Murphy, Chap. 14, this volume). Helping people shift from hostile self-criticism into compassionate self-support is crucial to the therapeutic journey, although CFT involves many other processes.

Conclusion

This chapter looked at an evolution-informed, biopsychosocial approach to schizotypy and compassion. It highlights that both the internal world (self-criticism) and the external world (social trust) can be experienced as threat-focused. When this happens, the individual is cut off from important affect-regulating systems that evolved with attachment and caring behavior. Because our brains have evolved to be highly social, these systems are vital for the maturation of processes such as the frontal cortex that facilitate integrative executive functions (Schore, 2019). As a result of trauma or for other reasons, if these systems do not mature to function optimally, individuals can be vulnerable to a range of mental health difficulties. They can struggle with the way motives, emotions, and competencies are integrated and with the ability to use safeness processing systems for social navigation. This chapter suggests, therefore, that we cannot decontextualize certain techniques such as self-compassion without understanding it is linked to the ability to receive compassion and also at times to be compassionate to others. Sometimes, self-compassion cannot proceed until the client has experienced some form of compassion from the therapist and can learn to trust compassion experiences, particularly if s/he has not experienced them before.

To date, tailored compassion-focused therapy for conditions like schizotypy is still in the developmental stages (see Heriot-Maitland & Murphy, Chap. 14, this volume). The greater clarity there is into the processes and four functions of mind underpinning conditions like stereotypy, the more fine-tuned and tailored interventions can become.

References

Abbass, A. (2015). *Reaching through resistance: Advanced psychotherapy techniques*. Seven Leaves Press.

Barkow, J. H. (1989). *Darwin, sex, and status*. University of Toronto Press.

Barkus, E., & Badcock, J. C. (2019). A transdiagnostic perspective on social anhedonia. *Frontiers in Psychiatry, 10*, 216.

Baron-Cohen, S. (2011). *Zero degrees of empathy: A new theory of human cruelty*. Penguin.

Baron-Cohen, S. (2020). *The pattern seekers: A new theory of human invention*. Allen Lane.

Beck, A. T., Emery, G., & Greenberg, R. L. (1985). *Anxiety disorders and phobias: A cognitive approach*. Basic Books.

Birchwood, M., Meaden, A., Trower, P., Gilbert, P., & Plaistow, J. (2000). The power and omnipotence of voices: Subordination and entrapment by voices and significant others. *Psychological Medicine, 30*, 337–344.

Bowlby, J. (1980). *Attachment and loss, Vol. 3: Loss: Sadness and depression*. Hogarth Press.

Braehler, C., Gumley, A., Harper, J., Wallace, S., Norrie, J., & Gilbert, P. (2013). Exploring change processes in compassion focused therapy in psychosis: Results of a feasibility randomized controlled trial. *British Journal of Clinical Psychology, 52*, 199–214.

Breitenbecher, K. H. (2006). The relationships among self-blame, psychological distress, and sexual victimization. *Journal of Interpersonal Violence, 21*(5), 597–611.

Bronchain, J., & Chabrol, H. (2020). Exploring the relationship between schizotypal traits and dispositional mindfulness from a network perspective. *Journal of Nervous and Mental Disease, 208*(8), 608–612.

Brown, L. H., Silvia, P. J., Myin-Germeys, I., Lewandowski, K. E., & Kwapil, T. R. (2008). The relationship of social anxiety and social anhedonia to psychometrically identified schizotypy. *Journal of Social and Clinical Psychology, 27*(2), 127–149.

Brown, K. W., Creswell, J. D., & Ryan, R. M. (Eds.). (2015). *Handbook of mindfulness: Theory, research, and practice*. Guilford Press.

Brown, P., Waite, F., Rovira, A., Nickless, A., & Freeman, D. (2020). Virtual reality clinical-experimental tests of compassion treatment techniques to reduce paranoia. *Scientific Reports, 10*, 8547.

Buss, D. M. (2019). *Evolutionary psychology: The new science of the mind* (6th ed.). Routledge.

Byrne, R. W. (2016). *Evolving insight: How it is we can think about why things happen*. Oxford University Press.

Camilleri, T., Rockey, S., & Dunbar, R. (2023). *The social brain: The psychology of successful groups*. Cornerstone Press.

Carvalho, C. B., Sousa, M., da Motta, C., & Cabral, J. M. (2019). The role of shame, self-criticism and early emotional memories in adolescents' paranoid ideation. *Journal of Child and Family Studies, 28*, 1337–1345.

Carver, C. S., & Ganellen, R. J. (1983). Depression and components of self-punitiveness: High standards, self-criticism, and overgeneralization. *Journal of Abnormal Psychology, 92*(3), 330–337. https://doi.org/10.1037/0021-843X.92.3.330

Cassidy, J., & Shaver, P. R. (2016). *Handbook of attachment: Theory, research and clinical applications* (3rd ed.). Guilford Press.

Castilho, P., Pinto-Gouveia, J., & Duarte, J. (2015). Exploring self-criticism: Confirmatory factor analysis of the FSCRS in clinical and nonclinical samples. *Clinical Psychology & Psychotherapy, 22*(2), 153–164.

Cheli, S. (2023). An evolutionary look at oddity and schizotypy: How the rise of social brain informs clinical practice. *New Ideas in Psychology, 68*, 100993.

Clarke, M., McEwan, K., Ness, J., Waters, K., Basran, J., & Gilbert, P. (2016). A descriptive study of feelings of arrested escape (entrapment) and arrested anger in people presenting to an emergency department following an episode of self-harm. *Frontiers in Psychiatry, 7*, 155. https://doi.org/10.3389/fpsyt.2016.00155

Cox, B. J., MacPherson, P. S., Enns, M. W., & McWilliams, L. A. (2004). Neuroticism and self-criticism associated with posttraumatic stress disorder in a nationally representative sample. *Behaviour Research and Therapy, 42*(1), 105–114.

Davey, G. C. (2018). Motivation. In D. G. Davey (Ed.), *Psychology* (pp. 206–261). JBPS Textbooks/Wiley.

Dell, P. F., & O'Neil, J. A. (2009). *Dissociation and the dissociative disorders: DSM-V and beyond*. Routledge.

Depue, R. A., & Morrone-Strupinsky, J. V. (2005). A neurobehavioral model of affiliative bonding. *Behavioral and Brain Sciences, 28*, 313–395.

Di Bello, M., Ottaviani, C., & Petrocchi, N. (2021). Compassion is not a benzo: Distinctive associations of heart rate variability with its empathic and action components. *Frontiers in Neuroscience, 15*, 223.

Dickey, C. C., Panych, L. P., Voglmaier, M. M., Niznikiewicz, M. A., Terry, D. P., Murphy, C., et al. (2011). Facial emotion recognition and facial affect display in schizotypal personality disorder. *Schizophrenia Research, 131*(1–3), 242–249.

Dunbar, R. I. (2022). *Friend: Understanding the power of our most important relationships*. Abacus.

Dunkley, D. M., Zuroff, D. C., & Blankstein, K. R. (2003). Self-critical perfectionism and daily affect: Dispositional and situational influences on stress and coping. *Journal of Personality and Social Psychology, 84*, 234–252.

Ellenberger, H. F. (1970). *The discovery of the unconscious: The history and evolution of dynamic psychiatry* (Vol. 1, pp. 280–281). Basic Books.

Epstein, S. (2003). Cognitive-experiential self-theory of personality. In T. Million & M. J. Lerner (Eds.), *Comprehensive handbook of psychology* (Vol. 5, pp. 159–184). Wiley.

Ferster, C. B. (1973). A functional analysis of depression. *American Psychologist, 28*(10), 857–870.

Freud, S. (1917). Mourning and melancholia. In *Complete psychological works* (Vol. 14, Standard ed., J. Strachey, Trans. and Ed.). Hogarth Press.

Gilbert, P. (1989). *Human nature and suffering*. Lawrence Erlbaum Associates.

Gilbert, P. (1992). *Depression: The evolution of powerlessness*. Lawrence Erlbaum Associates.

Gilbert, P. (1995). Biopsychosocial approaches and evolutionary theory as aids to integration in clinical psychology and psychotherapy. *Clinical Psychology & Psychotherapy, 2*, 135–156.

Gilbert, P. (1998). Evolutionary psychopathology: Why isn't the mind better designed than it is? *British Journal of Medical Psychology, 71*, 353–373.

Gilbert, P. (2000a). Social mentalities: Internal 'social' conflicts and the role of inner warmth and compassion in cognitive therapy. In P. Gilbert & K. G. Bailey (Eds.), *Genes on the couch: Explorations in evolutionary psychotherapy* (pp. 118–150). Psychology Press.

Gilbert, P. (2000b). Varieties of submissive behaviour: Their evolution and role in depression. In L. Sloman & P. Gilbert (Eds.), *Subordination and defeat. An evolutionary approach to mood disorders* (pp. 3–46). Lawrence Erlbaum Associates.

Gilbert, P. (2001a). Evolutionary approaches to psychopathology: The role of natural defences. *Australian and New Zealand Journal of Psychiatry, 35*, 17–27.

Gilbert, P. (2001b). Depression and stress: A biopsychosocial exploration of evolved functions and mechanisms. *Stress: The International Journal of the Biology of Stress, 4*, 121–135.

Gilbert, P. (2005). Compassion and cruelty: A biopsychosocial approach. In P. Gilbert (Ed.), *Compassion: Conceptualisations, research and use in psychotherapy* (pp. 3–74). Routledge.

Gilbert, P. (2006). Evolution and depression: Issues and implications [Invited review]. *Psychological Medicine, 36*, 287–297.
Gilbert, P. (2010). *Compassion focused therapy* (The CBT distinctive features series). Routledge.
Gilbert, P. (2014). The origins and nature of compassion focused therapy. *British Journal of Clinical Psychology, 53*, 6–41. https://doi.org/10.1111/bjc.12043
Gilbert, P. (2015). An evolutionary approach to emotion in mental health with a focus on affiliative emotions. *Emotion Review*. [Special issue: Normal and abnormal emotion. K. Scherer (Ed.)), *7*, 230–237. https://doi.org/10.1177/1754073915576552
Gilbert, P. (2017). Compassion as a social mentality: An evolutionary approach. In P. Gilbert (Ed.), *Compassion: Concepts, research and applications* (pp. 31–68). Routledge.
Gilbert, P. (2019). *Living like crazy* (2nd ed.). Annwyn House.
Gilbert, P. (2020a). Compassion: From its evolution to a psychotherapy. *Frontiers in Psychology, 11*, 3123.
Gilbert, P. (2020b). Evolutionary functional analysis: The study of social mentalities, social rank and caring-compassion. In J. N. Kirby & P. Gilbert (Eds.), *Making an impact on mental health* (pp. 4–42). Routledge.
Gilbert, P. (2022a). Chapter 2: Compassion focused therapy as an evolution informed, biopsychosocial science of the mind: History and challenge. In P. Gilbert & G. Simos (Eds.), *Compassion focused therapy: Clinical practice and applications* (pp. 24–89). Routledge.
Gilbert, P. (2022b). Chapter 5: Internal shame and self-disconnection: From hostile self-criticism to compassionate self-correction and guidance. In P. Gilbert & G. Simos (Eds.), *Compassion focused therapy: Clinical practice and applications* (pp. 164–206). Routledge.
Gilbert, P., & Allan, S. (1998). The role of defeat and entrapment (arrested flight) in depression: An exploration of an evolutionary view. *Psychological Medicine, 28*, 584–597.
Gilbert, P., & Choden. (2013). *Mindful compassion*. Constable Robinson.
Gilbert, P., & Irons, C. (2005). Focused therapies and compassionate mind training for shame and self-attacking. In P. Gilbert (Ed.), *Compassion: Conceptualisations, research and use in psychotherapy* (pp. 263–325). Routledge.
Gilbert, P., & Mascaro, J. (2017). Compassion: Fears, blocks, and resistances: An evolutionary investigation. In E. M. Seppälä, E. Simon-Thomas, S. L. Brown, M. C. Worline, L. Cameron, & J. R. Doty (Eds.), *The Oxford handbook of compassion science* (pp. 399–420). Oxford University Press.
Gilbert, P., & Simos, G. (Eds.). (2022). *Compassion focused therapy: Clinical practice and applications*. Routledge.
Gilbert, P., Birchwood, M., Gilbert, J., Trower, P., Hay, J., Murray, B., Meaden, A., Olsen, K., & Miles, J. N. V. (2001). An exploration of evolved mental mechanisms for dominant and subordinate behaviour in relation to auditory hallucinations in schizophrenia and critical thoughts in depression. *Psychological Medicine, 31*, 1117–1127.
Gilbert, P., Allan, S., Brough, S., Melley, S., & Miles, J. (2002). Relationship of anhedonia and anxiety to social rank, defeat and entrapment. *Journal of Affective Disorders, 71*, 141–151.
Gilbert, P., Clarke, M., Hempel, S., Miles, J. N. V., & Irons, C. (2004). Criticizing and reassuring oneself: An exploration of forms, styles and reasons in female students. *British Journal of Clinical Psychology, 43*(1), 31–50. https://doi.org/10.1348/014466504772812959
Gilbert, P., Irons, C., McEwan, K., Bhundia, R., Christie, R., & Broomhead, C. (2010). Self-harm in a mixed clinical population: The roles of shame, forms and functions of self-criticism and social rank. *British Journal of Clinical Psychology, 49*, 563–576.
Grant, K. A., Shively, C. A., Nader, M. S., Ehrenkaufer, R. L., Line, S. W., Morton, T. E., Gage, H. D., & Mach, R. H. (1998). Effects of social status on striatal dopamine D_2 receptor binding characteristics in cynomolgus monkeys assessed with positron emission tomography. *Synapse, 29*, 80–83.
Halamová, J., Kanovský, M., Gilbert, P., Troop, N. A., Zuroff, D. C., Hermanto, N., Petrocchi, N., Sommers-Spijkerman, M., Kirby, J. N., Schhar, B., Krieger, T., Martos, M., Asano, K., Yu, F., Basran, J., & Kupeli, N. (2018). The factor structure of the forms of self-criticising/attack-

ing & self-reassuring scale in thirteen distinct populations. *Journal of Psychopathology and Behavioral Assessment, 40*, 736–751.

Harris, D. L., & Ho, A. H. (Eds.). (2023). *Compassion-based approaches in loss and grief*. Taylor & Francis.

Heriot-Maitland, C., & Longden, E. (2022). *Relating to voices using compassion focused therapy: A self-help companion*. Taylor & Francis.

Heriot-Maitland, C., McCarthy-Jones, S., Longden, E., & Gilbert, P. (2019). Compassion focused approaches to working with distressing voices. *Frontiers in Psychology, 10*, 152.

Hickey, T., Nelson, B., Enticott, J., & Meadows, G. (2022). The potential role of self-criticism in distress related to attenuated psychotic symptoms and implications for clinical trajectory. *Schizophrenia Research, 243*, 298–299. https://doi.org/10.1016/j.schres.2020.06.023

Horton, L. E., Barrantes-Vidal, N., Silvia, P. J., & Kwapil, T. R. (2014). Worries about being judged versus being harmed: Disentangling the association of social anxiety and paranoia with schizotypy. *PLoS One, 9*(6), e96269.

Huang, J. Y., & Bargh, J. A. (2014). The selfish goal: Autonomously operating motivational structures as the proximate cause of human judgment and behavior. *Behavioral and Brain Sciences, 37*, 121–175.

Jia, L. X., Ye, J. Y., Cui, J. F., Shi, H. S., Yang, T. X., & Wang, Y. (2023). Proactive and reactive cognitive control for emotional conflict in individuals with high schizotypy: An ERP study. *Clinical Neurophysiology, 145*, 36–44.

Keltner, D., Kogan, A., Piff, P. K., & Saturn, S. R. (2014). The sociocultural appraisals, values, and emotions (SAVE) framework of prosociality: Core processes from gene to meme. *Annual Review of Psychology, 65*, 425–460. https://doi.org/10.1146/annurev-psych-010213-115054

Keltner, D., Oatley, K., & Jenkins, J. M. (2018). *Understanding emotions*. Wiley Global Education.

Kessler, S. E. (2020). Why care: Complex evolutionary history of human healthcare networks. *Frontiers in Psychology, 11*, 199. https://doi.org/10.3389/fpsyg.2020.00199

Kim, J. J., Parker, S. L., Doty, J. R., Cunnington, R., Gilbert, P., & Kirby, J. N. (2020). Neurophysiological and behavioural markers of compassion. *Scientific Reports, 10*(1), 1–9.

Kline, N. K., Berke, D. S., Rhodes, C. A., Steenkamp, M. M., & Litz, B. T. (2021). Self-blame and PTSD following sexual assault: A longitudinal analysis. *Journal of Interpersonal Violence, 36*(5–6), NP3153–NP3168.

Kucerova, B., Levit-Binnun, N., Gordon, I., & Golland, Y. (2023). From oxytocin to compassion: The saliency of distress. *Biology, 12*(2), 183.

Laithwaite, H., O'Hanlon, M., Collins, P., Doyle, P., Abraham, L., Porter, S., & Gumley, A. (2009). Recovery after psychosis (RAP): A compassion focused programme for individuals residing in high security settings. *Behavioural and Cognitive Psychotherapy, 37*(5), 511–526.

Langdon, R., Michie, P. T., Ward, P. B., McConaghy, N., Catts, S. V., & Coltheart, M. (1997). Defective self and/or other mentalising in schizophrenia: A cognitive neuropsychological approach. *Cognitive Neuropsychiatry, 2*(3), 167–193.

Larøi, F., Van der Linden, M., & Aleman, A. (2008). Associations between dimensions of alexithymia and psychometric schizotypy in nonclinical participants. *Journal of Nervous and Mental Disease, 196*(12), 927–930.

LeDoux, J. E. (2020). Thoughtful feelings. *Current Biology, 30*(11), R619–R623.

LeDoux, J. E. (2022). As soon as there was life, there was danger: The deep history of survival behaviours and the shallower history of consciousness. *Philosophical Transactions of the Royal Society B, 377*(1844), 20210292.

Lee, D. A. (2022). Chapter 25: Using compassion focused therapy to work with complex PTSD. In P. Gilbert & G. Simos (Eds.), *Compassion focused therapy: Clinical practice and applications* (pp. 565–583). Routledge.

Legg, L., & Gilbert, P. (2006). A pilot study of gender of voice and gender of patient in psychotic voice hearers. *Psychology and Psychotherapy, 79*, 517–527.

Longe, O., Maratos, F. A., Gilbert, P., Evans, G., Volker, F., Rockliffe, H., & Rippon, G. (2010). Having a word with yourself: Neural correlates of self-criticism and self-reassurance. *NeuroImage, 49*, 1849–1856.

Luyten, P., Campbell, C., Allison, E., & Fonagy, P. (2020). The mentalizing approach to psychopathology: State of the art and future directions. *Annual Review of Clinical Psychology, 16*, 297–325.

Mascaro, J. S., Florian, M. P., Ash, M. J., Palmer, P. K., Frazier, T., Condon, P., & Raison, C. (2020). Ways of knowing compassion: How do we come to know, understand, and measure compassion when we see it? *Frontiers in Psychology, 11*, 547241.

Mayhew, S., & Gilbert, P. (2008). Compassionate mind training with people who hear malevolent voices: A case series report. *Clinical Psychology & Psychotherapy, 15*, 113–138.

Petrocchi, N., Di Bello, M., Cheli, S., & Ottavianni, C. (2022). Chapter 10: Compassion focused therapy and the body: How physiological underpinnings of prosociality informed clinical practise. In P. Gilbert & G. Simos (Eds.), *Compassion focused therapy: Clinical practice and applications* (pp. 345–359). Routledge.

Porges, S. W. (2017). Vagal pathways: Portals to compassion. In E. M. Seppälä, E. Simon-Thomas, S. L. Brown, & M. C. Worline (Eds.), *The Oxford handbook of compassion science* (pp. 189–202). Oxford University Press.

Porges, S. W. (2021). Polyvagal theory: A biobehavioral journey to sociality. *Comprehensive Psychoneuroendocrinology, 7*, 100069.

Schore, A. N. (2019). *Right brain psychotherapy*. Norton.

Sears, R. W., Tirch, D. D., & Denton, R. B. (2011). *Mindfulness in clinical practice*. Professional Resource Press.

Seligman, M. E. P. (1975). *Helplessness: On depression, development and death*. Freeman.

Seppälä, E. M., Simon-Thomas, E., Brown, S. L., Worline, M. C., Cameron, C. D., & Doty, J. R. (Eds.). (2017). *The Oxford handbook of compassion science* (pp. 399–420). Oxford University Press.

Singer, T., & Engert, V. (2019). It matters what you practice: Differential training effects on subjective experience, behavior, brain and body in the ReSource Project. *Current Opinion in Psychology, 28*, 151–158.

Spikins, P. (2015). *How compassion made us human: The evolutionary origins of tenderness, trust and morality*. Spear and Sword Books.

Stevens, L. C., & Woodruff, C. C. (Eds.). (2018). *The neuroscience of empathy, compassion, and self-compassion*. Academic.

Suddendorf, T. (2018). Inside our heads: Two key features created the human mind. *Scientific American, 319*(3), 42–47.

Taylor, P. J., Gooding, P., Wood, A. M., & Tarrier, N. (2011). The role of defeat and entrapment in depression, anxiety, and suicide. *Psychological Bulletin, 137*(3), 391–420.

Török, E., & Kéri, S. (2022). The relationship among mentalization, mindfulness, working memory, and schizotypal personality traits in the general population. *Frontiers in Psychology, 13*, 682889.

Trower, P., Sherling, G., Beech, J., Horrop, C., & Gilbert, P. (1998). The socially anxious perspective in face to face interaction: An experimental comparison. *Clinical Psychology and Psychotherapy: An International Journal of Theory and Practice, 5*, 155–166.

Voruganti, L. N., & Awad, A. G. (2006). Subjective and behavioural consequences of striatal dopamine depletion in schizophrenia—Findings from an in vivo SPECT study. *Schizophrenia Research, 88*, 179–186.

Vrtička, P., Favre, P., & Singer, T. (2017). Compassion and the brain. In P. Gilbert (Ed.), *Compassion: Concepts, research and applications* (pp. 135–151). Routledge.

Waite, F., Knight, M. T., & Lee, D. (2015). Self-compassion and self-criticism in recovery in psychosis: An interpretative phenomenological analysis study. *Journal of Clinical Psychology, 71*(12), 1201–1217.

Watt, M. J., Roberts, C. L., Scholl, J. L., Meyer, D. L., Miiller, L. C., Barr, J. L., et al. (2014). Decreased prefrontal cortex dopamine activity following adolescent social defeat in male rats: Role of dopamine D_2 receptors. *Psychopharmacology, 231*, 1627–1636.
Werner, A. M., Tibubos, A. N., Rohrmann, S., & Reiss, N. (2019). The clinical trait self-criticism and its relation to psychopathology: A systematic review – Update. *Journal of Affective Disorders, 246*, 530–547.
Whelton, W. J., & Greenberg, L. S. (2005). Emotion in self-criticism. *Personality and Differences, 38*(7), 1583–1595.
White, R., Laithwait, H., & Gilbert, P. (2013). Negative symptoms in schizophrenia: The role of social defeat. In A. Gumley, A. Gillham, K. Taylor, & M. Schwannauer (Eds.), *Psychosis and emotion: The role of emotions in understanding psychosis, therapy and recovery*. Routledge.
Willner, P. (1993). Anhedonia. In C. G. Costello (Ed.), *Symptoms of depression* (pp. 63–84). Wiley.
Workman, I., Reader, W., & Barkow, J. H. (2020). *The Cambridge handbook of evolutionary perspectives on human behaviour*. Cambridge University Press.
Yang, H. X., Shi, H. S., Ni, K., Wang, Y., Cheung, E. F., & Chan, R. C. (2020). Exploring the links between alexithymia, empathy and schizotypy in college students using network analysis. *Cognitive Neuropsychiatry, 25*(4), 245–253.

Chapter 12
Interpersonal Diagnosis of Schizotypy

A. Esin Asan, Aaron L. Pincus, and Christopher J. Hopwood

Schizotypy is a class of psychopathology that reflects odd, eccentric, and disorganized cognitive, affective, and behavioral processes. Expressions of schizotypy significantly impact self and relational functioning, resulting in pervasive disinterest, discomfort, and dysfunction in interpersonal relationships, as well as variation in perceptions and representations of self and other. For example, previous research has broadly linked schizotypy to social withdrawal and flat affect (Tyrka et al., 1995), impairments in nonverbal interpersonal sensitivity (Miller & Lenzenweger, 2014), and self-referential hypermentalization (Wastler & Lenzenweger, 2019). The most widely accepted models of schizotypy are multidimensional, with distinct lower level factors including positive or cognitive-perceptual features (i.e., perceptual abnormalities, ideas of reference, and persecution), negative or socially detached features (i.e., avolition, flattened affect, and anergia), and disorganized features (i.e., formal thought disorder and grossly disorganized behavior; Kwapil et al., 2018; Raine et al., 1994). For detailed discussions of the neurodevelopment of schizotypy, its conceptualization across classification systems, and approaches to its assessment, see Part I of this book (Barrantes-Vidal & Kwapil, Chap. 6, this volume; Snyder et al., Chap. 1, this volume; Su & Cicero, Chap. 3, this volume). Suspiciousness and paranoia are core interpersonal components of positive schizotypy due to beliefs that others are threatening and malevolent (Horton et al., 2014). Negative schizotypy is associated with diminished social contact (Kwapil et al., 2020) and diminished interest in friendships and dating (Kemp et al., 2021). As many of these features involve interference with expressing, encoding, and responding to social cues, there are numerous interpersonal impacts of schizotypy.

A. E. Asan · A. L. Pincus
Pennsylvania State University, University Park, PA, USA

C. J. Hopwood (✉)
University of Zurich, Zurich, Switzerland

S. Cheli, P. H. Lysaker (eds.), *A Dimensional Approach to Schizotypy*,
https://doi.org/10.1007/978-3-031-41788-7_12

Previous research has consistently found moderate-to-large associations between features of schizotypal personality disorder and interpersonal coldness, vindictiveness, and social avoidance (Wright et al., 2012; Williams & Simms, 2016), and similar results are found for those at a clinically high risk for psychosis (Williams et al., 2022). A meta-analytic review of interpersonal dysfunction in personality disorders found that schizotypal personality disorder had a prototypical and distinctive interpersonal profile, reflecting a cold and distant interpersonal style overall (Wilson et al., 2017). However, due to its multidimensional nature, different dimensions of schizotypy are associated with distinct patterns of interpersonal impairment. Wright et al. (2012) suggested that psychoticism traits, analogous to positive schizotypy, are generally modestly associated with hostility and vindictiveness due to finding oneself at odds with and suspicious toward others due to discrepant realities. In contrast, detachment traits, analogous to negative schizotypy, specifically capture interpersonal separation, exhibiting strong associations with coldness and disaffiliation. Most recently, Asan and Pincus (2023) have confirmed that features of schizotypal pathology are prototypically and distinctively interpersonal constructs associated with cold and socially avoidant interpersonal problems and hypersensitivity to others' warmth and affection. To date, interpersonal research on schizotypal pathology has mainly focused on structural associations rather than unpacking how different structural features of schizotypal pathology manifest via patterns of interpersonal dynamics in social relationships. In this chapter, we demonstrate how interpersonal theory can be used as an integrative conceptual nexus to articulate the structural and dynamic features of schizotypy.

Contemporary Integrative Interpersonal Theory of Personality and Psychopathology

Interpersonal theory emerged from the relational psychoanalytic movement (e.g., Sullivan, 1953) and was advanced by the classic works of several founding scholars of the interpersonal tradition (e.g., Carson, 1969; Kiesler, 1996; Leary, 1957; Wiggins, 2003). Importantly, interpersonal theory has had a continuous reciprocal relationship with clinical practice since its inception (e.g., Anchin & Kiesler, 1982; Cain & Pincus, 2016; Pincus & Cain, 2008). This evolving theory of personality and psychopathology has also kept pace with major advances in psychological science over the past 70 years, leading to contemporary integrative interpersonal theory (CIIT; Dawood et al., 2018; Hopwood et al., 2021; Pincus, 2005). The CIIT provides an evidenced-based model of personality structure linked with dynamic social–cognitive, affective, and behavioral processes that offer a scientifically grounded framework for conceptualizing and empirically investigating personality (Roche & Cain, 2021), psychopathology (Wright et al., 2022, 2023), and psychotherapy (Cain et al., in press). The underlying assumptions of CIIT are captured by six principles.

Six Principles of CIIT

Fundamentally important functional expressions of personality and psychopathology typically occur in interpersonal situations. CIIT focuses on interpersonal functioning, which is broadly construed and organized within the "interpersonal situation" as a basic unit of analysis for personality, psychopathology, and psychotherapy (Hopwood et al., 2019; Pincus et al., 2020c). CIIT defines the interpersonal situation as "the experience of a pattern of relating self with other associated with varying levels of anxiety (or security) in which learning takes place that influences the development of self-concept and social behavior" (Pincus & Ansell, 2003, p. 210). Therefore, it is the dynamically unfolding context in which social learning takes place across the life span, promoting personality organization, development, and adjustment. CIIT conceptualizes psychological functions as dynamic interactions between self and other (Pincus et al., 2020a) and focuses on recurrent self-other patterns within and across interpersonal situations (Pincus & Wright, 2011). Critically, this encompasses direct proximal interactions and internal mental representations of interactions. While some clinical problems or symptoms manifest in prototypical interpersonal patterns, others can manifest via multiple patterns of interpersonal expression reflecting interpersonal pathoplasticity (Pincus et al., 2010).

Interpersonal functioning can be organized using the dimensions of agency and communion. The "metaconcepts" of agency and communion (Bakan, 1966; Wiggins, 1991) underlie an empirically validated circular structure referred to as the interpersonal circumplex (IPC) that is used to derive descriptive and explanatory concepts at different levels of specificity (Fig. 12.1 – Top). Agency refers to getting ahead and being in control versus being passive and seeking guidance from others. Communion refers to getting along and being close to others versus being socially cold and distant from others. The IPC provides conceptual coordinates for describing and measuring interpersonal dispositions (Fig. 12.1 – Bottom) that imply enduring patterns of perceiving, thinking, feeling, and behaving aggregated across time, place, and relationships. Finally, the IPC also specifies behaviors enacted within interpersonal situations (Moskowitz, 2005). The IPC is a "key conceptual map" (Kiesler, 1996, p. 172) for an interpersonal description of personality structures and personality processes.

The same structure organizes functioning across levels of experience. The IPC operationalizes data across different levels of inquiry using the same underlying agentic and communal dimensions, facilitating rich multilevel formulations (Leary, 1957; Dawood & Pincus, 2016; Pincus et al., 2020b). Figure 12.1 (Top) depicts three levels: motives, traits, and behaviors. Other potential levels, measurable via existing interpersonal instruments, include values, problems, sensitivities, influence tactics, and strengths (Locke, 2011).

Satisfying agentic and communal motives drives interpersonal behavior. Interpersonal behavior aims to satisfy agentic and communal motives (Horowitz et al., 2006; Sullivan, 1953). The CIIT posits that satisfaction of motives leads to decreased negative affect and vulnerability, increased positive affect, felt security,

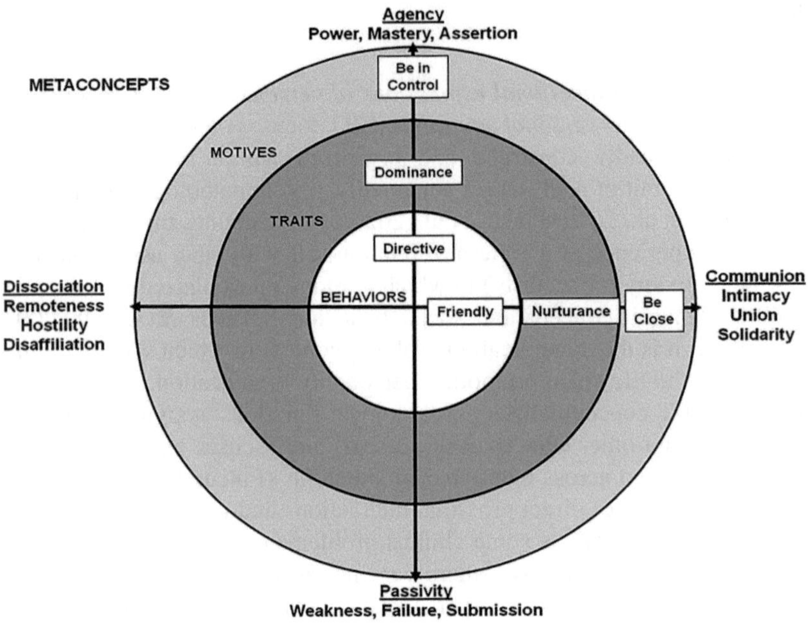

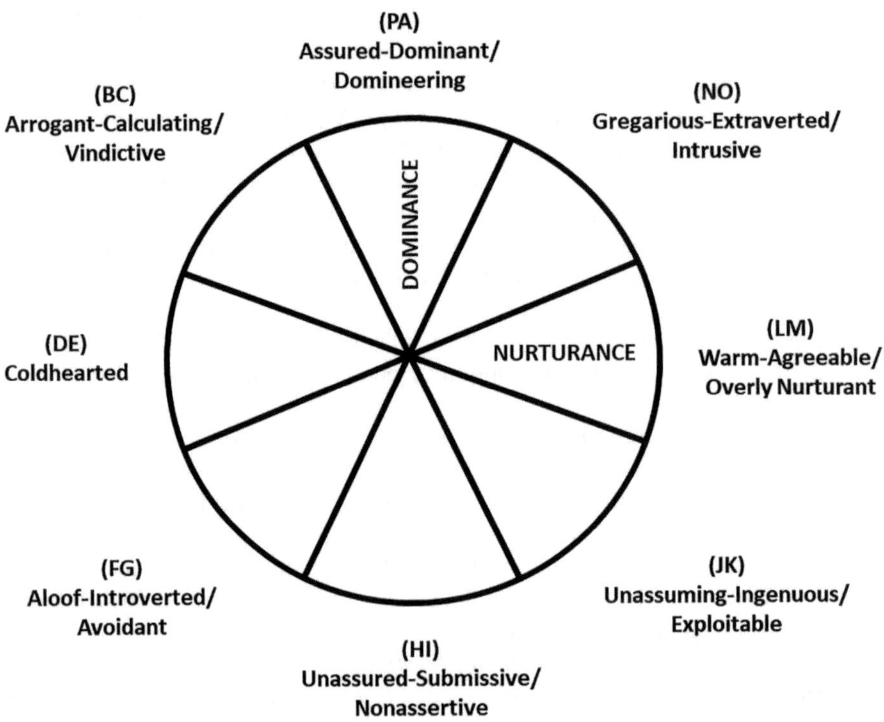

Fig. 12.1 Agency and communion meta-framework (Top); interpersonal circumplex (Bottom). (From Cain & Pincus, 2016. Reprinted with permission from Guilford Press)

and self-esteem, whereas frustration of motives leads to the opposite. These contingencies serve to reinforce/maintain or punish/modify specific behaviors in the short and long terms and explicitly link the interpersonal and affective domains. Individuals differ from each other in their average levels of these motives based on the interactions of innate biology and life experiences. In addition, individuals differ dynamically from themselves moment to moment and across situations as they encounter different opportunities for motive satisfaction.

The "interpersonal transaction cycle" provides probabilistic expectations for patterns of behavior and falsifiable predictions about behavioral sequences. The CIIT seeks to formulate reliable temporally dynamic patterns relating self with other that can describe an individual's personality and psychopathology (Pincus & Hopwood, 2012; Pincus & Wright, 2011; Wright et al., 2023). These patterns reflect interpersonal transaction cycles rooted in probabilistic functional connections between motivation, perception, construal, affect, and behavior of individuals interacting with one another and the situations contextualizing the interaction (Fig. 12.2). The basic components of an interpersonal transaction are (1) Person A's overt behavior toward Person B, (2) Person B's covert experience and construal in response to Person A's action, (3) Person B's overt behavioral response to Person A, and (4) Person A's covert experience and construal of Person B. These four components are parts of an ongoing transactional chain of event cycling toward mutual satisfaction, further negotiation, or disintegration. CIIT identifies important patterns built upon evidence-based processes that describe normative interpersonal behavior. The most well-established of these is complementarity or the prediction that

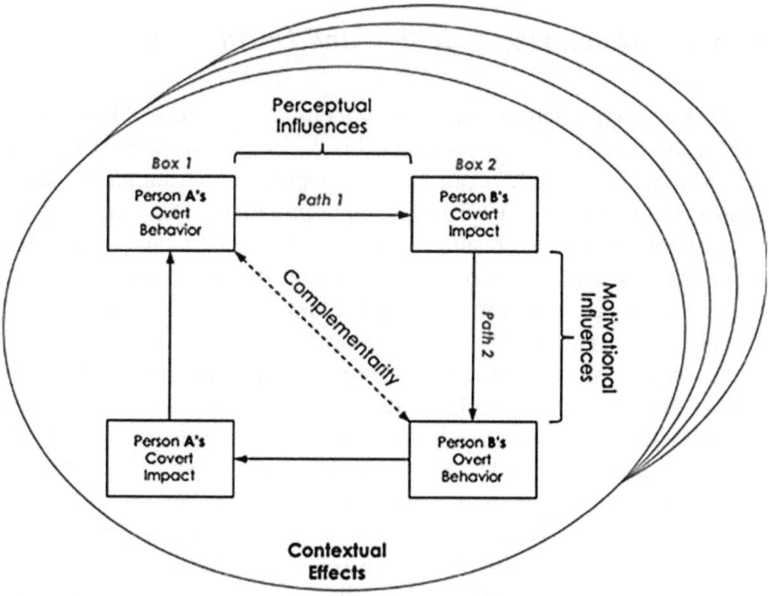

Fig. 12.2 The interpersonal transaction cycle

dominant behavior tends to elicit or invite submissive behavior (and vice versa), whereas warm behavior tends to elicit or invite warm behavior and cold behavior tends to elicit or invite cold behavior (Sadler et al., 2011). The complementarity principle can be elaborated and combined with key components of other psychological domains within interpersonal situations (e.g., motivation, perception, construal, affect, and behavior) to describe characteristic, recurring patterns of interpersonal dynamics in transaction cycles of personality (Halberstadt et al., in press), development (Skowron et al., 2010), psychopathology (Hopwood, 2018), and psychotherapy (Cain & Pincus, 2016).

Sustained deviations from these expected patterns (likely) reflect psychopathology. Deviations from complementary interpersonal exchanges, such as cold responses to others' warmth or dominant responses to others' dominance, are more likely to disrupt interpersonal relations (Kiesler, 1983) and may be indicative of pathological functioning (Benjamin, 1993; Pincus et al., 2010). Chronic deviations from culturally and developmentally normative social processes suggest impairments in recognizing the consensual understanding of interpersonal situations, adaptively communicating one's own interpersonal needs and motives, and comprehending the needs of others and the intent of their interpersonal behavior. Between-person comparisons communicate how a given patient tends to be different from others, such as being colder and/or more domineering than the average person. Within-person comparisons help identify important contexts, such as when there is a particularly strong link between other people's interpersonal behavior and a patient's experience of anger (e.g., Lewis & Ridenour, 2020; Roche et al., 2014).

Interpersonal Diagnosis: Function and Dysfunction

The interpersonal approach to diagnosis (Pincus & Wright, 2011) fundamentally differs from the common descriptive psychiatric approach of the Diagnostic and Statistical Manual of Mental Disorders (DSM) and the International Classification for Diseases (ICD). Rather than placing people into diagnostic categories based on descriptive characteristics or presumed etiology, the interpersonal approach focuses on interpersonal dynamics as a useful transdiagnostic and pantheoretical lens for conceptualizing human behavior, maladaptive and adaptive (Hopwood et al., 2023; Wright et al., 2023). This lens is useful because humans are highly social animals; thus, social learning shapes patterns of interpersonal dynamics, and those patterns can connect developmental origins with current functioning, maladaptive with adaptive characteristics, and behavior inside and outside of the consulting room. Interpersonal diagnosis provides an integrative conceptual nexus (Pincus et al., 2010) to describe and conceptualize how any kind of problem or symptom manifests in relationships. Some problems (e.g., social phobia) can be defined nearly completely in terms of patterns of interpersonal dynamics, whereas others (e.g., Alzheimer's disease) clearly have features that are not directly interpersonal, but nevertheless have interpersonal implications and manifest in interpersonal situations. Still other problems, including most of the patterns traditionally diagnosed as personality disorders, carry such severe interpersonal dysfunction and distortion that managing the relationship between the clinician and the patient is the main priority in treatment (Wright et al., 2022).

Interpersonal diagnosis provides a highly flexible system for conceptualizing different kinds of problems through an integrative and a clinically useful lens. As we describe later, schizotypy has some features that can be fully defined by patterns of interpersonal dynamics and other features arising from dysfunction in other systems such as cognitive impairments that have interpersonal implications. Thus, all features of schizotypy can disrupt interpersonal relations, and the content and processes outlined in CIIT provide valuable insights into an individual's manifestation of schizotypy.

CIIT principles can be used to define adaptive and maladaptive psychological functioning. Adaptive functioning reflects the sustained ability to engage interpersonally in ways that coordinate and satisfy the agentic and communal needs of self and other, relatively consistent with one's developmental stage and sociocultural context, through the flexible, stable, and effective regulation of self, affect, and interpersonal behavior. In CIIT, adaptive functioning is not defined by dispositional levels: rather, it is defined by the ability to stably yet flexibly coordinate and satisfy self and others' motives within the contexts of developmental, sociocultural, and situational demands. Accordingly, dysfunction is defined as the sustained breakdown in any of the processes that support and maintain the flexible, stable, and effective regulation of self, affect, and/or interpersonal behavior. Examples of contributing processes include impairments, biases, or instability of perceptions of self and other; over-reliance or under-reliance on perceptions of self and other; overvalued or extreme motivations or beliefs; interpersonal repertoire/skills deficits; idiosyncratic, deviant, inconsistent, or rigidly applied behavioral rules, such as overvalued or disavowed goals; and exaggerated links among perceptions, affect, and behavior (e.g., rejection sensitivity). Any one of these breakdowns could disrupt the successful mutual navigation of interpersonal transaction cycles by fueling distortions in the perception and construal of self, other, and context in interpersonal situations. Sustained breakdowns would tend to evoke self, affect, and behavioral dysregulation and ultimately unstable, dissatisfying, even destructive interpersonal relations.

The Interpersonal Situation

The interpersonal situation framework integrates the structural and process assumptions of CIIT. First, interpersonal situations involve two or more people (proximal or mentally represented) and are among the most influential situations we experience in life. Second, the important psychological characteristics of interpersonal situations are the perceptions of agentic (dominant–submissive) and communal (warm–cold) motives and behaviors of self and other, and their concomitant affects, within and across social interactions. The interpersonal situation reflects the dynamically unfolding contexts of human experience across the life span where social learning takes place that promotes adaptive or maladaptive self-concepts and relational patterns. Thus, the interpersonal situation characterizes how features of schizotypy impact the development and maintenance of maladaptive patterns of motivation, perception, construal, affect, and behavior in relational functioning.

In both proximal interactions and mental representations, the affective valence associated with an interpersonal situation is a function of one's ability to satisfy agentic and communal motives. When these motives are satisfied, the interaction is pleasant and the behavior is reinforced; when they are frustrated, it is unpleasant, prompting dysregulation, self-protective motives, and a need to cope and adapt (Horowitz et al., 2006; Pincus & Hopwood, 2012; Wright et al., 2023).

In Fig. 12.3, both self and other include their own self and affect systems. The self-system is organized by underlying agentic and communal interpersonal motives (Horowitz et al., 2006) that lead to schemas, behavioral styles, aversions, problems, and capabilities via social learning. Identity, self-concept, and self-worth vary per the degree to which interpersonal motives are satisfied. The affect system, structured by affective arousal and valence (Posner et al., 2005), has a reciprocal relationship with the self-system indicated by bidirectional arrows between the interpersonal and affective circles within self and other. Emotional experiences provide critical feedback regarding motive satisfaction that can intensify, dull, or change the course of interpersonal behavior. In turn, interpersonal behavior modulates affective experiences via the achievement of interpersonal goals.

The interpersonal field encapsulates the relationship between the self and other (Wiggins & Trobst, 1999) and is the arena for social exchange and learning (Carson, 1969). Each person's independent perceptions of self (curved arrows) and other (unidirectional arrows) are represented as inputs, perceived and construed in terms

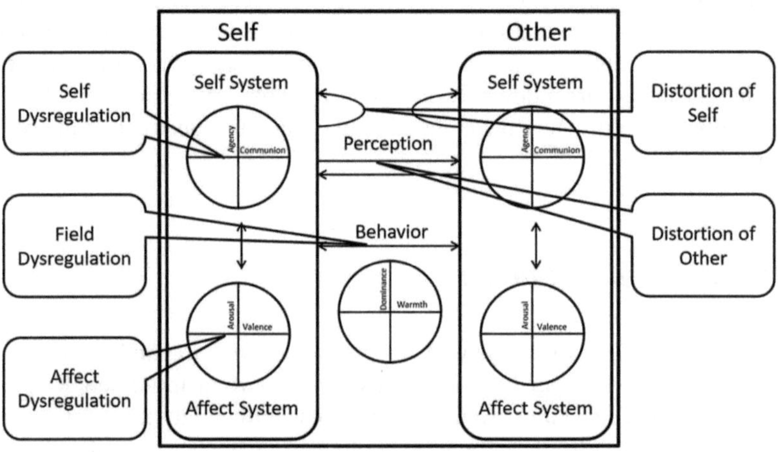

Fig. 12.3 The interpersonal situation. (From Hopwood, C. J., Wright, A. G., & Pincus, A. L. (2018, December 29). The Interpersonal Situation. https://doi.org/10.17605/OSF.IO/QJSCD)

of their agentic and communal behaviors and impacts. The specific agentic (dominant versus submissive) and communal (warm versus cold) behaviors enacted within the field are indicated by the bidirectional arrow between self and other (serving simultaneously as input and output). Overall, the integration of structure and process of the interpersonal field is best captured by the entirety of the interpersonal situation. Within the interpersonal field, perceptual and construal processes moderate the functioning of the self-system, affect system, and behavior (Hopwood et al., 2019; Pincus et al., 2020c).

Schizotypy Features from a Contemporary Interpersonal Perspective

In this chapter, we discuss schizotypy through the interpersonal situation framework using six different key features that are most relevant to interpersonal functioning: (1) referential thinking (i.e., aberrant salience), (2) persecutory thinking (i.e., suspiciousness/paranoia), (3) social disinterest, (4) inability to perceive and express social cues, (5) aberrant perceptions, and (6) disorganization. We chose to focus on these six specific features as we believe they have the most significant implications for an interpersonal diagnosis. We argue that, from a contemporary interpersonal lens, these impairments are linked to over-reliance or under-reliance on the construal of self or other in the interpersonal situation, self-protective motives, and perceptual and behavioral deficits, all of which give rise to dysregulation and distortion within the interpersonal situation. These features all coalesce around chronic deviations from expected patterns of expressing, encoding, and responding to interpersonal cues. We provide a general explanation of the six features, review prior research on how they impact social functioning, and examine how they influence direct proximal interactions and internal mental representations of interactions. Finally, we map these features onto the interpersonal situation framework, dynamically articulating where and how each feature gives rise to disturbed interpersonal relations. Supplementary figures depicting how each of these features unfolds in the interpersonal situation may be found at this link: https://osf.io/qrthk.

Feature 1: Self-Referential Thinking (Aberrant Salience)

Individuals with schizotypic traits tend to incorrectly interpret causal incidents, external events, and behaviors of others as having special meaning for the self (Lenzenweger et al., 1997). Even though referential thinking is a transdiagnostic construct, it is frequently described as a manifestation of schizotypy and schizotypal personality disorder (American Psychiatric Association, 2013; Meyer & Lenzenweger, 2009). Referential thinking in schizotypic individuals has previously been linked to aberrant salience and mentalization deficits, specifically hypermentalization errors (Cicero et al., 2010; Wastler & Lenzenweger, 2019). Ideas of reference can manifest in multiple different ways, ranging from "simple" ideas like others are taking special notice of the self, to "guilty" ideas like being associated with something blameworthy. Referential thinking can refer to both negatively valenced thoughts, such as "*when I notice something is wrong, I think that others are blaming me for it*," and positively valenced thoughts, such as "*when I hear a new song, I often think it was written about me*" (Cicero & Kerns, 2011).

Although ideas of reference and ideas of persecution (suspiciousness/paranoia) are strongly correlated (Meyer & Lenzenweger, 2009; Stefanis et al., 2004) and both are linked to mentalizing deficits, they are distinct features (Cicero & Kerns, 2011) and may therefore have distinct dynamics within the interpersonal situation. Cicero and Kerns (2011) attributed this distinction to *aberrant salience* exhibiting stronger associations with referential thinking compared to suspiciousness/paranoia. Aberrant salience is defined as the over-attribution of salience to otherwise personally irrelevant events, which may lead to either pleasant or unpleasant referential thoughts, when combined with high or low self-esteem, respectively (Kapur, 2003). Therefore, to differentiate self-referential thinking from persecutory thinking, we emphasize aberrant salience while explaining the interpersonal perspective on self-referential thinking.

From the perspective of CIIT, self-referential thinking arises from a rigid concept of the self as inordinately relevant across interpersonal situations, and there is evidence that aberrant salience in one situation carries over to subsequent experiences in daily life (Meyer et al., 2022). The perception of the self as unduly salient leads to a false belief that others perceive the self similarly, creating an over-reliance on the perception of the self by others when making interpersonal interpretations. Further, this perspective is supported by the strong link between hypermentalization and referential thinking (Wastler & Lenzenweger, 2019). For example, due to rigidly self-referent and excessive interpretations of others' mental states, a schizotypic individual might misperceive an innocuous behavior to mean that an interaction partner is angry with *them*, leading to mutual frustration of communal motives and eventual social alienation. Later, the same schizotypic individual might misperceive a neutral behavior to mean that an interaction partner is infatuated with *them*, leading to attempts to reciprocate misperceived communal overtures and inappropriate behavioral responses.

The interpersonal situation framework offers a dynamic exploration of how self-referential thinking plays out within an interpersonal transaction cycle: (1) a rigid self-concept as unduly salient and a distorted perception of the self as overly relevant in the interpersonal situation promote (2) the belief that the other perceives the self similarly, leading to (3) affect that is either negatively valenced (e.g., shame, if it is believed that the other is perceiving the self negatively) or positively valenced (e.g., happiness, if it is believed that the other is perceiving the self positively), which influences (4) the behavior that varies according to affective valence. If the schizotypic individual is ashamed, their subsequent behavior may be cold and submissive (i.e., withdrawn). If the schizotypic individual is happy, their subsequent behavior may be warm and dominant (i.e., extraverted). Distortions drive responding to otherwise neutral interpersonal cues with excessive withdrawal or extraversion causing deviation from the expected complementary patterns of interpersonal behavior, promoting dysregulation in the interpersonal situation.

Feature 2: Persecutory Thinking (Suspiciousness/Paranoia)

Interpersonal suspiciousness or paranoia, also referred to as persecutory thinking, is defined as the tendency to be inappropriately suspicious of other people's motives and behaviors, therefore perceiving them as intending to harm or mistreat the self (American Psychiatric Association, 2013; Fenigstein & Vanable, 1992). Although suspiciousness/paranoia is a transdiagnostic symptom, it is considered as one of the hallmark cognitive–perceptual symptoms of the psychosis continuum and therefore schizotypy and schizotypal personality disorder.

Theories of the structural mechanisms behind persecutory thinking have proposed low self-esteem and attributing negative beliefs about the self to others as potential causal pathways and hypothesized that paranoia serves a defensive function (see Bentall et al., 2001). However, research on these mechanisms has been inconclusive due to inconsistencies in theory and method. In terms of its social impact, interpersonal paranoia has been associated with problems with psychosocial functioning starting from adolescence (Wong & Raine, 2018). In adulthood, persecutory thinking has been linked to social dysfunction when coupled with the theory of mind deficits (Phalen et al., 2017). Although this is unsurprising, the interpersonal perspective can unpack the how this plays out dynamically between the self and the other.

From the perspective of CIIT, within the self-system, persecutory thinking arises from trait suspiciousness and self-protective interpersonal motives and is supported by an over-reliance on the self's perception of the other in the interpersonal situation, leading to errors in comprehending the needs of others and the intent of their interpersonal behavior. Due to ongoing hypervigilance to interpersonal threat, a rigid and distorted perception of others' intentions as hostile, and a global attribution of external stimuli as dangerous to the self, pursuit of interpersonal contact is perceived as risky and therefore distressing and bothersome. Consistent with this, a recent study found that multiple measures of interpersonal suspiciousness were strongly positively associated with elevated interpersonal distress and interpersonal hypersensitivity (Asan & Pincus, 2023). This study also showed that interpersonal suspiciousness was most strongly related to finding warm and dominant behaviors bothersome, likely due to distortion of other people's intentions and behaviors as hostile or vindictive.

The dynamics of suspiciousness/paranoia in the interpersonal situation unfold as follows: (1) Self-protective, cold, and submissive motives drive (2) the tendency to interpret interpersonal cues with suspicion, leading to (3) any type of behavior of the other being perceived as hostile or harmful, resulting in (4) either distant (e.g., ignoring and socially isolating) or cold and dominant behaviors (e.g., yelling and blaming). The perception of the other as hostile also leads to (5) negatively valenced and positively aroused affect (i.e., fear, anxiety, and anger), which reinforces both the (1) self-protective motives and (4) cold and distant behavior that varies in dominance. Overall, schizotypic suspiciousness/paranoia interferes with interpersonal complementarity, where the suspicious/paranoid self responds to any behavior of the other with coldness and distance, even when most people would perceive the other's behavior as warm or innocuous. Chronic distortions of the other by the paranoid/suspicious person will frustrate the others' interpersonal motives, leading to dysregulation in the interpersonal situation and disturbed interpersonal relations.

Feature 3: Social Disinterest

Negative schizotypy is characterized by impoverished or indifferent social experiences including social anhedonia, lack of close friends, and flat affect (American Psychiatric Association, 2013; Kwapil & Barrantes-Vidal, 2015; Raine et al., 1994). Experience sampling studies find that negative schizotypy is primarily expressed in daily life through *social disinterest*, specifically decreased likelihood to place importance on events that involve other people, greater social distance when with others, diminished feelings of closeness, an increased desire to be alone when with others, and a decreased desire to be with others when alone (Kwapil et al., 2012, 2020). Notably, unlike neuroticism and anxiety that are characterized by increased negative affect and affective instability, social disinterest is characterized by diminished positive affect. Social disinterest is especially relevant to daily social interactions, and the associated interpersonal dynamics can be well described within the interpersonal situation.

From the CIIT perspective, social disinterest may be defined as deficits in interpersonal motives and values, leading to a systematic under-reliance on the perception of other in relation to the self and the self in relation to the other. Within the interpersonal situation, the self-system of an individual with schizotypic social disinterest would be characterized by neither agentic nor communal motives and dispositions.

The dynamics of social disinterest in the interpersonal situation unfold as follows: (1) The relative absence of interpersonal motives and values leads to multiple outcomes, such as (2) inattention to or an under-reliance on the perception of the other, (3) deficient interpersonal behavioral engagement, and (4) flat affectivity that is low in arousal and neutral in valence. This lack of interpersonal engagement may lead to others perceiving the schizotypic individual as coldhearted, arrogant/calculated or aloof/avoidant (variations in low communion). Unsurprisingly, social disinterest would result in unmet interpersonal needs of interaction partners, who may avoid future interactions with schizotypic individuals, further intensifying their alienation. Lack of interpersonal motives and failure to value interpersonal relations as important manifest as deficits in interpersonal behavior (i.e., lack of responsiveness) and an underdeveloped social skills repertoire.

Feature 4: Inability to Perceive and Express Social Cues

Adaptive social interactions are a product of self and others' ability to convey behavioral and emotional cues to elicit mutually desired responses from each other. Chronic inability to perceive and express social cues results in a sustained breakdown within the interpersonal field, leading to dysregulation in the interpersonal situation and disturbed interpersonal relations. Independent of cognitive ability, schizotypic individuals have difficulties understanding the intentions, affects, and behavior of others, and communicating social cues that draw desired responses from others, or, more simply, "reading" other people and responding accordingly (Miller & Lenzenweger, 2014; Toomey et al., 1999).

From the CIIT perspective, the inability to successfully exchange social cues manifests within the interpersonal situation as deficits in (1) understanding (i.e., perception) and (2) communicating (i.e., behavior), leading others to (3) misunderstand the self, as well. In fact, this feature may be understood as an endophenotype of schizophrenia that underlies many symptoms of schizotypy. Further, the inability to perceive and express social cues is distinct from rigidly distorting perception of others in a particular way (e.g., suspiciousness/paranoia), and its subsequent effects on other components of the interpersonal situation arise from the deficits in perception and expression themselves.

Feature 5: Aberrant Perceptions

Perceptual aberrations experienced by schizotypic individuals are expressions of positive or cognitive–perceptual schizotypy and may be described as milder forms of psychotic symptoms experienced by patients with schizophrenia spectrum disorders, such as auditory and visual hallucinations and full-blown delusions (Kwapil et al., 2018). Like the inability to follow and express social cues, perceptual aberrations can also be characterized as an endophenotype of schizophrenia and therefore a broad process that underlies many different features of schizotypy (Lenzenweger, 2021). Although perceptual aberrations comprise previously discussed features of referential and persecutory thinking, we discuss it separately as it includes other symptoms like magical thinking, bizarre/supernatural beliefs, and unusual perceptual and somatic experiences and thus may have broader implications for interpersonal functioning. As an example, a schizotypic individual may believe that they possess extrasensory perception and therefore behave more dominantly in interpersonal situations in order to warn others of their apocalyptic visions or become more distant from others who do not heed their dire warnings.

From the CIIT perspective, aberrant perceptions manifest within the interpersonal situation as (1) deficits in perceptions of the self and (2) perceptions of the other and external stimuli, leading to (3) behavioral expressions of abnormal thoughts, beliefs, and experiences. These may be met with expressions of confusion and discomfort from interaction partners, leading them to distance themselves from the schizotypic individual. For the schizotypic individual who may be expressing aberrant perceptions driven by communal motives to seek closeness or submissive motives to seek care/protection, withdrawal from interaction partners is likely to lead to motive dissatisfaction, sadness, and alienation. In fact, an experience sampling study found that positive schizotypy was associated with negative affect and the attribution that being alone was due to being unwanted by others (Kwapil et al., 2012). Overall, aberrant perceptions are likely to result in dysregulation in the interpersonal situation and disturbed interpersonal relations.

Feature 6: Disorganization

Disorganization is one of the three main dimensions of schizotypy. It is characterized by disruptions in the ability to organize, understand, and express thoughts, emotions, and behavior and encompasses symptoms such as confusion, racing thoughts, loose associations, disrupted speech, and slowness of thought (Kemp et al., 2023). Disorganized schizotypy is positively associated with neuroticism, elevated negative affect, and elevated interpersonal distress and is negatively associated with conscientiousness (Asan & Pincus, 2023; Kemp et al., 2018; Kwapil et al., 2018). From the CIIT perspective, disorganization reflects broad behavioral dysfunction within the interpersonal situation. Due to their unpredictable nature, expressions of disorganized schizotypy may commonly interfere with complementary social exchanges in numerous ways, leading others to perceive the schizotypic individual as unreliable, odd, and inconsistent. Others may quickly wish to distance themselves from interpersonal interactions that are difficult to navigate. Overall, disorganization is likely to result in chronic self and relational dysfunction. Consistent with prior research linking disorganized schizotypy with affect dysregulation (Kemp et al., 2023), it is likely that social alienation and maladaptive relational patterns contribute to the intensity of negative affect experienced by disorganized individuals.

Integration of Features

In Fig. 12.4, we present an integration of the interpersonal dynamics of schizotypy manifested across interpersonal situations, which unfolds as follows: (1) self-protective, socially disinterested, and socially distancing motives that vary in agency, in addition to (2) a systematically suspicious perception of others, coupled

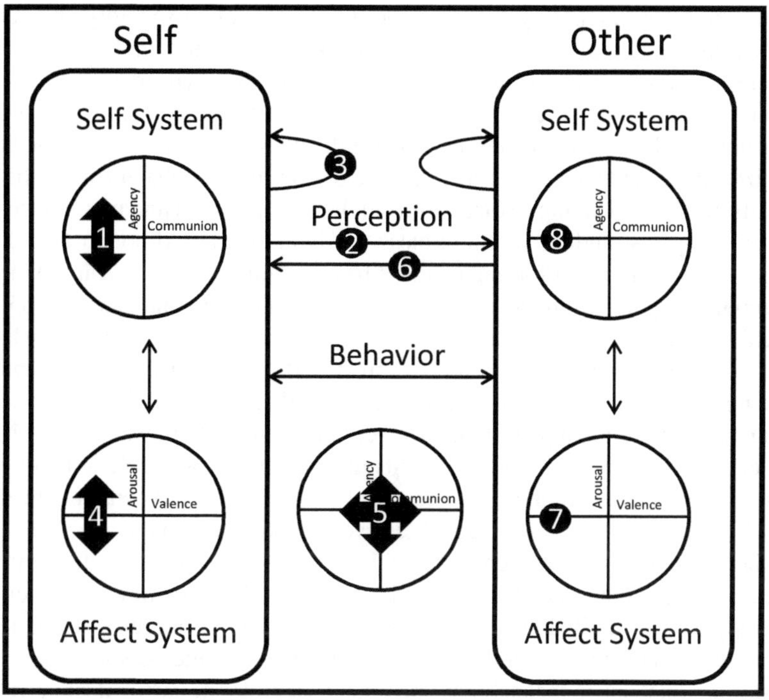

Fig. 12.4 Schizotypy within the interpersonal situation

with (3) inaccurate perceptions of self (aberrant salience) contribute to (4) negative affects about social interactions that vary from anxiety to apathy. This manifests as (5) inconsistent interpersonal behavior, which is (6) perceived by others as unpredictable and confusing, leading them to (7) feel dysregulated themselves and (8) desire to distance themselves from the schizotypic person, reinforcing (1) self-distancing motives and (3) the suspicious perception of others. In this chapter, for heuristic reasons, we illustrate the interpersonal dynamics of schizotypy features as orderly sequences. However, realistically, these dynamics may not play out sequentially, and each step may influence one another within and across interpersonal situations.

Implications for Clinical Practice

This chapter uses CIIT as a transdiagnostic and pantheoretical lens to conceptualize key features of schizotypy and provide an interpersonal diagnosis. CIIT offers guidance for case conceptualization and treatment planning for schizotypic clients by detailing processes that threaten the flexible, stable, and effective regulation of self, affect, and/or interpersonal behavior, leading to disturbed interpersonal relations.

Overall, the interpersonal dysfunction and dissatisfaction of schizotypic clients are fundamentally related to self-protective and self-distancing motives, along with deficient interest in relationships. Socially, these motives will inevitably be threatened due to inaccurate perceptions of the self as overly salient and others as hostile or threatening. This dynamic has specific implications for early therapeutic alliance as schizotypic clients may view any agentic or communal behavior from the therapist with suspicion, leading to discomfort in the therapy room and motives to protect themselves by responding with coldness and withdrawal. Although the clinician may be compelled to pull for engagement from the client via increasing their agentic (encouraging disclosure and asking questions) and communal (expressing empathy and concern) behaviors, they must (i) be sensitive to moments when the schizotypic client is likely to perceive threat and (ii) be cautious not to push for more engagement than the client can tolerate. Otherwise, the clinician risks reinforcing the dysfunctional pattern of social coldness and withdrawal. In addition, due to deficient motivation, schizotypic clients may appear to have little or no interest in building a therapeutic alliance. This can lead to the clinician to construe the schizotypic client as resistant or unreachable, even evoking complementary disinterest from the clinician. Further, even if the schizotypic client expresses interest in building relationships, they may have difficulty understanding or expressing social cues in therapy and in daily life. The ongoing challenges for alliance formation and ongoing treatment involve finding the right balance of interpersonal engagement and interpersonal space that schizotypic clients can tolerate, while decoupling from the complementary pulls of schizotypic clients' coldness, withdrawal, and social deficits that can evoke clinicians' reciprocal coldness toward and disinterest in the client and even pessimism about treatment itself. An interpersonal diagnosis of schizotypy highlights these issues and provides an empirically supported framework for case conceptualization and treatment planning (Hopwood et al., 2019).

References

American Psychiatric Association. (2013). *Diagnostic and statistical manual of mental disorders* (5th ed.). https://doi.org/10.1176/appi.books.9780890425596

Anchin, J. C., & Kiesler, D. J. (1982). *Handbook of interpersonal psychotherapy*. Pergamon Press.

Asan, A. E., & Pincus, A. L. (2023). Examining schizotypal personality scales within and across interpersonal Circumplex surfaces. *Assessment*, 10731911221143354. Advance online publication. https://doi.org/10.1177/10731911221143354

Bakan, D. (1966). *The duality of human existence: Isolation and communion in Western man*. Beacon Press.

Benjamin, L. S. (1993). Every psychopathology is a gift of love. *Psychotherapy Research, 3*(1), 1–24. https://doi.org/10.1080/10503309312331333629

Bentall, R. P., Corcoran, R., Howard, R., Blackwood, N., & Kinderman, P. (2001). Persecutory delusions: A review and theoretical integration. *Clinical Psychology Review, 21*(8), 1143–1192. https://doi.org/10.1016/s0272-7358(01)00106-4

Cain, N. M., & Pincus, A. L. (2016). Treating maladaptive interpersonal signatures. In W. J. Livesley, G. S. Dimaggio, & J. F. Clarkin (Eds.), *Integrated treatment for personality disorder: A modular approach* (pp. 305–324). Guilford Press.

Cain, N. M., Hopwood, C. J., & Pincus, A. L. (in press). Psychotherapy through the lens of contemporary integrative interpersonal theory. In F. Leong (Ed.), *APA handbook of psychotherapy*. American Psychological Association.

Carson, R. C. (1969). *Interaction concepts of personality*. Aldine.

Cicero, D. C., & Kerns, J. G. (2011). Unpleasant and pleasant referential thinking: Relations with self-processing, paranoia, and other schizotypal traits. *Journal of Research in Personality, 45*(2), 208–218. https://doi.org/10.1016/j.jrp.2011.02.002

Cicero, D. C., Kerns, J. G., & McCarthy, D. M. (2010). The aberrant salience inventory: A new measure of psychosis proneness. *Psychological Assessment, 22*(3), 688–701. https://doi.org/10.1037/a0019913

Dawood, S., & Pincus, A. L. (2016). Multi-surface interpersonal assessment in a cognitive-behavioral therapy context. *Journal of Personality Assessment, 98*, 449–460.

Dawood, S., Dowgwillo, E. A., Wu, L. Z., & Pincus, A. L. (2018). Contemporary integrative interpersonal theory of personality. In V. Zeigler-Hill & T. Shackleford (Eds.), *The SAGE handbook of personality and individual differences – Vol. 1: The science of personality and individual differences* (pp. 171–202). Sage.

Fenigstein, A., & Vanable, P. A. (1992). Paranoia and self-consciousness. *Journal of Personality and Social Psychology, 62*(1), 129–138. https://doi.org/10.1037/0022-3514.62.1.129

Halberstadt, A. L., Pincus, A. L., Mogle, J., & Ansell, E. B. (in press). Interpersonal complementarity and affect in daily life. *Motivation and Emotion*.

Hopwood, C. J. (2018). Interpersonal dynamics in personality and personality disorders. *European Journal of Personality, 32*, 499–524.

Hopwood, C. J., Pincus, A. L., & Wright, A. G. C. (2019). The interpersonal situation: Integrating personality assessment, case formulation, and intervention. In D. B. Samuel & D. R. Lynam (Eds.), *Using basic personality research to inform personality pathology* (pp. 94–121). Oxford University Press.

Hopwood, C. J., Pincus, A. L., & Wright, A. G. C. (2021). Six assumptions of contemporary integrative interpersonal theory of personality and psychopathology. *Current Opinion in Psychology, 41*, 65–70.

Hopwood, C. J., Pincus, A. L., & Wright, A. G. (2023). A clinically useful model of psychopathology must account for interpersonal dynamics. *World Psychiatry, 22*(1), 152. https://doi.org/10.1002/wps.21044

Horowitz, L. M., Wilson, K. R., Turan, B., Zolotsev, P., Constantino, M. J., & Henderson, L. (2006). How interpersonal motives clarify the meaning of interpersonal behavior: A revised circumplex model. *Personality and Social Psychology Review, 10*, 67–86.

Horton, L. E., Barrantes-Vidal, N., Silvia, P. J., & Kwapil, T. R. (2014). Worries about being judged versus being harmed: Disentangling the association of social anxiety and paranoia with schizotypy. *PLoS One, 9*(6), e96269. https://doi.org/10.1371/journal.pone.0096269

Kapur, S. (2003). Psychosis as a state of aberrant salience: A framework linking biology, phenomenology, and pharmacology in schizophrenia. *The American Journal of Psychiatry, 160*(1), 13–23. https://doi.org/10.1176/appi.ajp.160.1.13

Kemp, K. C., Gross, G. M., Barrantes-Vidal, N., & Kwapil, T. R. (2018). Association of positive, negative, and disorganized schizotypy dimensions with affective symptoms and experiences. *Psychiatry Research, 270*, 1143–1149. https://doi.org/10.1016/j.psychres.2018.10.031

Kemp, K. C., Bathery, A. J., Barrantes-Vidal, N., & Kwapil, T. R. (2021). Positive, negative, and disorganized schizotypy predict differential patterns of interview-rated schizophrenia-Spectrum symptoms and impairment. *Assessment, 28*(1), 141–152. https://doi.org/10.1177/1073191119900008

Kemp, K. C., Sperry, S. H., Hernández, L., Barrantes-Vidal, N., & Kwapil, T. R. (2023). Affective dynamics in daily life are differentially expressed in positive, negative, and disorganized

schizotypy. *Journal of Psychopathology and Clinical Science, 132*(1), 110–121. https://doi.org/10.1037/abn0000799
Kiesler, D. J. (1983). The 1982 Interpersonal Circle: A taxonomy for complementarity in human transactions. *Psychological Review, 90*(3), 185–214.
Kiesler, D. J. (1996). *Contemporary interpersonal theory and research: Personality, psychopathology, and psychotherapy*. Wiley.
Kwapil, T. R., & Barrantes-Vidal, N. (2015). Schizotypy: Looking back and moving forward. *Schizophrenia Bulletin, 41*(Suppl 2), S366–S373. https://doi.org/10.1093/schbul/sbu186
Kwapil, T. R., Brown, L. H., Silvia, P. J., Myin-Germeys, I., & Barrantes-Vidal, N. (2012). The expression of positive and negative schizotypy in daily life: An experience sampling study. *Psychological Medicine, 42*(12), 2555–2566. https://doi.org/10.1017/S0033291712000827
Kwapil, T. R., Gross, G. M., Silvia, P. J., Raulin, M. L., & Barrantes-Vidal, N. (2018). Development and psychometric properties of the multidimensional schizotypy scale: A new measure for assessing positive, negative, and disorganized schizotypy. *Schizophrenia Research, 193*, 209–217. https://doi.org/10.1016/j.schres.2017.07.001
Kwapil, T. R., Kemp, K. C., Mielock, A., Sperry, S. H., Chun, C. A., Gross, G. M., & Barrantes-Vidal, N. (2020). Association of multidimensional schizotypy with psychotic-like experiences, affect, and social functioning in daily life: Comparable findings across samples and schizotypy measures. *Journal of Abnormal Psychology, 129*(5), 492–504. https://doi.org/10.1037/abn0000522
Leary, T. (1957). *Interpersonal diagnosis of personality*. Ronald Press.
Lenzenweger, M. F. (2021). Schizotypy 17 years on: Psychotic symptoms in midlife. *Journal of Abnormal Psychology, 130*(4), 399. https://doi.org/10.1037/abn0000680
Lenzenweger, M. F., Bennett, M. E., & Lilenfeld, L. R. (1997). The referential thinking scale as a measure of schizotypy: Scale development and initial construct validation. *Psychological Assessment, 9*(4), 452–463. https://doi.org/10.1037/1040-3590.9.4.452
Lewis, K. C., & Ridenour, J. M. (2020). The integration of EMA and single-occasion multimethod assessment data for a complex psychiatric patient. *Assessment, 27*, 1532–1546.
Locke, K. D. (2011). Circumplex measures of interpersonal constructs. In L. M. Horowitz & S. Strack (Eds.), *Handbook of interpersonal psychology: Theory, research, assessment, and therapeutic interventions* (pp. 313–324). Wiley.
Meyer, E. C., & Lenzenweger, M. F. (2009). The specificity of referential thinking: A comparison of schizotypy and social anxiety. *Psychiatry Research, 165*(1–2), 78–87. https://doi.org/10.1016/j.psychres.2007.10.015
Meyer, M. S., Cohn, J. R., Hayashi, K., & Cicero, D. C. (2022). Momentary assessment of aberrant salience, anomalous self-experiences, and psychotic-like experiences. *Personality Disorders, Theory, Research, and Treatment, 13*(6), 641–653.
Miller, A. B., & Lenzenweger, M. F. (2014). Schizotypy, social cognition, and interpersonal sensitivity. *Translational Issues in Psychological Science, 1*(S), 106–119. https://doi.org/10.1037/2332-2136.1.S.106
Moskowitz, D. S. (2005). Unfolding interpersonal behavior. *Journal of Personality, 73*, 1607–1632.
Phalen, P. L., Dimaggio, G., Popolo, R., & Lysaker, P. H. (2017). Aspects of theory of mind that attenuate the relationship between persecutory delusions and social functioning in schizophrenia spectrum disorders. *Journal of Behavior Therapy and Experimental Psychiatry, 56*, 65–70. https://doi.org/10.1016/j.jbtep.2016.07.008
Pincus, A. L. (2005). A contemporary integrative interpersonal theory of personality disorders. In M. Lenzenweger & J. F. Clarkin (Eds.), *Major theories of personality disorder* (2nd ed., pp. 282–331). Guilford.
Pincus, A. L., & Ansell, E. B. (2003). Interpersonal theory of personality. In T. Millon & M. Lerner (Eds.), *Handbook of psychology: Personality and social psychology* (Vol. 5, pp. 209–229). Wiley.
Pincus, A. L., & Cain, N. M. (2008). Interpersonal psychotherapy. In D. C. S. Richard & S. K. Huprich (Eds.), *Clinical psychology: Assessment, treatment, & research* (pp. 213–245). Academic.

Pincus, A. L., & Hopwood, C. J. (2012). A contemporary interpersonal model of personality pathology and personality disorder. In T. A. Widiger (Ed.), *Oxford handbook of personality disorders* (pp. 372–398). Oxford University Press.

Pincus, A. L., & Wright, A. G. C. (2011). Interpersonal diagnosis of psychopathology. In L. M. Horowitz & S. Strack (Eds.), *Handbook of interpersonal psychology: Theory, research, assessment, and therapeutic interventions* (pp. 359–381). Wiley.

Pincus, A. L., Lukowitsky, M. R., & Wright, A. G. C. (2010). The interpersonal nexus of personality and psychopathology. In T. Millon, R. F. Krueger, & E. Simonsen (Eds.), *Contemporary directions in psychopathology: Scientific foundations for DSM-5 and ICD-11* (pp. 523–552). Guilford.

Pincus, A. L., Cain, N. M., & Halberstadt, A. L. (2020a). Importance of self and other in defining personality pathology. *Psychopathology, 53*, 133–140.

Pincus, A. L., Hopwood, C. J., & Dawood, S. (2020b). A contemporary interpersonal reassessment of Madeline G. In C. J. Hopwood & M. Waugh (Eds.), *Personality assessment paradigms and methods: A collaborative reassessment of Madeline G* (pp. 112–131). Routledge.

Pincus, A. L., Hopwood, C. J., & Wright, A. G. C. (2020c). The interpersonal situation: An integrative framework for the study of personality, psychopathology, and psychotherapy. In D. Funder, J. F. Rauthmann, & R. Sherman (Eds.), *Oxford handbook of psychological situations* (pp. 124–142). Oxford University Press.

Posner, J., Russell, J. A., & Peterson, B. S. (2005). The circumplex model of affect: An integrative approach to affective neuroscience, cognitive development, and psychopathology. *Development and Psychopathology, 17*, 715–734.

Raine, A., Reynolds, C. A., Lencz, T., Scerbo, A., Triphon, N., & Kim, D. (1994). Cognitive-perceptual, interpersonal, and disorganized features of schizotypal personality. *Schizophrenia Bulletin, 20*(1), 191–201. https://doi.org/10.1093/schbul/20.1.191

Roche, M. J., & Cain, N. M. (2021). Interpersonal theory and personality processes. In J. F. Rauthmann (Ed.), *The handbook of personality dynamics and processes* (pp. 669–688). Elsevier/Academic.

Roche, M. J., Pincus, A. L., Rebar, A. L., Conroy, D. E., & Ram, N. (2014). Enriching psychological assessment using a person-specific analysis of interpersonal processes in daily life. *Assessment, 21*, 515–528.

Sadler, P., Ethier, N., & Woody, E. (2011). Interpersonal complementarity. In L. M. Horowitz & S. Strack (Eds.), *Handbook of interpersonal psychology: Theory, research, assessment, and therapeutic interventions* (pp. 123–142). Wiley.

Skowron, E. A., Kozlowski, J. M., & Pincus, A. L. (2010). Differentiation, self-other representations, and rupture-repair processes: Predicting child maltreatment-risk. *Journal of Counseling Psychology, 57*, 304–316.

Stefanis, N. C., Smyrnis, N., Avramopoulos, D., Evdokimidis, I., Ntzoufras, I., & Stefanis, C. N. (2004). Factorial composition of self-rated schizotypal traits among young males undergoing military training. *Schizophrenia Bulletin, 30*(2), 335–350. https://doi.org/10.1093/oxfordjournals.schbul.a007083

Sullivan, H. S. (1953). *The interpersonal theory of psychiatry*. Norton.

Toomey, R., Seidman, L. J., Lyons, M. J., Faraone, S. V., & Tsuang, M. T. (1999). Poor perception of nonverbal social–emotional cues in relatives of schizophrenic patients. *Schizophrenia Research, 40*(2), 121–130. https://doi.org/10.1016/S0920-9964(99)00036-5

Tyrka, A. R., Cannon, T. D., Haslam, N., Mednick, S. A., Schulsinger, F., Schulsinger, H., & Parnas, J. (1995). The latent structure of schizotypy: I. Premorbid indicators of a taxon of individuals at risk for schizophrenia-spectrum disorders. *Journal of Abnormal Psychology, 104*(1), 173–183. https://doi.org/10.1037/0021-843X.104.1.173

Wastler, H. M., & Lenzenweger, M. F. (2019). Self-referential hypermentalization in schizotypy. *Personality Disorders, Theory, Research, and Treatment, 10*(6), 536–544. https://doi-org.ezaccess.libraries.psu.edu/10.1037/per0000344

Wiggins, J. S. (1991). Agency and communion as conceptual coordinates for the understanding and measurement of interpersonal behavior. In D. Cicchetti & W. M. Grove (Eds.), *Thinking clearly about psychology: Essays in honor of Paul E. Meehl, Vol. 2: Personality and psychopathology* (pp. 89–113). University of Minnesota Press.

Wiggins, J. S. (2003). *Paradigms of personality assessment*. Guilford Press.

Wiggins, J. S., & Trobst, K. K. (1999). The fields of interpersonal behavior. In L. Pervin & O. P. John (Eds.), *Handbook of personality: Theory and research* (2nd ed., pp. 653–670). Guilford.

Williams, T. F., & Simms, L. J. (2016). Personality disorder models and their coverage of interpersonal problems. *Personality Disorders, 7*(1), 15–27. https://doi.org/10.1037/per0000140

Williams, T. F., Ellman, L. M., Schiffman, J., & Mittal, V. A. (2022). Employing contemporary integrative interpersonal theory to understand dysfunction in those at clinical high risk for psychosis. *Schizophrenia Bulletin Open, 3*(1), sgac015. https://doi.org/10.1093/schizbullopen/sgac015

Wilson, S., Stroud, C. B., & Durbin, C. E. (2017). Interpersonal dysfunction in personality disorders: A meta-analytic review. *Psychological Bulletin, 143*(7), 677–734. https://doi.org/10.1037/bul0000101

Wong, K. K., & Raine, A. (2018). Developmental aspects of schizotypy and suspiciousness: A review. *Current Behavioral Neuroscience Reports, 5*, 94–101. https://doi.org/10.1007/s40473-018-0144-y

Wright, A. G. C., Pincus, A. L., Hopwood, C. J., Thomas, K. M., Markon, K. E., & Krueger, R. F. (2012). An interpersonal analysis of pathological personality traits in DSM-5. *Assessment, 19*(3), 263–275. https://doi.org/10.1177/1073191112446657

Wright, A. G. C., Ringwald, W. R., Hopwood, C. J., & Pincus, A. L. (2022). It's time to replace the personality disorders with the interpersonal disorders. *American Psychologist, 77*, 1085–1099.

Wright, A. G. C., Pincus, A. L., & Hopwood, C. J. (2023). Contemporary integrative interpersonal theory: Integrating structure, dynamics, temporal scale, and levels of analysis. *Journal of Psychopathology and Clinical Science, 132, 263.*

Part III
Integrated Interventions

Chapter 13
Cognitive Behavioural Therapy for Schizotypy and Psychosis: The Role of Trauma

Douglas Turkington and Nina Cioroboiu

Introduction

Schizotypy has been regarded as a schizophrenia phenotype (Rado, 1953) unfolding on a continuum of psychotic-like features, including non-clinical and clinical traits predisposing to schizophrenia spectrum disorders (SSDs) (Kwapil et al., 2013). The schizotypy continuum includes individuals with schizotypal trait and those with schizotypal personality disorder (STPD) (Barrantes-Vidal & Kwapil, Chap. 6, this volume). As a multidimensional construct, schizotypy comprises positive and negative symptoms, both prone to convert to psychosis under certain conditions (Kwapil et al., 2013). Positive schizotypy has been described as a maladaptive form of openness (Straub & Kerns, 2021) characterised by thoughts and behaviours outside of cultural norms. These include peculiar beliefs, magical thinking, odd speech, cognitive and perceptual anomalies, ideas of reference, paranoid ideation, suspiciousness and affective dysregulation (Kemp et al., 2021), all below the threshold for a schizophrenia diagnosis. Negative schizotypy is characterised by trait-like diminished capacity for positive affect, reduced motivation, anhedonia and withdrawal (Kemp et al., 2021). Although the trajectories of symptom development indicate distinct phenotypes, both positive schizotypy and negative schizotypy are associated with functional impairment (Kwapil et al., 2013). One of the hallmarks of schizotypy is a reduced interest and capacity for close relationships, but some studies found that only positive schizotypy was associated with excessive social anxiety, depression, low self-esteem, negative schemas (Barrantes-Vidal et al., 2013) and psychotic experiences (Kwapil et al., 2008). These symptoms make positive schizotypy suitable for modified cognitive behavioural therapy for psychosis (CBTp). CBTp is a structured psychological treatment based on a combination of Beck's cognitive

D. Turkington (✉) · N. Cioroboiu
CNTW NHS Foundation Trust, Newcastle, UK
e-mail: Douglas.Turkington@cntw.nhs.uk; Nina.Cioroboiu@cntw.nhs.uk

S. Cheli, P. H. Lysaker (eds.), *A Dimensional Approach to Schizotypy*,
https://doi.org/10.1007/978-3-031-41788-7_13

strategies and behavioural homework exercises. It relies upon a collaborative formulation informed by the cognitive model (Beck, 1979). Key techniques include deciding upon an agenda and a goal for the session, the use of guided discovery, feedback, various questioning strategies, reality testing, the generation of coping strategies, schema change and relapse prevention.

On the more severe end of the spectrum, persistent and significantly distressing schizotypal traits are clustered under STPD (Su & Cicero, Chap. 3, this volume), presenting high conversion rates to schizophrenia (Debbané et al., 2015; Woods et al., 2009; Şahin et al., 2013). Although STPD generally manifests without psychotic episodes, some individuals may have brief psychotic-like experiences such as hallucinations and delusions. When these symptoms occur, they tend to be less distressing, infrequent and short-lived. For this reason, they often go undiagnosed even though signs of STPD can be identified in early childhood or during adolescence (Hans et al., 2009). In general, people with STPD seek professional help for associated difficulties (e.g. anxiety and depression) and not for the personality disorder itself, but triggering life events may worsen symptoms, leading to decompensation and psychosis.

The dynamic relationship between genetic and environmental factors appears to play an essential role in the development of schizotypy (Snyder et al., Chap. 1, this volume). First-degree relatives of people diagnosed with a Cluster A personality disorder or a schizophrenia spectrum disorder were found to have a higher incidence of STPD (Battaglia et al., 1995), pointing towards a genetic component. Twin studies have supported the heritability of the condition and suggested that environmental factors are strongly linked to the development of STPD (Torgersen et al., 2000). Specifically, those experiencing childhood trauma, especially sexual abuse, residence in a children's home and homelessness, were at an increased risk of developing schizotypy and a psychotic disorder (Bebbington et al., 2004; Green et al., 2014). A growing body of evidence suggests that traumatic exposure plays a crucial role in the development of severe personality disorders. Schürhoff et al. (2009) found an association between childhood trauma and schizotypy scores in relatives of people with schizophrenia, but not bipolar disorder. This suggests that the interaction between schizophrenia-predisposing genes and the severe stress of childhood trauma leads to positive schizotypal traits. In a recent systematic review (Toutountzidis et al., 2022), abuse and neglect were significantly associated with total schizotypy scores. Interestingly, different types of abuse correlated with specific aspects of schizotypy. Early emotional abuse was linked to more ideas of reference, hallucinations and aberrant salience. Meanwhile, physical abuse was associated with more delusions and unusual perceptual experiences. One explanation for how early life adversity affects people links trauma to increased stress sensitivity through a change in the body's reaction to dopamine (Bebbington et al., 2004; Spauwen et al., 2006). Chun et al. (2019) found that when dopamine-mediated processes are disturbed, aberrant attribution of salience towards external events has been observed. More precisely, findings suggested that hyper-attribution could lead to positive schizotypy, while negative symptoms could be a symptom of hypo-attribution (Chun et al., 2019).

From a developmental perspective, people's attachment styles also influence proneness to psychotic phenomenology. Insecure attachment resulting from inadequate bonding with the caregivers was associated with increased symptoms of positive and negative schizotypy (Korver-Nieberg et al., 2014; Gumley et al., 2014; Berenbaum et al., 2003). Insecure attachment is also associated with problems in metacognition (Lysaker & Wiesepape, Chap. 8, this volume). Childhood trauma can have a lasting impact with significant negative consequences on later life development. Unfortunately, the nature of the condition may also attract bullying, thus increasing the risk of children being ostracised and unable to form friendships with their peers. In adults, adverse life events were linked to increased schizotypy, with around 50% of individuals with STPD reporting being attacked with the intention to kill or injure, of which 39.7% developed PTSD (Yen et al., 2002).

Our understanding of why only some people develop schizophrenia is still limited due to the scarcity of longitudinal studies. Conversion rates vary between studies depending on the follow-up time, with longer duration associated with an increased risk of breakdown. In a systematic review, Kirchner et al. (2018) found that conversion to SSDs ranged between 20% and more than 40%. Factors predicting an increased risk of conversion to psychosis are male gender (Nordentoft et al., 2006), poor socio-economic status, discrimination (Patel & Saxena, 2014), adverse life events, substance misuse and a lack of personal relationships (Flückiger et al., 2016). There are mixed results on whether positive or negative schizotypy is linked to a higher risk of conversion, with some finding that positive schizotypy was uniquely associated with psychosis (Kwapil et al., 2008), while others identifying anhedonia as a predictor of deterioration (Flückiger et al., 2016). Although longitudinal research is needed to understand these risk factors better, both dimensions of schizotypy were linked to social isolation, which is a key factor in the later development of psychosis. In this chapter, we describe how modified CBT techniques were used successfully with a client with psychosis, positive schizotypy and a trauma history.

Evidence Base for CBT for Psychosis

All national guidelines have endorsed CBT as a treatment for the overall symptom burden of SSDs when delivered as an adjunct to antipsychotic medication. These include the guidelines of the Schizophrenia Patient Outcomes Research Team (Schizophrenia PORT) (Kreyenbuhl et al., 2010) and the American Psychiatric Association (Keepers et al., 2020). The ongoing debate on evidence concerning the specific benefit of CBT for hallucinations and delusions has recently been clarified. In a review of meta-analyses where positive symptoms were the primary outcome of a CBT intervention, McKenna et al. (2019) concluded that CBT was effective for hallucinations and delusions in schizophrenia with an effect size of 0.2. This effect size relates to the efficacy of CBTp when added to antipsychotic medication and compared to another psychosocial intervention, such as professional befriending.

The effect size of CBTp is small but adds to the moderate effect size of antipsychotic medication (0.4) and that of family therapy (0.2). Taken all together, a comprehensive biopsychosocial intervention for schizophrenia should have a strong effect in terms of initiating a recovery trajectory. There is also evidence that CBTp can improve adherence to antipsychotic medication (Velligan & Weiden, 2006) and that families learn to use basic CBT-informed care techniques (Kopleovich et al., 2021). There is not sufficient meta-analytical evidence to comment on the efficacy of CBTp for negative symptoms, cognitive deficits or thought disorder. However, negative symptoms have been shown to be responsive to a longer course of CBTp with durable effects at follow-up (Grant et al., 2012). CBTp prevents and delays relapse, reduces time spent in hospital and is cost-effective (Malik et al., 2009). One small, randomised trial on clients with schizophrenia spectrum disorder who had refused antipsychotics showed CBTp to be acceptable with an effect size of 0.4 (Morrison et al., 2014). Unfortunately, schizotypy measures were unavailable in any of these studies, so comments cannot be made on whether the effect size would be different in clients with schizotypy who develop an SSD. This subject is covered in the case description and in the discussion that follows.

Treatment of Schizotypal Personality Disorder

The standard approach combines help with suitable work placement and social treatments, supportive psychotherapy and antipsychotic medication. To date, there are no NICE or the US Food and Drug Administration (FDA)-approved medications or psychosocial treatments for STPD and no large trials to support any specific psychotherapeutic interventions for STPD. However, several lines of research suggest that CBT, social skills training, positive psychological interventions, metacognitive interventions (Morris & Hasson-Ohayon, Chap. 15, this volume; Dimaggio & Popolo, Chap. 16, this volume) and psychodynamic supportive psychotherapy may improve functioning and reduce the risk of conversion to psychosis. Research on differences between healthy individuals and those at higher risk of deterioration suggested that mindfulness interventions might help reduce suspiciousness (McDonald et al., 2021), while targeting sleep hygiene (e.g. using CBT for insomnia) might increase the quality of life (O'Kane et al., 2022).

Social skills training gained attention, showing some benefits when targeting the interpersonal difficulties of people with schizotypy (McKay & Neziroglu, 1996; Nordentoft et al., 2006; Ryan et al., 2013; McClure et al., 2019). In 1996, McKay et al. used social skills training and exposure with response prevention for a person with STPD and obsessive–compulsive disorder (OCD). Although symptoms persisted at 6-month follow-up, general functioning had improved. Similarly, a randomised control trial (RCT; $N = 79$) concluded that a combination of social skills training, psychoeducation for the patient and relatives or friends and a multidisciplinary approach to treatment reduced transition to psychosis by 50% compared with standard care (Nordentoft et al., 2006). McClure et al. (2019) also found that social skills training was beneficial, especially in combination with computerised cognitive remediation (targeting attention, psychomotor skills, memory and executive function) and guanfacine.

Illustrative Case Study: CBT for Psychosis and Schizotypy

History

Gemma was 26 years old when referred for urgent psychiatric assessment and treatment by a psychosis expert (Douglas Turkington). The referral was urgently phoned though by the Crisis Response Team who had been delivering intensive home support and treatment over the previous five evenings. On each occasion, Gemma had needed treatment at the local Accident and Emergency (A&E) department due to lacerations and other injuries to her arms. This urgent situation had been of recent onset as Gemma had just returned to live with her parents after experiencing marriage problems. From the time of her childhood, Gemma had always seen and felt the presence of ghosts in the family home. She mainly had regarded them as harmless and non-intrusive although at times she would feel the need to pass on a message to others. Prior to her marriage, Gemma had worked in a call centre (where she met her best friend Cathy) and had attended Church groups but had been fairly socially isolated otherwise. She had married her first boyfriend after a whirlwind romance, but there were problems straight. Her husband reported that Gemma seemed 'lost in her own thoughts a lot of the time' and seemed very uncomfortable with alcohol, parties and intimacy. On return home, her father who was a lay preacher in a local fundamentalist church was viewed as being critical of Gemma after the marriage break-up. On the first day back, Gemma reported that the ghosts were much more agitated than she remembered. She was sitting sadly reflecting on certain stressful events in the marriage, when suddenly she saw a ghost appear and move towards her. She described the ghost as looking like a Victorian school teacher. Gemma said that the ghost lectured her about being a failure both as a daughter and as a wife for about 10 min while wagging her finger in her face. The ghost continued to speak out loud and asked the other ghosts what punishment Gemma should receive. She then demanded that Gemma go to the kitchen and bring back a sharp knife and cut her wrists as a punishment. In a very distressed, ashamed and saddened state, Gemma did so and started to cut. Gemma noticed that when the blood started to flow, the ghost would back off and leave her alone. On the first night after cutting her arm, Gemma was found by her mother, who sent for an urgent help from the neighbours and phoned an ambulance. Her mother was very supportive, but her father appeared to be critical and indicated that what she was describing indicated demonic possession and that an exorcism should be organised urgently.

On the sixth night of agitation, distress, family upheaval and shame, she was assessed for psychosocial management (a modified form of CBT with a family intervention). The Crisis Response Team indicated that if progress was not made quickly, an admission under the Mental Health Act would be needed to ensure her safety and initiate antipsychotic medication.

Gemma and her family were totally against this idea as they viewed psychiatric disorder as a spiritual matter that would only respond to prayer and the laying on of hands. Similarly, no family member had ever accepted medication of any kind.

Sessions 1–5

Gemma was lowered in mood when seen and deeply ashamed. She reported a paranoid delusion that when she tried to visit her friend Cathy for support, she was being followed by police cars. She said they were trying to catch her to put her in prison but did not know why. She said that the critical voice telling her to cut herself seemed to come in the evening when she was feeling bored and lonely and that her father was criticising her too and had told her that the voice and ghost were from an avenging demon 'Baal'. Gemma was reasonably easy to engage in CBT, and her father agreed to support the use of a talking treatment but not medication. I began by using self-disclosure of having hallucinated the sound of a cardiac arrest page going off after leaving the cardiology job. I explained that the job had been very stressful as I was sleep deprived, and the cardiac arrest page kept going off in the middle of the night. So even psychiatrists could hear things when they were stressed and sleep deprived. Gemma smiled at this and asked me if I was not frightened. I said no, as I knew that my mind was 'playing tricks' on me and that I had been stressed. I explained that the human brain very easily hallucinated and that more than 90% of voices went away again. So, I asked if she had been sleep-deprived or stressed. Gemma said that she had not felt safe in the marriage and so had been sleeping very poorly. On the first night, it was agreed that Gemma would try and keep busy and use normalising explanations to reduce distress if the voices started. Unfortunately, this did not work, and a trip to A&E for an emergency dressing was needed. We next decided that Gemma needed the support of her friend Cathy who knew about the marital problems and 'wasn't scared of ghosts'. We decided to reality-test the paranoid delusion. We went out to walk the route to her friend's house and gather information. Gemma saw three cars that she thought were police, but none were marked as police; the drivers were not looking in our direction and none slowed down to ask questions or ask for identification. This information was discussed, and Gemma agreed that they might not be police cars and that she could look for evidence whenever she was concerned about a car. The plan for that evening was to walk to Cathy's house where they would watch television (TV) together and cook some dinner. Cathy was fully aware of the situation. On the way, Gemma was to keep a diary of information about any cars that she thought might be police. Unfortunately, she became too frightened to leave the house and the same scenario (a visit to the Emergency Department for a wound dressing) occurred again.

Sessions 6–10

A Morrison maintenance formulation (Fig. 13.1) was collaboratively produced to further make sense of the situation. This is a circular formulation including idiosyncratic triggers, psychotic symptoms (hallucinations or delusions), catastrophic appraisal and emotional and behavioural consequences including safety behaviours (Morrison, 1998). The collaborative genesis of this model very often leads to increased optimism and insight as to how the distressing symptoms can be dealt with. We agreed that we needed to do something to change the relationship with the voice that demanded that she cut herself. It was decided that I would role-play the voice and behaviours of the ghost and that Gemma would use normalising explanations and rational responses to defend herself. When I started criticising her using the ghost's words, Gemma became extremely distressed and dissolved in tears. A role reversal was attempted with Gemma playing the role of the ghost, but Gemma found herself unable to utter the words. She said that she often thought these critical things about herself inside her head but would never say such things to another person. I asked her why, and Gemma said that it was 'bullying…plain and simple…and

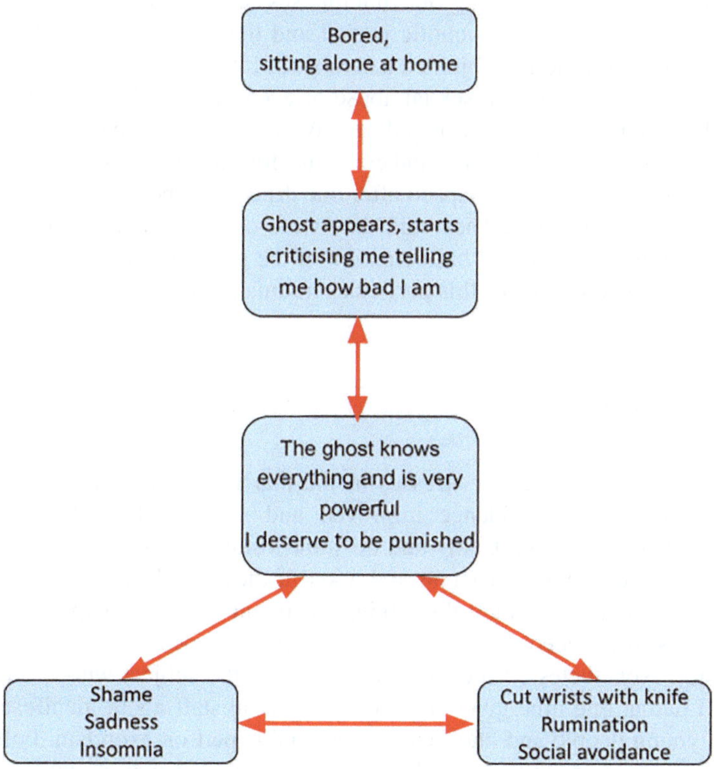

Fig. 13.1 Morrison formulation of Gemma's voices and self-harm

it's not right'. We developed rational responses for her own critical thinking and then used these in relating to the voice. Gemma also realised that she had seen this ghost before when she was a child, and it was not bullying her at that time. Practice proceeded with Gemma becoming more convincing as she spoke back to the ghost 'I've seen you before…no one should tell someone to cut themselves…it's not humane…I might not have been a perfect wife but then nobody is…maybe you could say something kind and sympathetic for a change?…Cathy, mum and dad never speak this way to me'. This approach, combined with activities and parental support, led to increasing confidence and a change in the relationship with the voice.

Sessions 11–15

By now, self-injury had stopped, and Gemma was visiting her friend regularly. We began to work on a timeline. While walking past the bus stop where she had gotten off the bus after leaving her marriage, another visual hallucination was seen. It was 8 feet tall and carrying an axe with a skeleton for a face. She thought it was the grim reaper. Gemma ran for home but called the police to report the vision and how frightened she was by it. During our timeline session the day before, Gemma had been talking about the pre-psychotic period and the fact that she had attended a party, became unconscious and joined a number of intoxicated people in a bedroom.

She disclosed her fear that sexual abuse or even rape might have occurred and that her husband might have drugged her. We explored the memory further and some of the people she recognised and could ask for information. Two of the people contacted said that she had collapsed after one drink, and they had put her on a bed and were looking after her. They said they were confident that she had not been abused in any way. The visual hallucination of the grim reaper was not seen again and seemed to be symbolic of this particular trauma memory.

Sessions 16–20

During these sessions, further stresses in the marriage were discussed and were emotions processed. Confidence improved and mood stabilised, and Gemma decided to share a flat with Cathy and do some voluntary work. Gemma's parents seemed delighted with her progress and asked if they could speak to me privately. Her father said that he thought the talking treatment had been helpful, but that an exorcism was still needed. I said this was an interesting idea but outwith my area of competence. Nonetheless, I did know an expert in the subject who could give an opinion. I had at one time given a lecture to clerical staff about manifestations of PTSD in young people and had met the regional expert on exorcism. Following a telephonic discussion with my colleague, it was decided that a simple saying of prayers would be adequate in Gemma's case. Gemma never started antipsychotic or other mood-stabilising medication and at 5-year follow-up had not relapsed. She was back at work and sharing accommodation with Cathy. The ghost who had been so critical had returned to being friendly and supportive. There had been a mutually agreed divorce, and Gemma did not pursue any further romantic relationships. One interesting development was a change in Gemma's schizotypy. She had developed more control over her perception of ghosts and their occasional communications with her and began to use this gift to help others. Gemma joined a Spiritualist Church where she became a highly valued member of the congregation.

Discussion

Modifying CBT for Clients with Schizotypy and Psychosis

The most crucial elements of modification would appear to be engaging, normalising, reality-testing and changing the relationship with visual and auditory hallucinations before moving on to identify and process traumatic experiences. Engaging required a clear description of role, an explanation of confidentiality and regular feedback. A social element was included to overcome the previous sense of social isolation. In an ideal world (without crisis), a couple of sessions of professional befriending to socialise the client would be very useful in developing the therapeutic alliance (Turkington et al., 2017). Clients with schizotypy are often concerned about meeting a mental health professional. It seems crucial to equalise the power balance using a period of socialisation and personal disclosure around issues such as sporting events, the weather or hobbies. The therapeutic alliance is enhanced by a slow pace of interaction with summary and regular feedback.

Personal disclosure was very important to establish a rapport and normalise how stressful work and relationships can be. I disclosed that after a long period of on-call and lack of sleep I began to have bad dreams about work and even to hear the phone ringing when it had not done so.

Normalising is described as the antidote to stigma. In schizotypy, there is stigma linked to perceptual experiences and unusual ideas, but also to the emergence of psychosis. The CBT therapist might normalise the experience of seeing ghosts, which is 33% among 18- to 34-year-olds (Kingdon et al., 1994). Normalising might also include the fact that most first marriages are unsuccessful and end in divorce. Normalising might cover the subject of imaginary friends, how common these are and how often an imaginary friend can 'turn nasty' after an emotionally difficult experience. Voices are also extremely common and temporary experiences, usually triggered by grief or other loss. In the presence of schizotypy and psychosis, more time is spent engaging and normalising. Success experiences are essential to demonstrate that improvement is possible. This might be achieved by reality-testing any paranoid delusion or hallucination that is present. In Gemma's case, this involved working with a delusion about the police but could involve testing out an auditory hallucination, for example, if she moved away from the ghost as it spoke, did it get quieter and if she put noise cancelling headphones on, did it stop? If not, could the voices be something else and have a more down-to-earth explanation? Romme et al. (1992) showed that those who perceive themselves to be stronger than the voice and set more limits to voice activity cope better with voice hearing. In schizotypy, the typical attitude to voice hearing is passivity, and unusual beliefs are not often reality-tested, nor is any evidence gathered. Modifications of CBTp are needed to change the relationship with the voice. In this case, role-playing the voice was the crucial intervention, which catalysed recovery and prevented inpatient admission. Working on transforming the aggressive image of the ghost back to the previously friendly appearance might also have been beneficial. We could have drawn the previous image and practised working with the image and the types of things that used to be said. Processing trauma memories was achieved by incorporating Ehlers and Clark's approach by repeatedly moving between experiencing the emotion linked to the trauma memory and the linked automatic thoughts and rational responses (Ehlers & Clark, 2000). This recovery which was durable after 18 months was achieved with a standard number of sessions, but it would appear likely that an increased number of sessions might be needed (perhaps up to 30 sessions including boosters). CBT-informed care is available as an online and live training modality and can support family members involved in therapy by allowing them to listen to audio recordings and helping with homework. This kind of family involvement can be beneficial but requires consent, and certain sessions may not be appropriate to share. Recovery was impressive and sustained and led to improved relationships and change in social activities. It would appear that modified CBTp is a viable intervention for schizotypy and psychosis and that further research is needed.

How Does Modified CBTp Compare and Contrast with Other Interventions?

CBTp, in this case, was used to change thinking, behavioural and emotional style in relation to trauma-triggered psychosis in schizotypy. More support for a CBT intervention came from a review of treatment options for adolescents with STPD. Ryan et al. (2013) proposed that the best line of treatment would be a combination of standard CBT, cognitive remediation, substance misuse management and omega-3 supplements. Standard CBT was used to explore ways of changing dysfunctional safety behaviours while reducing comorbid anxiety and depression (Ryan et al., 2013), while cognitive remediation was used to correct and compensate for cognitive deficits associated with social functioning. Again further research is needed to discover the most effective approach or combination of therapies.

Other studies targeted metacognitive deficits with promising results (Cheli et al., 2019; Cheli, 2020; Dmitryeva et al., 2021). However, only a course of treatment with a cognitive behavioural component proved beneficial. In a two-case series,

Cheli et al. (2019) reported a reduction in psychotic and paranoia in two patients with STPD randomly allocated to receive either metacognitive reflection and insight therapy (MERIT) or metacognitive interpersonal therapy (MIT). Both therapies aim to increase the client's capacity to understand mental states and create meaningful relationships through increased self-awareness and metacognitive capacity. MERIT aims to increase self-reflection, understanding of self and others, insight into personal challenges and ways to cope. MIT is a cognitive behavioural intervention focused on dysfunctional schemas, leading to problematic relationships. Drawing on this study, Cheli (2020) assessed the feasibility of a metacognitive intervention for STPD. A 12-month mixed intervention (i.e. 6-month MERIT followed by 6-month MIT) improved general symptoms of STPD and increased metacognition. This was achieved by increasing awareness of self and others through MERIT and employing the cognitive behavioural approach of MIT.

In a single case study, Ridenour argued that psychodynamic supportive psychotherapy is indicated for individuals diagnosed with STPD as a useful way to improve ego functioning and reality testing (Ridenour et al., Chap. 18, this volume). He also suggested that maintaining an attitude of analytic neutrality can help clinicians manage their intense and sometimes disorienting countertransference reactions and minimise the ego-boundary confusion commonly observed in individuals diagnosed with STPD (Stone, 1985). He particularly focused on some of the disorganised and cognitive perceptual symptoms of STPD, including paranoia, odd thinking and speech and magical thinking (Raine et al., 1994). Structured psychodynamic therapy may prove beneficial, but as Garrett and Turkington (2011) described, CBT approaches should be used first to strengthen the observing ego before moving on to psychodynamic work.

Implications

The impressive recovery as seen here supports the widespread use of modified CBT for psychosis in people with at-risk mental states, including those with schizotypal personality disorder. The client became more confident, returned to work and increased her quality of life without needing antipsychotic medication. This case study supports the conclusions of Ryan et al. (2013), recommending CBT tailored to the client's needs as a beneficial intervention for STPD. Importantly, our findings show that focusing on comorbid pathologies in people with elevated schizotypal traits is not enough. Instead, interventions must directly target positive and negative schizotypy. Until such time that we have a standardised, evidence-based treatment, early intervention consisting of low-intensity CBT integrating elements such as normalising and reality-testing may be useful in triggering a recovery trajectory. For this reason, in-depth training on working with people with schizotypal personality traits and trauma should be provided for mental health professionals working in at risk mental state services (ARMS).

Understanding schizotypy should not be limited to the mental health profession. As do people with other neurodivergent conditions such as autism or attention deficit hyperactivity disorder (ADHD), people on the schizotypy spectrum may feel ostracised by their peers. Adopting a social model when addressing the experience of people with schizotypy means acknowledging a different mode of being and changing the environment, for example, through destigmatising oddities and eccentricities, to allow people on the schizotypy spectrum to thrive. By raising awareness about living well with schizotypy and normalising this condition in schools and universities, we may prevent bullying and social isolation. As shown here, family and caregiver support and understanding are crucial in helping people with schizotypy in a crisis. This case study supports CBT-informed training aiming to increase the prosocial attitudes of carers and family members of people with schizotypy and psychosis (Psychosis REACH; Kopelovich et al., 2021). Therefore, public education campaigns may pave the way for those in need to be accepted and better supported in seeking help early to reduce the risk of conversion to psychosis.

References

Barrantes-Vidal, N., Gross, G. M., Sheinbaum, T., Mitjavila, M., Ballespí, S., & Kwapil, T. R. (2013). Positive and negative schizotypy are associated with prodromal and schizophrenia-spectrum symptoms. *Schizophrenia Research, 145*(1–3), 50–55.

Battaglia, M., Bernardeschi, L., Franchini, L., Bellodi, L., & Smeraldi, E. (1995). A family study of schizotypal disorder. *Schizophrenia Bulletin, 21*(1), 33–45.

Bebbington, P. E., Bhugra, D., Brugha, T., Singleton, N., Farrell, M., Jenkins, R., et al. (2004). Psychosis, victimisation and childhood disadvantage: Evidence from the second British National Survey of psychiatric morbidity. *The British Journal of Psychiatry, 185*(3), 220–226.

Beck, A. T. (Ed.). (1979). *Cognitive therapy of depression*. Guilford Press.

Berenbaum, H., Valera, E. M., & Kerns, J. G. (2003). Psychological trauma and schizotypal symptoms. *Schizophrenia Bulletin, 29*(1), 143–152.

Cheli, S. (2020). Assessment and treatment planning for schizotypal personality disorder: A metacognitively oriented point of view. *Psychiatric Rehabilitation Journal, 43*(4), 335.

Cheli, S., Lysaker, P. H., & Dimaggio, G. (2019). Metacognitively oriented psychotherapy for schizotypal personality disorder: A two-case series. *Personality and Mental Health, 13*(3), 155–167.

Chun, C. A., Brugger, P., & Kwapil, T. R. (2019). Aberrant salience across levels of processing in positive and negative schizotypy. *Frontiers in Psychology, 10*, 2073.

Debbané, M., Eliez, S., Badoud, D., Conus, P., Flückiger, R., & Schultze-Lutter, F. (2015). Developing psychosis and its risk states through the lens of schizotypy. *Schizophrenia Bulletin, 41*(suppl_2), S396–S407.

Dmitryeva, N., Chernov, N., Kostyuk, G., & Lysaker, P. H. (2021). Utilizing MERIT to promote recovery in schizotypal personality disorder: An illustrative case study. *Journal of Clinical Psychology, 77*(8), 1798–1806.

Ehlers, A., & Clark, D. M. (2000). A cognitive model of posttraumatic stress disorder. *Behaviour Research and Therapy, 38*(4), 319–345.

Flückiger, R., Ruhrmann, S., Debbané, M., Michel, C., Hubl, D., Schimmelmann, B. G., et al. (2016). Psychosis-predictive value of self-reported schizotypy in a clinical high-risk sample. *Journal of Abnormal Psychology, 125*(7), 923.

Garrett, M., & Turkington, D. (2011). CBT for psychosis in a psychoanalytic frame. *Psychosis, 3*(1), 2–13.

Grant, P. M., Huh, G. A., Perivoliotis, D., Stolar, N. M., & Beck, A. T. (2012). Randomized trial to evaluate the efficacy of cognitive therapy for low functioning patients with schizophrenia. *Archives of General Psychiatry, 69*, 121–127.

Green, M. J., Chia, T. Y., Cairns, M. J., Wu, J., Tooney, P. A., Scott, R. J., et al. (2014). Catechol-O-methyltransferase (COMT) genotype moderates the effects of childhood trauma on cognition and symptoms in schizophrenia. *Journal of Psychiatric Research, 49*, 43–50.

Gumley, A. I., Taylor, H. E. F., Schwannauer, M., & MacBeth, A. (2014). A systematic review of attachment and psychosis: Measurement, construct validity and outcomes. *Acta Psychiatrica Scandinavica, 129*(4), 257–274.

Hans, S. L., Auerbach, J. G., Nuechterlein, K. H., Asarnow, R. F., Asarnow, J., Styr, B., & Marcus, J. (2009). Neurodevelopmental factors associated with schizotypal symptoms among adolescents at risk for schizophrenia. *Development and Psychopathology, 21*(4), 1195–1210.

Keepers, G. A., Fochtmann, L. J., Anzia, J. M., Benjamin, S., Lyness, J. M., Mojtabai, R., et al. (2020). The American Psychiatric Association practice guideline for the treatment of patients with schizophrenia. *American Journal of Psychiatry, 177*(9), 868–872.

Kemp, K. C., Bathery, A. J., Barrantes-Vidal, N., & Kwapil, T. R. (2021). Positive, negative, and disorganized schizotypy predict differential patterns of interview-rated schizophrenia-spectrum symptoms and impairment. *Assessment, 28*(1), 141–152.

Kingdon, D., Turkington, D., & John, C. (1994). Cognitive behaviour therapy of schizophrenia: The amenability of delusions and hallucinations to reasoning. *The British Journal of Psychiatry, 164*(5), 581–587.

Kirchner, S. K., Roeh, A., Nolden, J., & Hasan, A. (2018). Diagnosis and treatment of schizotypal personality disorder: Evidence from a systematic review. *NPJ Schizophrenia, 4*(1), 1–18.

Kopelovich, S. L., Stiles, B., Monroe-DeVita, M., Hardy, K., Hallgren, K., & Turkington, D. (2021). Psychosis REACH: Effects of a brief CBT-informed training for family and caregivers of individuals with psychosis. *Psychiatric Services, 72*(11), 1254–1260.

Korver-Nieberg, N., Berry, K., Meijer, C. J., & De Haan, L. (2014). Adult attachment and psychotic phenomenology in clinical and non-clinical samples: A systematic review. *Psychology and Psychotherapy: Theory, Research and Practice, 87*(2), 127–154.

Kreyenbuhl, J., Buchanan, R. W., Dickerson, F. B., & Dixon, L. B. (2010). The schizophrenia patient outcomes research team (PORT): Updated treatment recommendations 2009. *Schizophrenia Bulletin, 36*(1), 94–103.

Kwapil, T. R., Barrantes-Vidal, N., & Silvia, P. J. (2008). The dimensional structure of the Wisconsin schizotypy scales: Factor identification and construct validity. *Schizophrenia Bulletin, 34*(3), 444–457.

Kwapil, T. R., Gross, G. M., Silvia, P. J., & Barrantes-Vidal, N. (2013). Prediction of psychopathology and functional impairment by positive and negative schizotypy in the Chapmans' ten-year longitudinal study. *Journal of Abnormal Psychology, 122*(3), 807.

Malik, N., Kingdon, D., Pelton, J., Mehta, R., & Turkington, D. (2009). Effectiveness of brief cognitive-behavioural therapy for schizophrenia delivered by mental health nurses: Relapse and recovery at 24 months. *Journal of Clinical Psychiatry, 70*(2), 201–207.

McClure, M. M., Graff, F., Triebwasser, J., Perez-Rodriguez, M., Rosell, D. R., Koenigsberg, H., et al. (2019). Guanfacine augmentation of a combined intervention of computerized cognitive remediation therapy and social skills training for schizotypal personality disorder. *American Journal of Psychiatry, 176*(4), 307–314.

McDonald, H., Babunashvili, M., Finn, A., Willard, A., Valmaggia, L., Chadwick, P., & Antonova, E. (2021). Positive schizotypy and the experience of creativity: The distinctive roles of suspiciousness and dispositional mindfulness. *Schizophrenia Research, 228*, 151–158.

Mckay, D., & Neziroglu, F. (1996). Social skills training in a case of obsessive-compulsive disorder with schizotypal personality disorder. *Journal of Behavior Therapy and Experimental Psychiatry, 27*(2), 189–194.

McKenna, P., Leucht, S., Jauhar, S., Laws, K., & Bighelli, I. (2019). The controversy about cognitive behavioural therapy for schizophrenia. *World Psychiatry, 18*(2), 235.

Morrison, A. (1998). A cognitive analysis of the maintenance of auditory hallucinations: Are voices to schizophrenia what bodily sensations are to panic? *Behavioural and Cognitive Psychotherapy, 26*, 289–302.

Morrison, A., Turkington, D., Pyle, M., Spencer, H., Brabban, A., Dunn, G., Christodoulides, T., Dudley, R., Chapman, N., Callcott, P., Grace, T., Lumley, V., Drage, L., Tully, S., Irving, K., Cummings, A., Byrne, R., Davies, L. M., & Hutton, P. (2014). Cognitive therapy for people with schizophrenia spectrum disorders not taking antipsychotic drugs: A single-blind randomised controlled trial. *The Lancet, 383*(9926), 1395–1403.

Nordentoft, M., Thorup, A., Petersen, L., Øhlenschlæger, J., Melau, M., Christensen, T. Ø., et al. (2006). Transition rates from schizotypal disorder to psychotic disorder for first-contact patients included in the OPUS trial. A randomized clinical trial of integrated treatment and standard treatment. *Schizophrenia Research, 83*(1), 29–40.

O'Kane, T. W., Sledjeski, E. M., & Dinzeo, T. J. (2022). The examination of sleep hygiene, quality of life, and schizotypy in young adults. *Journal of Psychiatric Research, 150*, 1–7.

Patel, V., & Saxena, S. (2014). Transforming lives, enhancing communities – Innovations in global mental health. *New England Journal of Medicine, 370*(6), 498–501.

Rado, S. (1953). Dynamics and classification of disordered behavior. *American Journal of Psychiatry, 110*(6), 406–416.

Raine, A., Reynolds, C., Lencz, T., Scerbo, A., Triphon, N., & Kim, D. (1994). Cognitive-perceptual, interpersonal, and disorganized features of schizotypal personality. *Schizophrenia Bulletin, 20*(1), 191–201.

Romme, M. A. J., Honig, A., Noorthoorn, E. O., & Escher, A. D. M. A. C. (1992). Coping with hearing voices: An emancipatory approach. *The British Journal of Psychiatry, 161*(1), 99–103.

Ryan, A., Macdonald, A., & Walker, E. (2013). The treatment of adolescents with schizotypal personality disorder and related conditions: A practice-oriented review of the literature. *Clinical Psychology: Science and Practice, 20*(4), 408.

Şahin, S., Yüksel, Ç., Güler, J., Karadayı, G., Akturan, E., Göde, E., et al. (2013). The history of childhood trauma among individuals with ultra high risk for psychosis is as common as among patients with first-episode schizophrenia. *Early Intervention in Psychiatry, 7*(4), 414–420.

Schürhoff, F., Laguerre, A., Fisher, H., Etain, B., Méary, A., Soussy, C., Szöke, A., & Leboyer, M. (2009). Self-reported childhood trauma correlates with schizotypal measures in schizophrenia but not bipolar pedigrees. *Psychological Medicine, 39*(3), 365–370.

Spauwen, J., Krabbendam, L., Lieb, R., Wittchen, H. U., & Van Os, J. (2006). Impact of psychological trauma on the development of psychotic symptoms: Relationship with psychosis proneness. *The British Journal of Psychiatry, 188*(6), 527–533.

Stone, M. (1985). Schizotypal personality: Psychotherapeutic aspects. *Schizophrenia Bulletin, 11*(4), 576–589.

Straub, K. T., & Kerns, J. G. (2021). Positive schizotypy, maladaptive openness, and openness facets. *Personality Disorders, Theory, Research, and Treatment, 12*(1), 51.

Torgersen, S., Lygren, S., Øien, P. A., Skre, I., Onstad, S., Edvardsen, J., et al. (2000). A twin study of personality disorders. *Comprehensive Psychiatry, 41*(6), 416–425.

Toutountzidis, D., Gale, T. M., Irvine, K., Sharma, S., & Laws, K. R. (2022). Childhood trauma and schizotypy in non-clinical samples: A systematic review and meta-analysis. *PLoS One, 17*(6), e0270494.

Turkington, D., Spencer, H., Lebert, L., & Dudley, R. (2017). Befriending: Active placebo or effective psychotherapy? *The British Journal of Psychiatry, 211*(1), 5–6.

Velligan, D. I., & Weiden, P. J. (2006). Interventions to improve adherence to antipsychotic medications. *Psychiatric Times, 23*(9), 50–50.

Woods, S. W., Addington, J., Cadenhead, K. S., Cannon, T. D., Cornblatt, B. A., Heinssen, R., et al. (2009). Validity of the prodromal risk syndrome for first psychosis: Findings from the North American Prodrome Longitudinal Study. *Schizophrenia Bulletin, 35*(5), 894–908.

Yen, S., Shea, M. T., Battle, C. L., Johnson, D. M., Zlotnick, C., Dolan-Sewell, R., Skodol, A. E., Grilo, C. M., Gunderson, J. G., Sanislow, C. A., & Zanarini, M. C. (2002). Traumatic exposure and posttraumatic stress disorder in borderline, schizotypal, avoidant, and obsessive-compulsive personality disorders: Findings from the collaborative longitudinal personality disorders study. *The Journal of Nervous and Mental Disease, 190*(8), 510–518.

Chapter 14
A Compassion-Focused Approach to Working with Problematic Belief Systems

Charles Heriot Maitland and Nicola Murphy

Introduction

- This chapter focuses on how compassion-focused therapy (CFT) can be used to work with unusual or problematic belief systems. CFT is a motivational, integrative and multimodal approach to human suffering, which has roots in neuroscience, evolutionary, social and developmental psychology (Gilbert, 2009; see section "Evolutionary Aspects of Schizotypy"). In clinical settings, unusual belief systems are often encountered among people who have a diagnosis of psychosis (i.e. the so-called 'delusions'); however, while this chapter refers frequently to the literature on CFT for psychosis, holding unusual beliefs is a transdiagnostic phenomenon, and indeed delusion-believing is found to exist on a continuum in the general population (Linscott & van Os, 2012; van Os et al., 2000). Unusual belief systems are linked to the dimension of 'positive schizotypy' and may range from magical thinking, to strongly held beliefs, to delusional ideation (Kemp et al., 2018). In the non-clinical population, beliefs constituting that of a delusion have been estimated at an annual prevalence rate of 5% (van Os et al., 2009). Bizarre delusions have been reported by around 2% of the general population, while paranoid delusions and delusions of having special powers had prevalence rates of 4–8% (Eaton et al., 1991). Magical thinking, the most common of which includes extra-sensory perception, precognitive dreams, contact with the dead or astrological beliefs, has been found to occur in 13–23% of the general population (Dagnall et al., 2016). People with intense spiritual or religious beliefs can have experiences akin to those diagnosed with

C. H. Maitland
Balanced Minds, Edinburgh, UK
e-mail: charlie@balancedminds.com

N. Murphy (✉)
Saint John of God Community Services, Dublin, Ireland

S. Cheli, P. H. Lysaker (eds.), *A Dimensional Approach to Schizotypy*,
https://doi.org/10.1007/978-3-031-41788-7_14

psychotic phenomena (Jackson & Fulford, 1997; Peters et al., 1999); however, in many cases, the experiences result in healthy and adaptive outcomes. Whether experiences meet clinical thresholds, or whether people seek help, can depend on factors such as level of intrusiveness, frequency and other forms of mental distress, together with personal and cultural factors such as coping, adaptive versus maladaptive appraisals, reasoning and cognitive biases, ability to process emotion, available social networks and societal acceptance/stigma (Heriot-Maitland & Peters, 2015; Johns & van Os, 2001). In this chapter, we regard the presence of unusual belief systems as being disconnected from pathology and that it is other biopsychosocial factors that determine pathology and clinical relevance.

Compassion as an Evolved Social Mentality

Social mentalities are the evolved motivational patterns that orientate our mind and body for certain *social* roles that are essential for survival (e.g. Gilbert, 1989/2016). In CFT, compassion is viewed as a social mentality, linked to the evolved motives for attachment and caring (Gilbert, 1989/2016), and is defined as a 'sensitivity to suffering in self and others with a commitment to try to relieve and prevent it' (Gilbert & Choden, 2013). Central to this definition are the two psychologies of compassion: (i) the motivation to notice and engage with the suffering in the self or another and (ii) the motivation to take action to prevent or alleviate suffering in oneself and others. Thus, in CFT, compassion is defined according to its underlying motivation, which can be thought of simply in terms of an 'if A then do B' algorithm, where 'A' would be some signal of distress or need and 'B' would be the supportive response (e.g. Gilbert, 2020). Like other motives, compassion can be switched on and cultivated. There is now considerable evidence that our brains and bodies flourish in environments where we feel cared for and about, and where we feel we can make a contribution that others value (e.g. Seppälä et al., 2017).

While we have physiological systems that facilitate compassion, we also possess physiological systems that facilitate threat perception, fight/flight responses and competitiveness. Of particular relevance to CFT models of psychosis are the social mentalities and systems that organise us in terms of social rank. When a social rank mentality is switched on, our minds become primed to detect information about the dominant, controlling or threatening intent of others. Where a person holds threat-based beliefs about others, the world or themselves, this may reflect their alignment to social-rank relationships. Low social rank is commonly linked to shame and submissive behaviour and can be associated with depression, anxiety (Birchwood et al., 2000) and 'positive symptoms' of psychosis (Wood & Irons, 2016). Shame may be focused internally (directed towards the self, e.g. 'I'm worthless') or externally ('I'm unacceptable to others'). Figure 14.1 illustrates a mentality organised by social rank, which organises attention, thinking, imagery, behaviour towards threat, danger and self-protection. This mentality may also focus memory on emotional

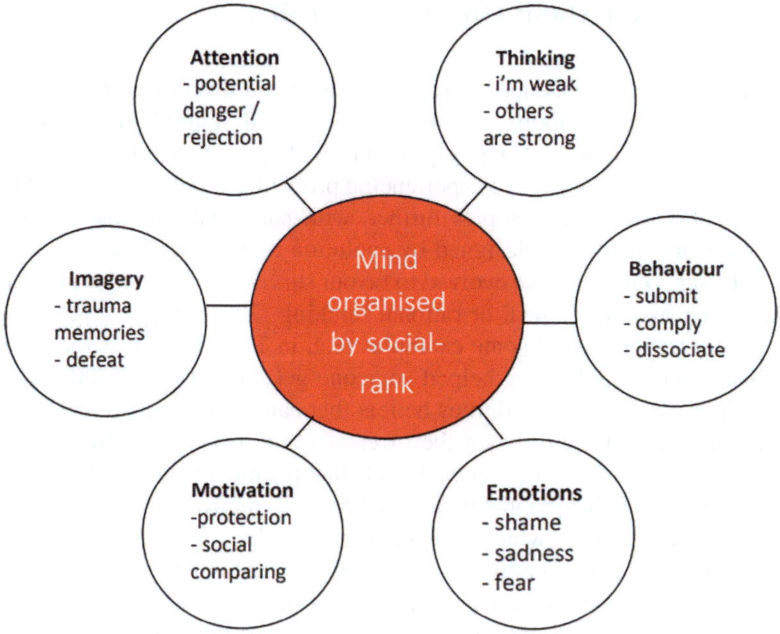
Attention
- potential
danger /
rejection
Thinking
- i'm weak
- others
are strong
Imagery
- trauma
memories
- defeat
Mind
organised
by social-
rank
Behaviour
- submit
- comply
- dissociate
Motivation
-protection
- social
comparing
Emotions
- shame
- sadness
- fear

Fig. 14.1 Social rank mentality. (© Charles Heriot-Maitland)

episodes of abuse and shame, increasing the possibility of sensory intrusions/ flashbacks.

Where care-based social mentalities are under-activated, under-developed or blocked (e.g. by experiences of early interpersonal trauma), threat-based social rank mentalities are likely to dominate. One of the key aims of CFT for psychosis is to help people to notice when their social rank patterns are switched on and to practice switching to (and training up) compassionate patterns. To achieve this, CFT seeks to understand and engage the various biological and psychological processes that support compassionate minds and compassionate relating to self and others (Heriot-Maitland, 2022). Studies looking at the application of CFT for people with psychosis suggest that this is a feasible and an acceptable therapeutic approach (Braehler et al., 2012; Mayhew & Gilbert, 2008). For the remainder of this chapter, we describe the key stages and processes of a CFT intervention for unusual or problematic belief systems, using case examples to illustrate CFT formulations of the possible function of beliefs, and the therapy techniques that might help to engage compassionate understanding and relating to the beliefs and what is behind them.

Psychoeducation About Our Tricky Brains

The standard CFT psychoeducation relating to an evolutionary understanding of the nature of 'tricky brains', 'loops', 'emotion systems' and 'multiple selves' (described fully in Gilbert & Simos, 2022) is helpful in providing a de-shaming context for the intervention. For people who are experiencing problematic belief systems, it may be useful to elaborate on these topics further, with particular examples of how our tricky brains are (naturally) designed by evolution to bias our thinking and frameworks of belief. Our brains are evolved to favour survival, safety and protection, and this will often override logical or rational thinking. The therapist might therefore ask the client to think about some examples (e.g. in TV shows, in stories or in real life) when a belief might have helped someone get through a difficult time. They may consider, for example, religious beliefs that can help someone feel a sense of guidance or companionship when they were feeling lost in their life (i.e. having faith). They may consider the magical beliefs that people often have after a bereavement, for example, believing that their loved one will return. They may consider the so-called 'placebo effect', which is an example of when a belief about receiving a treatment can itself lead to improved outcomes, even though no actual treatment has been received (i.e. the pill is just a sugar pill with no medicinal value). Another possible topic to consider may be the topic of visual illusions, which clearly demonstrate to us that what we experience as 'reality' is in fact constantly being constructed by our beliefs, expectations, predictions, motives and desires. Learning that our brains are tricky and that brains are forever bending and biasing our experiences and beliefs about the world should help the client to prepare for the formulation work (the next section) where that may start to become curious about the function (e.g. motivational or emotional function) of certain belief systems in the context of their lives. Importantly, throughout the psychoeducation, the message is not that our brains are broken or disordered, but that this is the very natural and normal operation of our evolved tricky brain, which is ultimately built for survival, rather than accuracy (better to be safe than sorry).

Formulation Focusing on the *Function* of Belief Systems

In CFT, we are interested in developing an understanding and empathy towards distress/suffering and the causes of this distress, and that is why CFT interventions are always built upon a solid psychoeducation and formulation that provide an understanding of the *function* of experiences, both in their evolutionary context (psychoeducation) and in the context of our personal lives (formulation). The psychoeducation helps us to understand how our brain patterns and emotions have evolved to perform certain functions, and the formulation helps us to understand some of the functional (often protective) strategies we have developed in our personal lives to deal with difficult experiences, challenges and threats. Together, the

CFT psychoeducation and formulation help to create an attitude of empathy and curiosity towards our distress and difficulties, which sees them as valid, functional and understandable. The idea of regarding difficulties (the so-called 'symptoms') as having a protective function also invites curiosity towards what we are being protected from, that is, the lived experiences, threats, memories and traumas that sit *behind* these strategies and are often driving them. Hence, the functional analysis approach in CFT formulation directs us towards the traumas, fears and vulnerabilities that are causing or underlying the distress – these are the parts that often need compassion the most. Heriot-Maitland (in press) has recently described some possible functions that certain belief systems may serve specifically in the context of trauma: (a) having an orientated and mobilised threat system, (b) managing overwhelming emotion and defeat states and (c) providing meaning and control. In this chapter, we touch on some of these themes as we discuss, with case illustrations, some examples of CFT formulations that focus on the possible function of belief systems:

When Rosie was 3 years old, she was diagnosed with tuberculosis. She was hospitalised for almost 2 years, mostly in isolation. Her parents were advised not to visit her to reduce the potential for 'unsettling' her. She frequently expressed emotional responses relating to terror, anger, despair and loneliness, which often resulting in her being strapped to the hospital bed until she 'calmed down' ('be a good girl'). Rosie learned that people were not to be trusted, that she should never display emotion and that she was better off alone. She struggled to form relationships with her peers, seeing danger in all social interactions….

External Threats: Belief Systems That Elicit Protective/ Submissive Responses to Avoid Harm from Other People

Common belief systems among clinical populations with psychosis involve paranoia or perception of threat or danger in objectively non-threatening situations. Where an individual's brain has been sensitised to social rank experiences through historical experiences of harm, danger or domination from others, it increases the likelihood that they will perceive the world as hostile and unsafe, priming them to perceptions of threat.

It is key to highlight that any threat-protective strategies the person developed to keep themselves safe (fight, flight, defeat, subordinate and freeze) should not be deemed pathological. Rather they were adaptive, in-built survival strategies that were engaged to enable their survival and safety. Also important to consider is that when faced with dominant, aggressive or frightening others, the person in the subordinate position will need to suppress the innate survival response to fight back in order to protect themselves from further harm (verbal or physical), avoid conflict and appease others (Pinto-Gouveia et al., 2014). Instead, a submissive, 'low rank', defensive response such as freeze/defeat is enacted, and a pattern can subsequently become established whereby the person suppresses their own healthy displays of anger in future confrontations (Gilbert & Irons, 2005). Rather than anger becoming directed outwards in retaliation to the other, it can get turned inwards, resulting in a highly critical inner world whereby danger and threat are inescapable. In CFT, anger is regarded as a healthy emotion to be honoured and felt, not soothed away or denied. Hence, the individual is supported to get in touch with healthy experiences and expressions of anger and to work through unprocessed rage towards those who have harmed them. This may help to 'unstick' the patterns of anger expression towards the self and reduce the likelihood that thwarted survival responses will keep getting played out in future encounters.

Internal Threats: Belief Systems That Orient the Mind and Avoid Difficult Emotions, Memories and Emotional Conflicts

For certain types of beliefs, as may be seen with grandiose beliefs, it is hypothesised that they may be psychologically adaptive, helping to manage overwhelmingly unpleasant emotions that would otherwise lead to depression and protect against negative self-perceptions and down-rank social comparisons with others (e.g. Bortoliotti, 2015). McKay and Dennett (2009) suggested that, in situations of extreme stress, people come to believe what they desire to be true and not what they have evidence for; it is not an evolutionary 'mistake'; rather, it is designed to avoid breakages that would have worse consequences for the person's self-esteem and well-being. The premise is that the person is already experiencing high levels of distress and can come to more serious harm unless her negative emotions are managed. Thus, the benefit here amounts to the prevention of more serious harm than the one the person is already experiencing. In other words, the adaptive misbelief is equivalent to an emergency response. This may be an effect of being overly located in the ranking system (Heriot-Maitland, 2022), in that if social motives such as caring and affiliation are not well developed, the individual has no other system available for processing social information, so getting pulled into a power dynamic.

Sometimes where beliefs are linked to ideas of reference, meaningful coincidences, synchronicities, some other spiritual ideas, magical thinking, etc., this might serve the function of providing a connection to a greater 'reality'. There may be a couple of things going on in such situations; first, this might be about having some direction and orientation in the world (to protect against disorientation/helplessness); second, there might be some comfort and reassurance in knowing that we are not alone (to protect against aloneness), we are connected to something greater, and we simply have to work out signs for how to access that desperately longed for truth and connection. Working with grief is a significant part of the CFT. Harris (2022) stressed the importance of addressing non-death losses (in the past and present), which may involve grieving the loss of hope, fantasies and ideals (Gilbert 2022). Gilbert highlighted the significance of grieving for unmet archetypal needs or archetypal relationships that were needed but never happened. Gilbert (1989/2016) referred to the yearning for social connectedness, safeness, to be wanted and to be loved. In the absence of the reality of such experiences, it may be that the person develops protective beliefs to protect them from the painful grief relating to the harsh reality of their relational experiences.

Milo's mother was diagnosed with schizophrenia before he was born and spent months in institutional care. His father walked out on them when he was 5 years old. Milo developed an active and a vivid fantasy world. As an adult, he developed a belief that his colleague at work, whom he hardly knew, had a deep love and attraction for him. When confronted, his colleague, who was shocked and perturbed, denied having any romantic feelings for him. Milo would not accept this and bombarded his colleague with text messages stating his belief that she loved him....

Naz's parents struggled financially, and both worked long hours to make ends meet. He and his siblings were expected to fend for themselves. Naz was a sensitive boy and often had nightmares at night. No one came to soothe him, and he often cried himself and went back to sleep. Naz was sexually abused by a neighbour when he was 10 years old. He came to believe that spirits would come and steal him away at night....

A key aspect of the CFT formulation is developing a curiosity about what might lies behind the belief system that the person holds, in terms of fears, avoidance and self-protective strategies. The kinds of prompt questions that might start to guide the process towards this direction are the following: What is this belief helping you with (now or in the past)? What was going on in your life when this belief started? If this belief was not there, what would you be left with? What would start to surface? What would be your concern if you could no longer have this belief system?

Within the CFT formulation, there is also a particular focus on incorporating the person's strengths and resiliency, making room for their own narrative.

CFT Processes to Prepare the Mind for Working with Problematic Belief Systems

Developing the Compassionate Self

Integral to any CFT/compassionate mind training (CMT) intervention is the development of a social mentality that holds the capacity to help rather than to harm. Significant investment is given to designing and cultivating the biopsychosocial conditions conducive to the provision of safeness, through the development of the concept of the 'compassionate self', a part of themselves that is sensitive to their distress and supports them to flourish. This, of course, relates to the care-giving mentality discussed earlier in this chapter. For those who have experienced little or no care or safety throughout their lives, or multiple experiences of harm, the concept of a 'compassionate mind' may seem alien or threatening. Working with the fears and blocks to compassion is a fundamental part of the work (Matos et al., 2022; Steindl et al., 2022), as discussed later in this chapter.

Clients are invited to engage in role-play, and method acting techniques are utilised to support the practice of 'stepping into' the compassionate self.

Figure 14.2 illustrates the ways in which a client can be supported to develop a compassionate mind set. The client is invited to work through each of the components to generate their own ways of growing and strengthening a 'compassionate mind'.

Establishing Safeness: Internal and External

The process of building safeness is ongoing throughout the therapy. When people are experiencing distressing beliefs, particularly when relational trauma is involved, supporting the development of social safeness is a key priority. We can cultivate social safeness externally (via relationships, social networks, connecting activities, such as dancing and singing and supportive environments) and/or internally (via self–self relating, together with supportive practices such as breath work, grounding, posture and imagery) (Heriot-Maitland, 2018). Disentangling 'safety' and 'safeness' is important in the CFT. Safety tends to relate to the threat system (protection from a potential harm, with attention focused on keeping ourselves safe). Safeness, however, occurs when there is a sense of feeling secure and safe in us, with an openness to experience and curiosity to explore. This is more linked to experiences of calm and groundedness in the soothing system. Clients are encouraged to recognise their strengths and blocks that arise within each of their flows of compassion and to develop them over the course of the therapy.

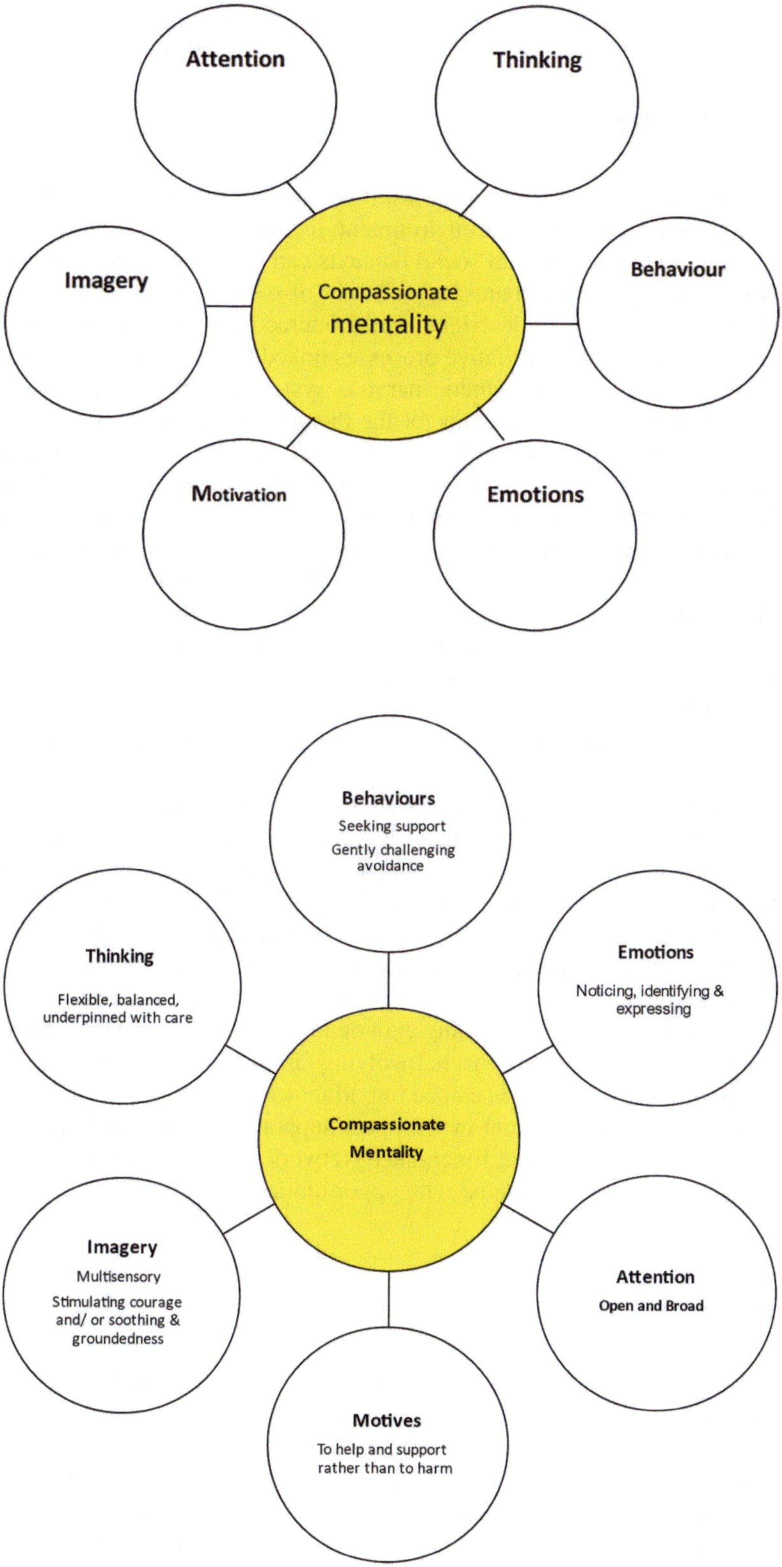

Fig. 14.2 A working example of a compassionate mentality. (© Charles Heriot-Maitland)

External Safeness

From the start of the therapeutic process, it can be helpful to consider the client's level of connectedness with their environment, including family, friends, peers and communities. Relationships and social contexts can be a key aspect of supporting the key CFT therapeutic mechanisms/processes of social safeness and compassion (Heriot-Maitland, 2018). As described, social interactions can help to stimulate the 'soothing system' through affiliative processes linked to attachment. Affiliation can help to activate the parasympathetic nervous system branch to support slowing, calming and settling. It is important for the therapist to be aware of when experiences of social attachment and affiliation may not activate soothing/safeness system, but rather the threat system. This may relate to the attachment system becoming associated with threat, due to conditioning in early life relationships, particularly where caregivers have been unavailable or a source of danger. In the CFT, the therapist may aim to support the person to increase their capacity for affiliative relating through gradual exposure to social connection. Some of the exercises described below aimed at supporting internal safeness may be very important from the outset, particularly if the person is very distressed or overwhelmed by their experiences. As discussed by Petrocchi et al. (2022), body-based practices, such as yoga and tai chi, may be helpful with assisting the development of prosocial intentions for both ourselves and others not only via increased vagal activity and self-regulation (Sullivan et al., 2018), but also through improved self-awareness and interoception (see Petrocchi et al., 2022). In addition, exposure to nature and green environments, such as forest bathing, may have a positive impact on the body's felt sense of safeness, for example, by influencing heart rate variability (HRV; Petrocchi et al., 2022).

Supporting the client to develop real-world opportunities to develop social safeness and connection is a key aspect of the CFT, building on the three flows of compassion. This relational context fits well with social network approaches designed for people with unusual or distressing experiences, such as Open Dialogue and the National Paranoia Network approach. Involving families, friends and other involved professionals in the intervention can be important for enhancing connectedness and social safeness. Linking a client in with peer support networks, such the Spiritual Crisis Network or the Spiritual Emergence Network, may be helpful for providing a normalising, de-shaming context with opportunities for connection.

Internal Safeness

Various body-based practices are used to support the building of physiological patterns involved in building a compassionate mind, often referred to in the CFT as 'using the body to support the mind'. Using exercises to tone up the vagus nerve can lead to a felt sense of safeness in the body. The myelinated vagus nerve is proposed to function as an active vagal brake that actively inhibits the sympathetic nervous system's influences on the heart and dampens hypothalamic–pituitary–adrenal (HPA) axis activity (see Porges, 2001). The vagal brake promotes self-soothing behaviours and calm states, facilitating the enactment of social engagement behaviours (Porges, 2007). Given that various muscles involved in facial expression, speech and breath work are connected with the vagus nerve, it is proposed that vagal tone can be improved by engaging the body in particular postures and practices, together with exploring the senses to bring grounding and presence.

Box 14.1 Developing Internal Safeness

Developing soothing rhythm breathing: A practice shown to increase heart rate variability (HRV). High HRV has been shown to be associated with improved emotion regulation, decision-making and attention (Thayer et al., 2009).

Experiment with body language, including posture, facial expressions, voice modulation and tone: Walking tall, head held high, bringing a friendly facial expression and openness to the chest to allow for greater ease of breathing. Imagining the body as strong and solid, like a mountain or a tall, rooted tree, with affect and voice tone to reflect care and concern.

Consider compassionate motives: We have compassion when we intentionally and knowingly choose to address suffering. Developing a compassionate self-identity involves making a choice to 'live to be helpful not harmful to self and others' (Gilbert, 2020).

Explore core qualities of compassion: With focus on wisdom, strength and courage. Having a compassionate mind set is not about being calm at all times, but rather to have the courage and strength to face what is challenging and the wisdom to make choices to support, not to harm.

Engagement and action skills: The 'compassionate self' can act as a vehicle through which to start to engage with the function of beliefs and provides a secure base from which to engage with and process memories and emotions associated with trauma.

Use of imagery: Images can be used to stimulate a felt sense of safeness to support the development of care-giving/care-receiving motives (See Irons & Beaumont, 2017), for example, calm place imagery, compassionate colour imagery & compassionate other/ perfect nurturer imagery (Lee, 2005).

The compassionate kitbag (Lucre & Corten, 2013; Lucre & Clapton, 2020): Developing a compassionate mind, with its associated motives, behaviours and practices, is not a set of skills that one acquires and then retains for life, but rather nurtures over one's lifetime. This may be supported through a collection of tangible and imaginal items, which can represent transitional objects for the client. The kitbag may contain concrete representations of items that stimulate soothing and slowing down, but also items that stimulate courage. Clients are invited to use all of the senses when identifying items, for example, crystals or pebbles, photographs of supportive figures, including pets, soft toys, fabrics, scents associated with pleasant memories (e.g. sun cream) or that ignite feelings of vigour (e.g. peppermint oil); supportive comments made by others; a cue to remind them of their compassionate other image or calm place; and playlists that stimulate energy and bravery or that calm and soothe.

Fears, Blocks and Resistances (FBRs)

As we have mentioned, the process of giving and receiving care can feel challenging for both the client and therapist at times. This is, in part, because caring strategies both evolved, and work best, in trusting environments. Often our clients come from environments that can be hostile, unpredictable or neglectful, where associations with both care provision and receiving can be negative and unpleasant (Gilbert, 2020). As such, FBRs can develop to particular emotions and motives. Moreover, there may be times when the therapist or CFT procedures may unwittingly trigger experiences of shame, self-consciousness or humiliation, as a consequence of activating an attachment system whereby safeness/care has been associated with harm or trauma (Matos et al., 2022). Understanding the client's FBRs to compassion is deemed essential to the success of the therapy and is key to preventing and repairing ruptures in the therapeutic relationship (Gilbert, 2020). Gilbert stressed that FBRs are 'protections rather than problems' to be solved (Gilbert, 2020). The downsides of avoiding FBRs, or indeed the cultivation of a compassionate mind set, are that clients are 'cut off from all of those potentially helpful emotion regulating processes linked to secure base, safe haven, and their physiological substrates' (Gilbert, 2020, p. 24). Recent studies (Matos et al. (2022) and Steindl et al. (2022)) have informed some preliminary guidelines for working with FBRs in the CFT, some of which are outlined in Box 14.2.

Box 14.2 Working with FBRs

- Before teaching the client about compassion, the therapist must begin their work with the client in the care and attachment system (Gilbert, 2020). Avoidant attachment styles close the care-seeking mentality down (Gilbert & Simos, 2022). A key aim is to cultivate safeness and connection within the therapeutic relationship, which can offer a powerful relational place for the client to feel valued and respected, where trust and courage can develop.
- The therapist's own ability to access feelings of safeness prior to and during therapeutic encounters is crucial. Developing one's own repertoire of self-regulatory strategies (e.g. through the use of supportive breath work, e.g. 'cyclic sighing' (Balban et al., 2023); compassionate imagery; and supportive body-based practices (e.g. Clapton & Hiskey, 2023; Cuddy, 2012; Dana, 2020)) can support a process of co-regulation with the client, whereby the therapist's presence will directly impact the client's felt sense of safeness.
- Developing a shared case formulation, including functions and origins of FBRs, can help to provide a validating and de-shaming context. Psychoeducation, particularly debunking myths around compassion as weak/self-indulgent/having to be nice/not getting angry, can support this process (see Irons & Beaumont, 2017).

- Addressing FBRs directly through experiential interventions, for example, increasing the felt sense of safeness and capacity for compassion through body-based and imagery-based practices, and then addressing FBRs directly through chair work, imagery, letter writing and method acting. For those from harsh or punitive backgrounds, interest and excitement can be difficult for them due to little exposure to playfulness, parental interest or enthusiasm. Gently bringing playfulness into the therapy room can be an important aspect of experiential interventions (Gilbert, 2022). The pacing of such experiential practices can be important, for example, using the metaphor of the "compassionate ladder" (see Irons & Beaumont, 2017).
- Crucially it may be important to stress that learning the abilities to feel compassion can take time. Gently highlighting (e.g. through psycho-education and multiple selves work) that this can be linked to the ability to tolerate sadness and to grieve (or rage) for the life/love/experiences they wanted but did not have can be important for working through their FBRs (Gilbert & Irons, 2005).

Preparing Our Compassionate Mind for What Is *Behind* the Belief System

In CFT, time and care is spent tuning up the psychophysiological systems and neural pathways associated with compassion. Often clients are reminded that just as physical fitness needs practice, commitment, fine-tuning and repetition, so too does the practice of compassion. In those who experience disturbing beliefs about the world, pre-existing patterns can be heavily shaped by threat and trauma and can take time and commitment to re-train compassionate patterns. Importantly, it is not just about training compassionate patterns and pathways, but also about reducing threat-protection/harm avoidance patterns.

As we have discussed, firmly held beliefs developed to serve an important protective function at some stage in the individual's life. It is vital to keep in mind that there may be a vulnerability lying behind the belief that the client is terrified to engage with.

Box 14.3 shows some examples of how the compassionate self may be used to engage with protective beliefs, with a particular attention paid to what is behind them. In the following section, we will return to demonstrate how the CFT uses therapy techniques such as chair work and imagery to support the process of compassionately relating to parts and to the threats/vulnerabilities that are being protected by the belief system.

Box 14.3 Compassion for Parts That Hold the Beliefs

Functions of belief system	Response from the 'compassionate self' to the part that holds the belief and the function
Beliefs to activate my threatdetection and response systems	*Engagement*: 'I can see why you've been holding on to this belief that keeps me alert to danger. People have been scary, and I needed protection.' *Action*: 'I can start to find the courage to trust people more and to learn how to set boundaries'.
Beliefs to provide orientation and a sense of control in the world	*Engagement*: 'Thank you for holding this belief when I felt so lost in the world; I know you were trying to help me to keep going in life with some purpose'. *Action*: 'I am starting to think about what I want in life, and what my goals are. I am ready to start choosing my own purpose and direction'.
Beliefs to protect against feelings of grief/loss	*Engagement*: 'I understand why you have been holding this belief because it was too early and painful, and I wasn't ready to grieve. It felt too much and as though it would overwhelm me'. *Action*: 'I will take time with this, there is no rush. And when I'm ready I will slowly start to feel into my pain and to grieve for my loss in order to heal'.

Credit to Heriot-Maitland (2022)

Case Examples: Bringing the Compassionate Mind to a Formulation

We now present three people (**Michael, Neenah** and **Layla**) to illustrate how CFT interventions might proceed directly from the formulation of different functions associated with their beliefs.

Michael

Michael, a 28-year-old man, presented to services due to feeling overwhelmed by distressing thoughts and isolation. He was fearful of close relationships. He did not share his innermost thoughts or feeling with anybody. He believed he had special powers or abilities, such as the capacity to read people's minds. He believed that aliens from other galaxies had shown him the gifts he possessed as part of a special mission he had been sent on to bring harmony to the lives of human beings.

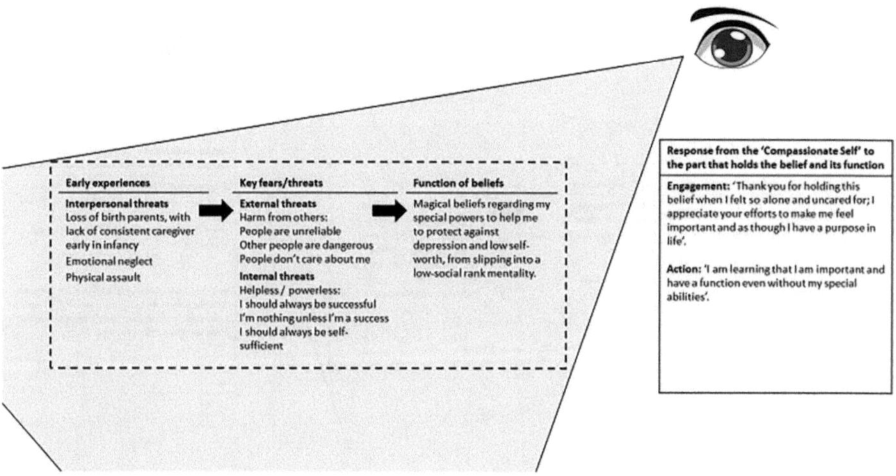

Fig. 14.3 Michael's CFT formulation, with responses from his compassionate self. (© Charles Heriot-Maitland)

Michael was adopted from an orphanage aged 8 months. His adoptive parents provided him with all he needed on a material level but lacked warmth. They did not like to talk about emotions and could be critical of his behaviour and choices. He was praised and held in high esteem when achieving; however, when he was not, he was shunned. Michael was physically assaulted during an unprovoked attack aged 20 years. He was so ashamed; he never spoke of it to anyone.

Michael's Formulation

We formulated how the establishment of Michael's beliefs may be linked to his key threats/fears (external: people leave me, people harm me, and trust no one; and internal: I'm nothing unless I'm achieving) that related to his early life experiences of being abandoned as an infant and being raised in a family where the only validation he received occurred when he was achieving. Michael developed an understanding that his beliefs were protective to him in some way to alert him to possible threats in the world and to protect him from difficult emotions. Figure 14.3 provides a summary of the formulation of the protective processes that may be operating within Michael's problematic beliefs. It also illustrates how Michael's compassionate self i) brings understanding and empathy to these functions (engagement) and ii) sets an intention to help (action), a process that may be facilitated through chair work, letter writing or imagery (see later in this chapter).

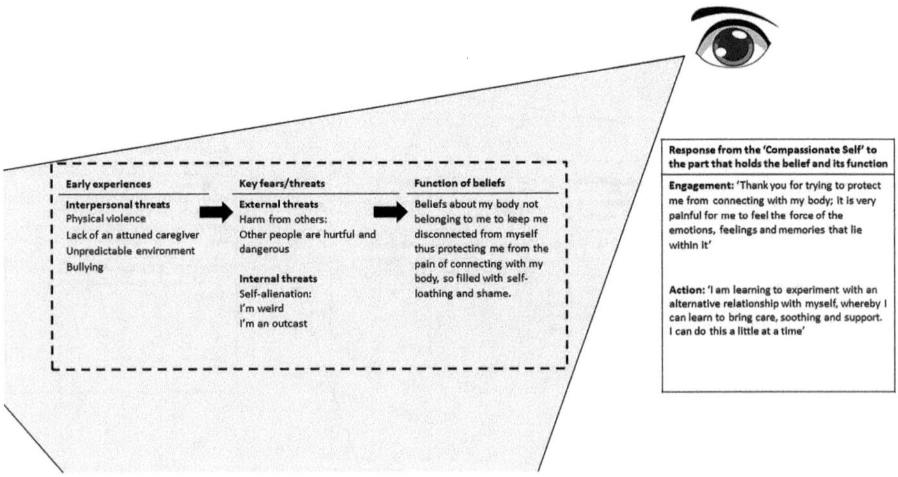

Fig. 14.4 Neenah's CFT formulation, with responses from her compassionate self

Neenah

Neenah, a 35-year-old woman, sought help for panic attacks relating to the belief that her body was no longer her own; parts of her body would disappear when she looked in the mirror.
Neenah's father was alcohol-dependent and violent. Her mother was kind but so fearful and preoccupied with her father's behaviour that she could afford little attunement to Neenah's needs. She was shy and struggled to form connections with people. Neenah was severely bullied throughout her childhood; she was told by her peers that she was weird, fat and ugly.

Neenah's Formulation

We formulated that Neenah's beliefs may be linked to her key threats/fears (external: people hurt and harm me, people are dangerous; and internal: 'I'm weird', 'I'm an outcast') that related to her early life experiences of not having been truly 'seen' or attuned to, together with being badly bullied by her peers. Neenah developed an understanding that her beliefs were protective to him in some way to alert her to possible threats in the world and to protect her from difficult emotions. Figure 14.4 provides a summary of the formulation of Neenah's problematic beliefs. It also outlines Neenah's compassionate engagement and action with her beliefs.

Layla

Layla is a 19-year-old young woman. She was highly self-critical and described herself as a 'loner', always having struggled to make friends. Social situations were anxiety-provoking for her, and yet, she was lonely. She was shy and mistrustful of others. She believed people, even strangers, treated her with suspicion and disdain, crossing the road to avoid her or averting their gaze when she looked at them. Sometimes she felt that the presence of other people caused her to feel physically weakened. She developed beliefs in a conspiracy to harm her, only to be offered protection by the presence of her dead mother whom she believed was not actually dead but had been sent away by her father.
Layla suffered significant interpersonal trauma. Her mother died when Layla was 9 years old, leaving her in the care of her father who quickly remarried. She felt unwanted and a 'misfit'. She ran away from home aged 12 years and subsequently spent time in the looked-after system where she struggled to form any meaningful connections.

Layla's Formulation

We formulated that the origins of Layla's beliefs may be linked to her key threats/fears (external: trust no one, people leave me; and internal: my feelings and experiences will overwhelm me; trust no one) that related to her early life experiences of parental death, bullying and a lack of a secure base/safe haven. Layla developed an understanding that her beliefs were protective to her in some way to alert him to possible threats in the world and to protect her from difficult emotions.

Figure 14.5 provides a summary of the formulation of the protective function of Layla's problematic beliefs, together with compassionate engagement and action with these beliefs.

CFT Techniques for Compassionate Relating

Multiple Selves and Parts Work

Rather than viewing the self as a unitary concept, in CFT, the self is regarded as a set of mixed motives, emotions and algorithms. Socratic questions are used to support the individual to start to identify their different parts (which may be emotions, beliefs or motives) through guided discovery. Often, we start with what Gilbert (2020) refers to as 'the big three' threat-based emotions of anger, anxiety and sadness, referring to these as the 'angry self', 'anxious self' and 'sad self', and about how these parts work together and conflict with each other, for example, 'How does sad self feel about angry self?' Over time, the client learns about the different

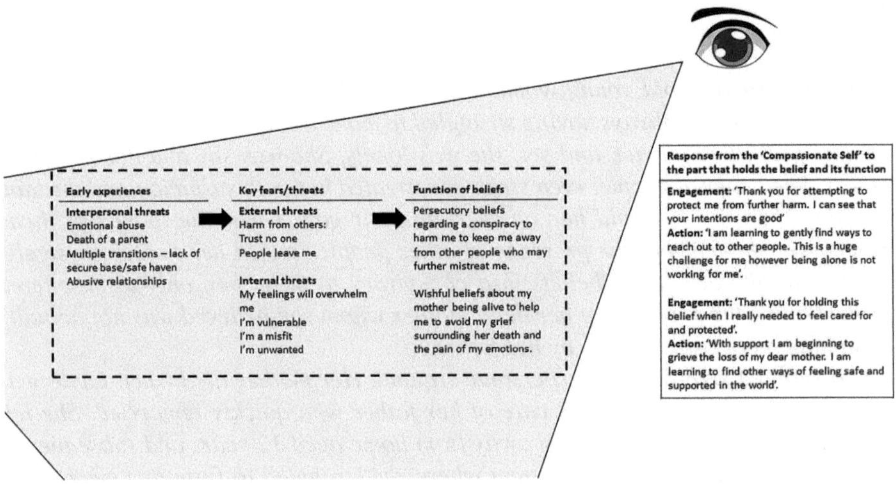

Fig. 14.5 Layla's CFT formulation, with responses from her compassionate self: © Charles Heriot-Maitland

functions of their emotional 'parts'. This process can be effectively facilitated though the use of chair work, whereby a different chair is used to represent each of the 'parts'. Some clients may be able to mentalise their different 'parts' using their imagination. Once different selves have been identified, they may be mapped out on a sheet of paper, which can be added to as different 'parts' are discovered over the course of the intervention (see Box 14.4).

For people who experience problematic belief systems, there may be conflicting parts of the self that are holding on tightly to a belief. It is important to note that these might also be parts of the self that have been split off/dissociated/avoided or parts that are being protected by the beliefs. There may be experiences of grief, rage, fear, shame or regret. Exploring these underlying emotions and corresponding motives and physiological patterns can be key to supporting the client to make sense of (and perhaps let go of) a belief system that is harming them.

Over time, the therapist will support the client to engage with their different 'parts' from the perspective of their compassionate self, for example, 'How would compassionate self support angry self/anxious self/sad self?'. The therapist tries to avoid instructing the client how to relate to their parts but rather uses socratic questioning and guided discovery to support them to generate their own ideas, from a place of wisdom and courage. Clients may be invited to imagine the different parts as guests at a dinner party, or crew members on a ship, with the compassionate self as the host or the captain. They may be asked to consider how the host or the captain may show up for and support each of its guests/crew, without trying to soothe away their pain.

Box 14.4 illustrates the use of a visual map to represent relationships between different parts.

This process of mapping, profiling and enquiring about the nature and function of the individual's experiences helps to support the development of a shift in mind set, away from threat and harm avoidance, towards a compassionate mentality.

Let us return to **Neenah**, whom we met earlier in the chapter, to help us to illustrate this process. Box 14.4 shows that a visual map was used to represent the relationships between Neenah's different parts. In Box 14.4a, you can see that her anxious self is big and close to her, highlighting how easily accessible anxiety is to her. Her angry self is smaller and further away, while her sad self is smaller still, representing the fact that anger and especially sadness are much harder for her to access. In Box 14.4b, the 'disconnected' and paranoid parts are shown to be protecting Neenah from accessing her traumatised part and feelings of grief. In Box 14.4c, the compassionate self is introduced. This is developed and practiced until it is ready to be positioned as the central 'self', from which the therapeutic work is directed. Box 14.4d illustrates how Neenah's multiple selves are arranged in a semicircle around her compassionate self. None of the parts are removed, but rather each is recognised and held in equal value; each has an important message to communicate, but no part is dominant or held in lower value. This exercise of mapping and profiling the different parts can support the client to hold a different relationship with their distressing experiences, shifting mind set from threat protection to empathic curiosity. This helps to pave the way for a shift in mind set/motivation towards compassion.

Box 14.4 Mapping Relationships Between Neenah's Parts (© Charles Heriot-Maitland)

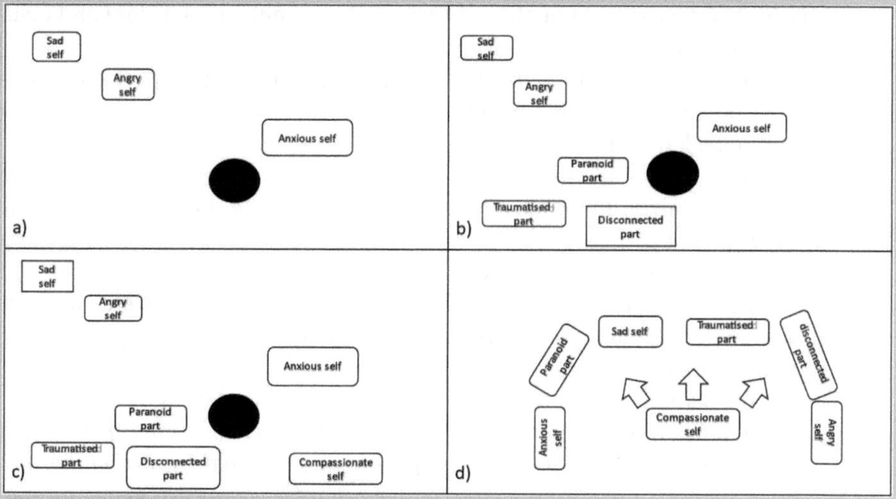

Compassionate Letter Writing

Compassionate letter writing is another method regularly utilised in CFT. In this instance, the individual may write from the position of their compassionate self to a particular troublesome belief, bringing empathy, wisdom and understanding for the reasons the belief(s) developed and highlighting the importance of its protective function. Some possible steps for this process have been outlined by Irons & Beaumont (2017). These steps are summarised in Box 14.5, incorporating ideas from our client, *Layla*.

Working with Trauma Memories/Traumatised Parts

Once the individual has a well-developed felt-sense of their compassionate self and has other imaginal (e.g. compassionate other/perfect nurturer image) and more tangible (e.g. the compassionate kitbag) methods of tapping psychological safeness, they may be ready to extend interventions to work with younger parts that have experienced trauma or to work with specific trauma-based memories. Without engaging with these parts and/or memories, the distressing beliefs may persist.

Box 14.5 Compassionate Letter Writing Steps

1. Engage compassionate mind (connect to compassionate self using posture, breathing, imagery).

Consider compassionate qualities of caring – commitment, wisdom and courage/strength.

2. Connect with motivation to write this letter, e.g. to bring support and understanding to the identified belief.
3. Begin the letter identifying the particular difficulty:

Dear Layla, I know that life feels tough for you right now as you have been struggling with these terrifying thoughts relating to a conspiracy to harm you.

4. Bring validation and empathy for the struggle:

It is understandable that you are finding things difficult. You were raised to believe people would leave you or harm you and that other people were not to be trusted.

5. Understanding of your attempts to manage your threat system:

It makes sense that you developed protective beliefs that served to keep you away from people to prevent you from being exposed to further harm. I know that you have been trying to avoid painful feelings of grief and sad-

ness by focusing all of your attention on making sense of this conspiracy. It is not your fault that you have been coping in this way – you were never taught how to deal with painful feelings.

6. Taking responsibility – tapping into strength and wisdom:

I can see that it is not your fault that you have avoided facing your grief; however, it is your responsibility now to begin to work through the issues that have caused you pain. Engaging your wisdom and strength may help you to think about and feel into how to do things differently.

7. Exploring how to help – compassionate thoughts and behaviours, Engaging the compassionate mind to generate ways to bring support:

I know you are hard on yourself for being so wary of people, but it is important to acknowledge that you are lonely and would like to feel a part of something different. Don't forget how much you achieved in your life despite the setbacks. Perhaps you might consider an evening class as a first step in being part of something in your community. Your therapist might help you to find a support group where you may meet others who have had experiences like you. Let's start small, and remember you are not alone.

8. Working with difficulties and setbacks:

There may be times when your worries about other people become too hard to tolerate. Remember that there are things you have learned that can support you, such as practicing soothing rhythm breathing and imagining your perfect nurturer. It may be helpful to share concerns with your therapist as they arise so that you do not fall back into the pattern of avoiding situations and painful emotions.

9. Compassionate commitment to change:

Hold in mind your caring commitment to look after yourself and bring about positive changes. I am here for you and will always be available for support and encouragement if you choose to engage with me. I wish you the best of luck, your loving compassionate self.

Compassionate letter writing may be used to write to younger, traumatised parts from the standpoint of the compassionate self or from angry self to the dominant/abusive other, supporting the client to connect with emotion that may have become dissociated during experiences of trauma. Alternatively, imagery re-scripting may be used with trauma memories whereby the compassionate self or the perfect nurturer image enters the visual scene to support the client in the way that they deserved but did not receive. Clients are encouraged to be a creative and fantastical as they wish with this process (see Lee, 2005).

Any trauma-focused intervention should be carefully planned, formulation-driven, with clear consideration regarding the readiness and necessity of the intervention at this stage in the therapy process.

Compassionate Relating in Every-Day Life

The goal of therapy is ultimately that the client's compassionate self becomes their own internal 'therapist' and guides in their own daily life. Flashcards, compassion diaries and embodied (compassionate self) practices can be a useful way of helping the client bring compassion into day-to-day situations (see Heriot-Maitland, 2018, 2022).

Summary

A common feature of schizotypy is the experience of holding belief systems that are unusual, distressing or problematic to the individual in terms of the impact they can have on their sense of connectedness with themselves and others. This chapter outlines how CFT can be used to work with such beliefs/thinking styles, in particular, to support the person to increase their understanding of the protective function of their beliefs, to develop internal and external experiences of 'safeness' and threat-regulatory capacity and to work with parts of themselves that have become split off, suppressed or over-inflated.

References

Balban, M.Y., Neri, E., Kogon, M.M., Weed, L., Nouriani, B., Jo, B., Holl, G., Zeitzer, J. M., Spiegel, D. & Huberman, A. D. (2023). Brief structured respiration practices enhance mood and reduce physiological arousal. *Cell Reports Medicine, 4*(1).

Birchwood, M., Meaden, A., Trower, P., Gilbert, P., & Plaistow, J. (2000). The power and omnipotence of voices: Subordination and entrapment by voices and significant others. *Psychological Medicine, 2*, 337–344.

Bortoliotti, L. (2015). The epistemic innocence of motivated delusions. *Consciousness and Cognition, 33*, 490–499.

Braehler, C., Gumley, A., Harper, J., Wallace, S., Norrie, J., & Gilbert, P. (2012). Exploring change processes in compassion focused therapy in psychosis: Results of a feasibility randomized controlled trial. *British Journal of Clinical Psychology, 52*, 199–214.

Clapton, N., & Hiskey, S. (2023). The way is in training: Martial arts-informed compassionate mind training to enhance CFT therapists' compassionate competencies. *OBM Integrative and Complementary Medicine, 8*(1), 19.

Cuddy, A. (2012). Your body language may shape who you are. *TED Conferences*. https://www.ted.com/talks/amy_cuddy_your_body_language_may_shape_who_you_are?utm_campaign=tedspread&utm_medium=referral&utm_source=tedcomshare

Dagnall, N. A., Drinkwater, K., Parker, A., & Clough, P. (2016). Paranormal experience, belief in the paranormal and anomalous beliefs. *Paranthropology, 7*, 4–15.

Dana, D. (2020). *Polyvagal exercises for safety and connection: 50 client-centered practices*. W. W. Norton & Co.

Eaton, W. W., Romanoski, A., Anthony, J. C., & Nestadt, G. (1991). Screening for psychosis in the general population with a self-report interview. *Journal of Nervous and Mental Disease, 179*(11), 689–693.

Gilbert, P. (1989/2016). *Human nature and suffering*. Routledge.
Gilbert, P. (2009). *The compassionate mind: A new approach to the challenge of life*. London: Constable & Robinson.
Gilbert, P. (2020). Evolutionary functional analysis: The study of social mentalities, social rank and caring-compassion. In J. N. Kirby & P. Gilbert (Eds.), *Making an impact on mental health* (pp. 4–42). Routledge.
Gilbert, P., & Choden. (2013). *Mindful compassion*. Constable and Robinson.
Gilbert, P. & Irons, C. (2005). Focused therapies and compassionate mind training for shame and self attacking. In P. Gilbert (Ed.), *Compassion: conceptualisations, research and use in Psychotherapy*, (pp. 263–325). London, UK: Routledge.
Gilbert, P., & Simos, G. (2022). *Compassion focused therapy: Clinical practice and applications* (1st ed.). Routledge.
Heriot-Maitland, C. (2018). *CFT for psychosis – Manual*. http://compassionforvoices.com/CFTpManual
Heriot-Maitland, C. (2022).Compassion focused therapy for voice hearing and delusions in psychosis. In P. Gilbert & G. Simos (Eds.), *Compassion Focused Therapy: Clinical Practice and Applications*, (1st ed., pp. 549–654). London, UK: Routledge.
Heriot-Maitland, C. (In press). Trauma and delusions, in K. Hardy and D. Turkington (Eds) Decoding delusions. American Psychiatric Association.
Heriot-Maitland, C., & Peters, E. R. (2015). Dimensional approaches to delusional beliefs. In O. Mason & G. Claridge (Eds.), *Series: Advances in mental health research*. Routledge.
Irons, C., & Beaumont, E. (2017). *The Compassionate Mind Workbook: A step-by-step guide to developing your compassionate self*. Robinson.
Jackson, M. C., & Fulford, K. W. M. (1997). Spiritual experience and psychopathology. *Philosophy, Psychiatry, and Psychology, 4*(1), 41–65.
Johns, C., & van Os, J. (2001). The continuity of psychotic experiences in the general population. *Clinical Psychology Review, 21*(8), 1125–1141.
Kemp, K. C., Gross, G. M., Barrantes-Vidal, N., & Kwapil, T. R. (2018). Association of positive, negative, and disorganized schizotypy dimensions with affective symptoms and experiences. *Psychiatry Research, 270*, 1143–1149.
Lee, D. A. (2005). The perfect nurturer. A model to develop a compassionate mind within the context of cognitive therapy. In P. Gilbert (Ed.), *Compassion: Conceptualisations, research and use in psychotherapy* (pp. 326–352). Routledge. eBook ISBN 9780203003459.
Linscott, R. J., & Van Os, J. (2012). An updated and conservative systematic review and meta-analysis of epidemiological evidence on psychotic experiences in children and adults: On the pathway from proneness to persistence to dimensional expression across mental disorders. *Psychological Medicine*, 1–17.
Lucre, K., & Clapton N. (2020). The compassionate kitbag: A creative and integrative approach to compassion-focused therapy. *Psychology and Psychotherapy, 94*(52), 497–516. e12291. https://doi.org/10.1111/papt.12291
Lucre, K. M., & Corten, N. (2013). An exploration of group compassion-focused therapy for personality disorder. *Psychology and Psychotherapy: Theory, Research and Practice, 86*(4), 387–400. https://doi.org/10.1111/j.2044-8341.2012.02068.x
Matos, M., Petrocchi, N., Irons, C., & Steindl, S. R. (2022). Never underestimate fears, blocks, and resistances: The interplay between experiential practices, self-conscious emotions, and the therapeutic relationship in compassion focused therapy. *Journal of Clinical Psychology*, 1–16. https://doi.org/10.1002/jclp.23474
Mayhew, S., & Gilbert, P. (2008). Compassionate mind training with people who hear malevolent voices: A case series report. *Clinical Psychology and Psychotherapy, 15*, 113–138.
McKay, R., & Dennett, D. (2009). The evolution of misbelief. *Behavioral and Brain Sciences, 32*(6), 493–561.
Peters, E., Day, S., McKenna, J., & Orbach, G. (1999). Delusional ideation in religious and psychotic populations. *The British Journal of Clinical Psychology, 38*(1), 83–96.

Petrocchi, N., Di Bello, M., Cheli, S., & Ottaviani, C. (2022). Compassion focused therapy and the body: How physiological underpinnings of prosociality inform clinical practice. In P. Gilbert & G. Simos (Eds.), *Compassion focused therapy: Clinical practice and applications* (1st ed., pp. 345–359). Routledge.

Pinto-Gouveia, J., Matos, M., Castilho, P., & Xavier, A. (2014). Differences between depression and paranoia: The role of emotional memories, shame and subordination. *Clinical Psychology and Psychotherapy, 21*(1), 49–61.

Porges, S. W. (2001). The polyvagal theory: Phylogenetic substrates of a social nervous system. *International Journal of Psychophysiology, 42*(2), 123–146. https://doi.org/10.1016/S0167-8760(01)00162-3

Porges, S. W. (2007). *The polyvagal perspective Biological Psychology, 74*(2), 116–143. https://doi.org/10.1016/j.biopsycho.2006.06.009

Seppälä, E. M., Simon-Thomas, E., Brown, S. L., Worline, M. C., Cameron, C. D., & Doty, J. R. (2017). *The Oxford handbook of compassion science*. Oxford University Press.

Steindl, S., Bell, T., Dixon, A., & Kirby, J. N. (2022). Therapist perspectives on working with fears, blocks and resistances to compassion in compassion focused therapy. *Counselling & Psychotherapy Research, 00*, 1–14. https://doi.org/10.1002/capr.12530

Sullivan, M. B., Erb, M., Schmalzl, L., Moonaz, S., Noggle Taylor, J., & Porges, S. W. (2018). Yoga Therapy and Polyvagal Theory: The convergence of traditional wisdom and contemporary neuroscience for self-regulation and resilience. *Frontiers in Human Neuroscience, 12*(67), 1–15. https://doi.org/10.3389/fnhum.2018.00067

Thayer, J. F., & Lane, R. D. (2009). Claude Bernard and the heart-brain connection: Further elaboration of a model of neurovisceral integration. *Neuroscience and Biobehavioral Reviews, 33*(2), 81–88.

van Os, J., Hanssen, M., Bijl, R. V., & Ravelli, A. (2000). Straus (1969) revisited: A psychosis continuum in the general population? *Schizophrenia Research, 45*, 11–20.

van Os, J., Linscott, R. J., Myin-Germeys, I., Delespaul, P., & Krabbendam, L. (2009). A systematic review and meta-analysis of the psychosis continuum: Evidence for a psychosis proneness-persistence impairment model of psychotic disorder. *Psychological Medicine, 39*, 179–195.

Wood, L., & Irons, C. (2016). Exploring the associations between social rank and external shame with experiences of psychosis. *Behavioural and Cognitive Psychotherapy, 44*(5), 527–538. https://doi.org/10.1017/S1352465815000570

Chapter 15
Addressing Schizotypy in Metacognitive Reflection and Insight Therapy

Courtney N. Wiesepape, Madyson Morris, and Ilanit Hasson-Ohayon

The construct of schizotypy is understood as a latent personality organization that harbors the liability for schizophrenia (Lenzenweger, 2018). Some individuals with schizotypy may go on to develop a psychotic disorder (e.g., schizophrenia); however, others may never experience or be diagnosed with a clinically significant disorder. Although schizotypy is a distinct construct, it is conceptually related to and sometimes discussed interchangeably with schizotypal personality disorder. In this chapter, we primarily focus on schizotypy; however, there is some overlap between these constructs in the literature reviewed.

Evidence supports that schizotypy is made up of three dimensions that map onto the symptom structure of schizophrenia, including positive, negative, and disorganized domains (Kwapil et al., 2018). The positive domain may include subthreshold psychotic symptoms such as magical thinking and paranoia, whereas the negative domain may involve avolition, anhedonia, and social disengagement. The disorganized dimension typically includes disruptions in one's thoughts and behaviors (Kwapil et al., 2018). Although some positive schizotypy traits have been found to be associated with an increased sense of well-being, in general, schizotypy features and subclinical psychotic symptoms are associated with decreased well-being (Fumero et al., 2018), suggesting that psychosocial treatment may be beneficial for people with schizotypy.

C. N. Wiesepape
Department of Psychiatry, Indiana University School of Medicine, Indianapolis, IN, USA

M. Morris
Department of Psychology, Indiana State University, Terre Haute, IN, USA

I. Hasson-Ohayon (✉)
Department of Psychology, Bar-Ilan University, Ramat Gan, Israel
e-mail: ilanit.hasson-ohayon@biu.ac.il

S. Cheli, P. H. Lysaker (eds.), *A Dimensional Approach to Schizotypy*,
https://doi.org/10.1007/978-3-031-41788-7_15

Existing Treatments for Schizotypy

Overall, existing treatments for schizotypy are limited and poorly covered in the literature. One systematic review focused on the use of antipsychotic medications in schizotypy and schizotypal personality disorder concluded that more high-quality studies were needed to determine whether antipsychotics were effective in treating these disorders (Jakobsen et al., 2017). However, some individual studies suggest that low-dose antipsychotics are effective in reducing symptom severity in schizotypal personality disorder specifically (Koenigsberg et al., 2003; Keshavan et al., 2004). Another systematic review that focused on both pharmacological and psychotherapy treatment for schizotypy and schizotypal disorder concluded that there is only limited evidence available to utilize in making treatment decisions for these individuals (Kirchner et al., 2018). One relevant randomized clinical trial found that integrated treatment (e.g., assertive community treatment, family involvement, and social skills training) postponed or prevented the onset of psychosis in a group of individuals with subthreshold psychotic symptoms or schizotypy (Nordentoft et al., 2006).

These existing treatments for schizotypy may offer pharmacological intervention or focus on skill-building aimed at reducing symptoms. However, they seem to neglect self-experience and personal recovery that are thought to be important to address in psychotic disorders and by extension in schizotypy populations (Parnas & Handest, 2003). Building upon accumulating literature on the effectiveness of metacognitive reflection and insight therapy (MERIT) among people with serious mental illness, including psychosis (e.g., Lysaker et al., 2020a), as well as some limited literature on this treatment approach in schizotypy-related disorders, the current chapter will discuss MERIT as an integrated treatment focused on one's subjective experience that could address self-experience and promote recovery in schizotypy. We will first introduce MERIT and evidence for its effectiveness. Then, we will discuss how MERIT can be applied in a schizotypy population. Finally, we will present a clinical case example using MERIT with a person with schizotypy.

Metacognitive Reflection and Insight Therapy: General Framework and Central Elements

Metacognitive reflection and insight therapy (MERIT) is an integrative form of individual psychotherapy focused on promoting one's ability to form increasingly complex ideas about self, others, and the world and to use this knowledge to find meaning in one's experience, make decisions about how to respond to psychosocial challenges, and reestablish connection in one's community (Lysaker & Klion, 2017). Inspired by research on the integrated model of metacognition and models of subjective recovery, MERIT was developed as a flexible, recovery-oriented approach designed to address metacognitive deficits in persons diagnosed with psychosis (Lysaker et al., 2018, 2020a). It provides a framework that fosters recovery by helping individuals to form a personally acceptable sense of their challenges and decide how to manage these challenges with their unique metacognitive knowledge (Lysaker et al., 2020b). Although MERIT was initially developed in the context of serious mental illness to address metacognitive deficits, its focus on recovery and self-experience highlights its transdiagnostic potential. Of note, MERIT is an integrative approach, offering a framework that can be adapted by therapists from a range of psychotherapy orientations and backgrounds to stimulate metacognition (Lysaker et al., 2018, 2020a).

MERIT is provided in the context of certain values that include (1) understanding patients as unique individuals who can recover; (2) understanding patients as being capable of directing their own path to recovery; (3) willingness to interact with patients in a nonhierarchical manner that supports recovery; (4) believing that the experience of psychosis (e.g., disorganization and delusions) can be understood; (5) accepting and being prepared for the idea that increased awareness may result in increased emotional distress; and finally, (6) understanding that stigma is a barrier to recovery, which can emerge from a variety of sources (Lysaker & Klion, 2017).

In addition to the implementation of these values, MERIT includes eight therapeutic elements that should be present during each psychotherapy session and are believed to interact to enhance metacognition (Lysaker et al., 2020a; Lysaker & Klion, 2017). These include four content elements, two process elements, and two superordinate elements. The content elements focus on the substance of each session and include (1) focus on the patient's agenda; (2) insertion of the therapist's mind; (3) eliciting narrative episodes from the patient's life; and (4) defining the psychological problem. Element one, or focus on the patient's agenda, involves the therapist and patient attending to and thinking together about what the patient may be trying to accomplish in the moment or hoping results from the session. Patient agendas may be contradictory, not readily apparent, or unrelated all together. Examples include wanting to feel less angry, confuse the therapist, or feel connected to someone. Element two concerns the insertion of the mind of the therapist. This may include the therapist sharing their thoughts or reactions to the patient and serves to establish the therapist as a partner in dialogue. Element three, or eliciting narrative episodes, involves attending to and reflecting on the narratives or stories from a patient's life and how they think about their experiences. Initially, with lower levels of metacognition, narratives may appear fragmented or difficult to follow. However, as metacognition increases, the ability to reflect upon and create coherent narratives within the flow of life is expected to improve. The final content element, or defining the psychological problem, asks the therapist to think together with the patient and jointly identify one or more psychological problems. Of note, psychological problems can vary drastically and change over time.

Process elements emphasize active reflection upon (5) the therapeutic relationship and (6) progress in psychotherapy within each therapy session. Because the therapeutic relationship is the context in which the four content elements are explored, it is important to jointly reflect upon the interpersonal processes that occur within the dyad in element five. Element six involves reflection on progress. This may include the patient's experience of therapy and how therapy has had an impact on them with focus on any changes the patient notices. Elements five and six occur as the patient and therapist reflect together about the process of therapy.

The final two superordinate elements involve using metacognitive interventions that aim to stimulate or increase (7) self-reflectivity and understanding of others and (8) mastery, or the ability to use metacognitive knowledge to respond to psychological problems. Within these elements, therapists should intentionally tailor interventions to a given patient's capacity to stimulate reflection of self and others as well as metacognitive mastery. To do this, practitioners of MERIT engage in ongoing assessment of patients' current metacognitive capacity using the Metacognition Assessment Scale-Abbreviated (MAS-A), as discussed below, and accordingly provide graded interventions to stimulate reflection to promote the development of higher levels of metacognition. The MAS-A is used in each session within this approach to both track progress and metacognitive growth over time.

Metacognition and the Metacognition Assessment Scale

In MERIT, metacognition is understood to refer to a spectrum of activities, including awareness of discrete cognitive, affective, and embodied acts and the synthesis of these into a broader and evolving sense of self and others as they relate to one another in the world. The integrated model of metacognition distinguishes between four domains of metacognitive functioning, including (1) self-reflectivity or the ability to reflect upon one's thoughts, emotions, and actions in increasingly complex and integrated ways; (2) understanding the mind of the other, or the ability to understand the thoughts, emotions, and behaviors of others in increasingly complex and integrated ways; (3) decentration, or the ability to notice that others in the world have complex lives and experiences that are unrelated to oneself; and (4) mastery, or the ability to use this metacognitive knowledge to respond to psychosocial challenges. Each of these domains can be assessed through a coding system using the Metacognition Assessment Scale-Abbreviated (MAS-A; Lysaker et al., 2005), which is based on the original Metacognition Assessment Scale (Semerari et al., 2003). On this measure, higher scores reflect more complex and integrated understandings of the self, others, and the surrounding world. Although each domain is assessed in isolation, they are also thought to interact with one another. Therapists use this coding system as a framework for ongoing assessment of their patient's level of metacognition during sessions and to tailor specific metacognitive interventions to patients' current level of functioning.

Evidence for MERIT Effectiveness in Psychosis

Despite its novelty, MERIT has a robust and growing research base linking metacognition to a number of clinical outcomes in prolonged and first-episode psychosis populations and a variety of other diagnoses (see Lysaker et al., 2020a). In an initial pilot study, nine participants completed 12 MERIT sessions, demonstrating that MERIT is an acceptable and a feasible intervention and providing evidence for metacognitive improvement (de Jong et al., 2016a).

Randomized trials have also been completed to assess the effectiveness of MERIT. In one trial, 20 individuals with early psychosis were randomized to 6 months of MERIT or 6 months of treatment as usual. It was found that individuals who completed 6 months of MERIT displayed significant improvements in insight in comparison with the treatment as a usual group (Vohs et al., 2018). In another randomized controlled trial, 18 participants diagnosed with schizophrenia completed 8 months of MERIT intervention. These participants showed significant improvements in metacognitive domains of self-reflectivity and mastery (de Jong et al., 2019). After participating this trial, one qualitative study showed that the majority of participants (10 of 14) reported that therapy was helpful in their recovery and improved their understanding of their thinking (de Jong et al., 2020). Participants tended to attribute this to the therapeutic relationship, self-expression, and taking an active role in therapy. Another randomized control trial of MERIT in a community clinic that included session-by-session assessment of adherence to elements, therapeutic alliance, and emotional experience showed increased metacognition and decreased symptoms (Hasson-Ohayon et al. submitted). In addition, the results of a controlled trial in an inpatient unit also showed improvements in metacognition and decrease in symptoms (Cohen-Hazani et al. submitted).

Further, in a session-by-session evaluation of MERIT which reviewed 221 sessions from ten individuals with schizophrenia, it was found that metacognition significantly improved in self-reflectivity and mastery domains (Lavi-Rotenberg et al., 2020). In addition, it was found that two MERIT elements, introducing the mind of the therapist and reflecting on progress, were associated with better outcomes the following week. In another session-by-session evaluation of 563 sessions from 37 individuals with schizophrenia, it was found that greater emotional experience, expression, and regulation in sessions were associated with better session outcomes, suggesting that emotion plays an important role in the MERIT (Igra et al., 2022). An additional study suggests that therapeutic improvements in recovery and metacognition after MERIT are maintained for 2 years post-treatment (Schweitzer et al., 2017).

In addition to findings from clinical trials, numerous case studies also provide evidence for MERIT effectiveness (Lysaker et al., 2020a). These case studies cover different diagnoses and clinical presentations, including first-episode psychosis with a focus on negative symptoms (Van Donkersgoed et al., 2016; Leonhardt et al., 2018), positive symptoms (Hillis et al., 2015; Leonhardt et al., 2016), and depression (Hasson-Ohayon et al., 2017) and prolonged schizophrenia spectrum disorders (e.g., schizophrenia and schizoaffective disorder) with a focus on demoralization (Arnon-Ribenfeld et al., 2018), disorganization (Arnon-Ribenfeld et al., 2018; Hamm & Firmin, 2016; de Jong et al., 2016b), paranoia (Buck & George, 2016), negative symptoms (George & Buck, 2018; Hamm & Leonhardt, 2016), trauma (Hillis et al., 2018), and substance abuse (James et al., 2018). Each case study reported overall increases in metacognition, including the ability to think about and reflect upon oneself and others and the ability to cope with psychological problems. Other positive outcomes were also observed, including increased self-compassion (Arnon-Ribenfeld et al., 2018), decreased symptoms (Van Donkersgoed et al., 2016; George & Buck, 2018; Hillis et al., 2018; James et al., 2018), improved interpersonal functioning (Hillis et al., 2018), and increased insight (Leonhardt et al., 2016). Taken together, this suggests that MERIT can be successfully applied to a range of psychological diagnoses and presentations by providers from different backgrounds and theoretical orientations.

Metacognition and Schizotypy

Although MERIT was established in a population of individuals diagnosed with serious mental illness and displaying metacognitive deficits, advances in research on MERIT have recently documented the presence of similar deficits in a range of other mental health diagnoses and thus established MERIT as a potential treatment for a range of diagnoses. Specific to schizotypy, the metacognitive domains of self-reflectivity and understanding others' minds as measured by the MAS-A have been shown to be correlated with schizotypy traits (Rabin et al., 2014). Similarly, Chan et al. (2015) found that higher self-reported schizotypy was associated with more dysfunctional metacognitive beliefs on the metacognitions questionnaire-30. Another study using the MAS-A found a significant relationship between negative schizotypy traits and metacognitive capacity; however, metacognition capacity was not able to differentiate between a schizotypy group and a non-schizotypy control group (Davis et al., 2020). Although more work is needed to establish specific metacognitive deficits in a schizotypy population, initial studies suggest that metacognition is a viable treatment target.

Evidence for MERIT in Schizotypy-Related Diagnoses

Although somewhat limited, there is research suggesting that MERIT is applicable to people with schizotypy and other similar populations. Broadly, MERIT has been utilized as a treatment for individuals with various personality disorders, suggesting that it can be successful with individuals with maladaptive personality organizations. For example, two case studies focused on emotional dysregulation in borderline personality disorder reported increases in metacognitive functioning following MERIT (Buck et al., 2018; Vohs & Leonhardt, 2016).

Other studies have focused more specifically on schizotypal and schizoid personality disorders. In a two-case series that implemented metacognitively oriented psychotherapy with two individuals diagnosed with schizotypal personality disorder over a period of 6 months, it was found that both individuals achieved a reduction in symptoms and a significant decrease in schizotypal features (Cheli et al., 2019). There were no reported adverse effects of this treatment, and both participating individuals reported a reduction in disturbing thoughts, improved functioning, and a richer understanding of self. In a more recent case study, similar results were reported. Specifically, MERIT was utilized with an individual diagnosed with schizotypal personality disorder over 3 months. At the end of treatment, this individual reported decreased symptoms and related distress and also demonstrated increases in metacognitive functioning (Dmitryeva et al., 2021). In another two case series, Cheli et al. (2022) integrated MERIT and compassion focused therapy with two individuals diagnosed with schizoid personality disorder. No adverse effects were reported, and decreases in symptomology and schizoid personality traits were observed. Taken together, these findings are encouraging and suggest that MERIT should be further explored as a treatment in a schizotypy population.

Clinical Case Example

Robert, a white male in his early 40s living in a mid-sized city in the Midwest, reported to psychotherapy after experiencing various difficulties in his life, including angry outbursts and difficulty understanding and relating to others. Robert had been married for over 10 years and had no children, although he expressed that he had wanted children in the past but ultimately decided against it based on his and his wife's psychiatric histories. Robert was unemployed but did receive financial compensation for a disability. Initially, Robert often discussed a desire to get a job to provide for his family; however, he never made any concrete effort (e.g., submitting applications) to find a job. He was highly educated with both a Master of Business Administration and Master of Arts. Robert discussed that he wanted to be a writer but also never attempted to publish or submit his work to local competitions. Although he could express various desires and wants, he seemed to be quite risk-averse and fearful of rejection. He often experienced avolition and some anhedonia. Robert did not endorse any overt psychotic symptoms but discussed a "mystical feeling" or a sense that something was not quite right. He displayed some magical thinking and endorsed mild disorganization, including feelings of confusion and lack of impulse control. Through clinical interviews and collaborative therapeutic conversations with his therapist, Robert was assessed to be experiencing schizotypy. Robert completed 12 months of MERIT with a trained therapist. Below, we discuss examples of elements as they arose during treatment.

Agenda: Although Robert presented with a range of agendas throughout treatment, one prominent agenda included Robert wanting to be seen as a competent and intelligent man. He often seemed to want to confirm that he was smarter than most people, including the therapist. He often spent time in session discussing his advanced degrees and the knowledge he had acquired through rigorous daily studying and reading about psychological topics. It was important to Robert that those he deemed worthy saw him in a specific light, independent of any psychological symptoms or challenges. This agenda was prominent and played a major role throughout therapy, including coloring the therapeutic relationship and narrative episodes from Robert's life.

Insertion of therapist's mind: After meeting with the patient for some time, the therapist noticed that Robert tended to display disorganized thought processes and hyper-focus on the clock at certain points in the session. The therapist's shared her interpretation of the situation such that the patient engaged in these behaviors to divert the conversation and make himself less understandable to the therapist when uncomfortable emotions began to emerge. This gave way to an open dialogue such that Robert reported that he attempted to "randomize" things when he did not want to talk or answer difficult questions. This randomizing often took the form of Robert saying inappropriate or sexual things to the therapist, attempting throw the therapist off track to avoid the therapist's mind when he was unable to tolerate the thoughts of the therapist and attempting to cut sessions short. Although initially unsuccessful, Robert and the therapist were eventually able to think together about why he "randomizes" things and how this also occurs in his other interpersonal relationships.

Narrative episodes: Robert was open to sharing various narrative episodes from this life; however, they often focused on either perceived wrongs from others and his explosive anger or his academic and intellectual accomplishments. Over time, Robert and the therapist were able to address themes of sensitivity to rejection, failure, and inadequacy woven throughout his narratives and make connections between different narratives from his life. By also eliciting narrative episodes unrelated to these themes, the therapist and Robert were able to expand their joint understanding of his life and how he wanted to move forward.

Psychological problem: The psychological problem proved to be a challenge to nail down. Robert did not endorse any overt psychotic symptoms but often discussed a sense of something being wrong or magical in his life. Eventually, Robert and the therapist were able to agree on a couple of psychological problems, including a lack of wider connection to the world and a prominent fear of being viewed as a failure or inadequate, leading to hesitancy to take risks in his life. Robert's psychological problem was significantly intertwined with his overarching agenda such that his deep fears of failure and inadequacy prompted him to engage in impression management throughout therapy.

Therapeutic relationship: The therapeutic relationship between Robert and therapist seemed to wax and wane over time. At one point during therapy, the therapist shared that she did not seem to leave much of a "residue" on Robert's mind such that his ideas about the therapist did not linger or continue once therapy sessions were over. Robert did not agree with this assessment but was able to reflect more deeply about his ideas about the therapeutic relationships after the therapist shared her thoughts via Element 2. Moreover, the therapeutic relationship tended to deteriorate during periods in which there were longer intervals between sessions (i.e., holidays). Following this, Robert would often become significantly more aloof and disorganized and display less positive verbal and nonverbal behavior toward the therapist. Robert and the therapist were able to collaboratively reflect on this pattern and explore the potential purposes of it and to examine how similar interpersonal patterns may have manifested in Robert's other relationships. Specifically, the therapist was able to think with Robert about his experiences of rejection sensitivity and difficulties connecting to others and their subsequent influence on his understanding of the therapist and the therapeutic relationship.

Progress: Overtime, Robert was able to share how his thoughts and emotions changed throughout the course of therapy. He noted that therapy helped him to better organize his thoughts and was able to discuss what role the therapy played for him. Although at times Robert and the therapist were unsure about what they were working toward, consistent joint reflection and dialogue allowed progress to become clearer. Notably, after some time in therapy, Robert noticed that he became more comfortable with genuine self-expression, experiencing and tolerating uncomfortable emotions, and the subjectivity and fallibility of his thoughts and perspectives.

Stimulation of self-reflectivity and understanding of others: Robert presented to therapy with the ability to understand a range of thoughts and emotions in himself; however, he did not seem to have a consistent ability to identify a range of thoughts and emotions in others which sometimes interfered with his ability to interact with others in a prosocial way. For example, Robert often lashed out when others did not share his same perspective (e.g., coronavirus disease-19 [COVID-19] precautions), leading to various negative consequences in his interpersonal relationships. With metacognitive intervention, including collaboratively exploring how Robert came to hold his specific belief systems with such conviction, as well as how he developed into someone who becomes irate with others over differences in perspective, Robert began to better understand that his thoughts could be wrong or change and that specific others have a diverse range of thoughts and emotions, which helped him to better interact with others. Throughout the therapy, Robert developed greater metacognitive knowledge of both himself and others.

Stimulation of mastery: Stimulating mastery in Robert proved challenging due his self-identified "lack of motivation." Once the psychological problems, as discussed above, had been identified, Robert seemed uncertain about how to move forward to understand and cope with these psychological problems. Over the course of therapy, Robert moved from gross avoidance of his psychological problems (e.g., avoiding being around other people and avoiding writing or taking risks) to changing his behavior to begin to address these challenges. Specifically, Robert began to spend more time with his family and friends without becoming irate or frustrated with them. Most notably, Robert began to write again and submitted a short story to a local writing competition. Throughout sessions, the therapist was able to use metacognitive interventions to promote mastery and help Robert understand how he wanted to move forward with his life as an agent.

Conclusion

A sense of personal recovery and self-experience are important concepts in the treatment of psychotic disorders, which extends to the experience of schizotypy or the latent personality organization that harbors the liability for schizophrenia. Metacognitive reflection and insight therapy (MERIT) is a recovery-oriented, integrative form of individual psychotherapy focused on promoting one's ability to form increasingly complex ideas about self, others, and the world and to use this knowledge to find meaning in one's experience, make decisions about how to respond to psychosocial challenges, and reestablish connection in one's community. This approach has a growing research base supporting its efficacy in treating psychotic disorders, and some research has also demonstrated support for this approach in personality disorders, including schizotypal personality disorder. We suggest that MERIT can be successfully utilized as a transdiagnostic psychotherapy for individuals experiencing schizotypy; however, more work is needed to establish this approach as evidence-based in this population.

References

Arnon-Ribenfeld, N., Bloom, R., Atzil-Slonim, D., Peri, T., de Jong, S., & Hasson-Ohayon, I. (2018). Metacognitive Reflection and Insight Therapy (MERIT) among people with schizophrenia: Lessons from two case studies. *American Journal of Psychotherapy, 71*(4), 175–185. https://doi.org/10.1176/appi.psychotherapy.20180037

Buck, K. D., & George, S. E. (2016). Metacognitive reflective and insight therapy for a person who gained maximal levels of metacognitive capacity and was able to terminate therapy. *Journal of Contemporary Psychotherapy, 46*(4), 187–196. https://doi.org/10.1007/s10879-016-9322-y

Buck, K. D., Vertinski, M., & Kukla, M. (2018). Metacognitive Reflection and Insight Therapy (MERIT): Application to a long-term therapy case of borderline personality disorder. *American Journal of Psychotherapy, 71*(4), 145–154. https://doi.org/10.1176/appi.psychotherapy.20180035

Chan, C. C., Spencer, C. C., West, C., Viegas, C., & Bedwell, J. S. (2015). Metacognitive processes in psychometrically defined schizotypy. *Psychiatry Research, 230*(2), 279–286. https://doi.org/10.1016/j.psychres.2015.09.006

Cheli, S., Lysaker, P. H., & Dimaggio, G. (2019). Metacognitively oriented psychotherapy for schizotypal personality disorder: A two-case series. *Personality and Mental Health, 13*(3), 155–167. https://doi.org/10.1002/pmh.1447

Cheli, S., Chiarello, F., & Cavalletti, V. (2022). A psychotherapy oriented by compassion and metacognition for schizoid personality disorder: A two cases series. *Journal of Contemporary Psychotherapy, 53*, 1–10.

Davis, B. J., Firmin, R. L., Lysaker, P. H., Salyers, M. P., McGrew, J., & Minor, K. S. (2020). An investigation of metacognition in schizotypy: Evidence of linkage with negative traits. *Translational Issues in Psychological Science, 6*(1), 81–91. https://doi.org/10.1037/tps0000221

de Jong, S., van Donkersgoed, R. J., Aleman, A., van der Gaag, M., Wunderink, L., Arends, J., Lysaker, P. H., & Pijnenborg, M. (2016a). Practical implications of metacognitively oriented psychotherapy in psychosis: Findings from a pilot study. *The Journal of Nervous and Mental Disease, 204*(9), 713–716. https://doi.org/10.1097/NMD.0000000000000564

de Jong, S., van Donkersgoed, R., Pijnenborg, G. H., & Lysaker, P. H. (2016b). Metacognitive Reflection and Insight Therapy (MERIT) with a patient with severe symptoms of disorganization. *Journal of Clinical Psychology, 72*(2), 164–174. https://doi.org/10.1002/jclp.22249

de Jong, S., van Donkersgoed, R. J. M., Timmerman, M. E., Aan Het Rot, M., Wunderink, L., Arends, J., van Der Gaag, M., Aleman, A., Lysaker, P. H., & Pijnenborg, G. H. M. (2019). Metacognitive reflection and insight therapy (MERIT) for patients with schizophrenia. *Psychological Medicine, 49*(2), 303–313. https://doi.org/10.1017/S0033291718000855

de Jong, S., Hasson-Ohayon, I., van Donkersgoed, R., Aleman, A., & Pijnenborg, G. H. M. (2020). A qualitative evaluation of the effects of Metacognitive Reflection and Insight Therapy: 'Living more consciously'. *Psychology and Psychotherapy, 93*(2), 223–240. https://doi.org/10.1111/papt.12212

Dmitryeva, N., Chernov, N., Kostyuk, G., & Lysaker, P. H. (2021). Utilizing MERIT to promote recovery in schizotypal personality disorder: An illustrative case study. *Journal of Clinical Psychology, 77*(8), 1798–1806. https://doi.org/10.1002/jclp.23239

Fumero, A., Marrero, R. J., & Fonseca-Pedrero, E. (2018). Well-being in schizotypy: The effect of subclinical psychotic experiences. *Psicothema, 30*(2), 177–182.

George, S., & Buck, K. D. (2018). Metacognitive reflection and insight therapy for persons with severe negative symptoms of schizophrenia. *American Journal of Psychotherapy, 71*(4), 135–144. https://doi.org/10.1176/appi.psychotherapy.20180036

Hamm, J. A., & Firmin, R. L. (2016). Disorganization and individual psychotherapy for schizophrenia: A case report of metacognitive reflection and insight therapy. *Journal of Contemporary Psychotherapy, 46*(4), 227–234. https://doi.org/10.1007/s10879-016-9326-7

Hamm, J. A., & Leonhardt, B. L. (2016). The role of interpersonal connection, personal narrative, and metacognition in integrative psychotherapy for schizophrenia: A case report. *Journal of Clinical Psychology, 72*(2), 132–141. https://doi.org/10.1002/jclp.2016.72.issue-2

Hasson-Ohayon, I., Arnon-Ribenfeld, N., Hamm, J., & Lysaker, P. H. (2017). Agency before action: The application of behavioral activation in psychotherapy with persons with psychosis. *Psychotherapy, 54*(3), 245–251. https://doi.org/10.1037/pst0000114

Hillis, J. D., Leonhardt, B. L., Vohs, J. L., Buck, K. D., Salvatore, G., Popolo, R., Dimaggio, G., & Lysaker, P. H. (2015). Metacognitive reflective and insight therapy for people in early phase of a schizophrenia spectrum disorder. *Journal of Clinical Psychology, 71*(2), 125–135. https://doi.org/10.1002/jclp.22148

Hillis, J. D., Bidlack, N., & Macobin, B. (2018). Metacognitive Reflection and Insight Therapy (MERIT) for persons with a schizophrenia spectrum disorder and interpersonal trauma. *American Journal of Psychotherapy, 71*(4), 186–195. https://doi.org/10.1176/appi.psychotherapy.20180031

Igra, L., Sened, H., Lavi-Rotenberg, A., Pijnenborg, M., Lysaker, P. H., & Hasson-Ohayon, I. (2022). Emotional experience and metacognition among people with schizophrenia: Analysis of session by session and outcome of metacognitive-oriented psychotherapy. *Journal of Psychiatric Research, 156*, 460–466. https://doi.org/10.1016/j.jpsychires.2022.10.048

Jakobsen, K. D., Skyum, E., Hashemi, N., Schjerning, O., Fink-Jensen, A., & Nielsen, J. (2017). Antipsychotic treatment of schizotypy and schizotypal personality disorder: A systematic review. *Journal of Psychopharmacology, 31*(4), 397–405. https://doi.org/10.1177/0269881117695879

James, A. V., Leonhardt, B. L., & Buck, K. D. (2018). Metacognitive Reflection and Insight Therapy for schizophrenia: A case study of a patient with a co-occurring substance use disorder. *American Journal of Psychotherapy, 71*(4), 155–163. https://doi.org/10.1176/appi.psychotherapy.20180038

Keshavan, M., Shad, M., Soloff, P., & Schooler, N. (2004). Efficacy and tolerability of olanzapine in the treatment of schizotypal personality disorder. *Schizophrenia Research, 71*(1), 97–101. https://doi.org/10.1016/j.schres.2003.12.008

Kirchner, S. K., Roeh, A., Nolden, J., & Hasan, A. (2018). Diagnosis and treatment of schizotypal personality disorder: Evidence from a systematic review. *Schizophrenia, 4*(1), 20. https://doi.org/10.1038/s41537-018-0062-8

Koenigsberg, H. W., Reynolds, D., Goodman, M., New, A. S., Mitropoulou, V., Trestman, R. L., Silverman, J., & Siever, L. J. (2003). Risperidone in the treatment of schizotypal personality disorder. *The Journal of Clinical Psychiatry, 64*(6), 628–634. https://doi.org/10.4088/jcp.v64n0602

Kwapil, T. R., Gross, G. M., Silvia, P. J., Raulin, M. L., & Barrantes-Vidal, N. (2018). Development and psychometric properties of the Multidimensional Schizotypy Scale: A new measure for assessing positive, negative, and disorganized schizotypy. *Schizophrenia Research, 193*, 209–217. https://doi.org/10.1016/j.schres.2017.07.001

Lavi-Rotenberg, A., Bar-Kalifa, E., de Jong, S., Igra, L., Lysaker, P. H., & Hasson-Ohayon, I. (2020). Elements that enhance therapeutic alliance and short-term outcomes in metacognitive reflection and insight therapy: A session-by-session assessment. *Psychiatric Rehabilitation Journal, 43*(4), 318–326. https://doi.org/10.1037/prj0000415

Lenzenweger, M. F. (2018). Schizotypy, schizotypic psychopathology and schizophrenia. *World Psychiatry, 17*(1), 25–26. https://doi.org/10.1002/wps.20479

Leonhardt, B. L., Benson, K., George, S., Buck, K. D., Shaieb, R., & Vohs, J. L. (2016). Targeting insight in first episode psychosis: A case study of metacognitive reflection insight therapy (MERIT). *Journal of Contemporary Psychotherapy, 46*, 207–216.

Leonhardt, B. L., Ratliff, K., & Buck, K. D. (2018). Recovery in first episode psychosis: A case study of metacognitive reflection and insight therapy (MERIT). *American Journal of Psychotherapy, 71*(4), 128–134. https://doi.org/10.1176/appi.psychotherapy.20180032

Lysaker, P. H., & Klion, R. E. (2017). *Recovery, meaning-making, and severe mental illness: A comprehensive guide to metacognitive reflection and insight therapy*. Routledge.

Lysaker, P. H., Carcione, A., Dimaggio, G., Johannesen, J. K., Nicolò, G., Procacci, M., & Semerari, A. (2005). Metacognition amidst narratives of self and illness in schizophrenia: Associations with neurocognition, symptoms, insight and quality of life. *Acta Psychiatrica Scandinavica, 112*(1), 64–71. https://doi.org/10.1111/j.1600-0447.2005.00514.x

Lysaker, P. H., Gagen, E., Moritz, S., & Schweitzer, R. D. (2018). Metacognitive approaches to the treatment of psychosis: A comparison of four approaches. *Psychology Research and Behavior Management, 11*, 341–351. https://doi.org/10.2147/PRBM.S146446

Lysaker, P. H., Gagen, E., Klion, R., Zalzala, A., Vohs, J., Faith, L. A., Leonhardt, B., Hamm, J., & Hasson-Ohayon, I. (2020a). Metacognitive Reflection and Insight Therapy: A recovery-oriented treatment approach for psychosis. *Psychology Research and Behavior Management, 13*, 331–341. https://doi.org/10.2147/PRBM.S198628

Lysaker, P. H., Kukla, M., Leonhardt, B. L., Hamm, J. A., Schnakenberg Martin, A., Zalzala, A. B., Gagen, E. C., & Hasson-Ohayon, I. (2020b). Meaning, integration, and the self in serious mental illness: Implications of research in metacognition for psychiatric rehabilitation. *Psychiatric Rehabilitation Journal*. https://doi.org/10.1037/prj0000436

Nordentoft, M., Thorup, A., Petersen, L., Ohlenschlaeger, J., Melau, M., Christensen, T. Ø., Krarup, G., Jørgensen, P., & Jeppesen, P. (2006). Transition rates from schizotypal disorder to psychotic disorder for first-contact patients included in the OPUS trial. A randomized clinical trial of integrated treatment and standard treatment. *Schizophrenia Research, 83*(1), 29–40. https://doi.org/10.1016/j.schres.2006.01.002

Parnas, J., & Handest, P. (2003). Phenomenology of anomalous self-experience in early schizophrenia. *Comprehensive Psychiatry, 44*(2), 121–134. https://doi.org/10.1053/comp.2003.50017

Rabin, S. J., Hasson-Ohayon, I., Avidan, M., Rozencwaig, S., Shalev, H., & Kravetz, S. (2014). Metacognition in schizophrenia and schizotypy: Relation to symptoms of schizophrenia, traits of schizotypy and social quality of life. *The Israel Journal of Psychiatry and Related Sciences, 51*(1), 44–53.

Schweitzer, R. D., Greben, M., & Bargenquast, R. (2017). Long-term outcomes of Metacognitive Narrative Psychotherapy for people diagnosed with schizophrenia. *Psychology and Psychotherapy, 90*(4), 668–685. https://doi.org/10.1111/papt.12132

Semerari, A., Carcione, A., Dimaggio, G., Falcone, M., Nicolo, G., Procacci, M., & Alleva, G. (2003). How to evaluate metacognitive function in psychotherapy? The Metacognition Assessment Scale its applications. *Clinical Psychology & Psychotherapy, 10*(4), 238–261. https://doi.org/10.1002/cpp.362

Van Donkersgoed, R. J., de Jong, S., & Pijnenborg, G. H. M. (2016). Metacognitive Reflection and Insight Therapy (MERIT) with a patient with persistent negative symptoms. *Journal of Contemporary Psychotherapy, 46*(4), 245–254. https://doi.org/10.1007/s10879-016-9333-8

Vohs, J. L., & Leonhardt, B. L. (2016). Metacognitive reflection and insight therapy for borderline personality disorder: A case illustration of an individual in a long term institutional setting. *Journal of Contemporary Psychotherapy, 46*(4), 255–264. https://doi.org/10.1007/s10879-016-9335-6

Vohs, J. L., Leonhardt, B. L., James, A. V., Francis, M. M., Breier, A., Mehdiyoun, N., Visco, A. C., & Lysaker, P. H. (2018). Metacognitive Reflection and Insight Therapy for early psychosis: A preliminary study of a novel integrative psychotherapy. *Schizophrenia Research, 195*, 428–433. https://doi.org/10.1016/j.schres.2017.10.041

Chapter 16
Metacognitive Interpersonal Therapy for Schizotypal Personality Disorder

Dario Catania, Giancarlo Dimaggio, and Raffaele Popolo

Introduction

The term "schizotypal" was first used by Rado (1953) to refer to a group of patients with a particular form of attenuated schizophrenia in the absence of frankly psychotic symptoms, that is, an attenuated phenotype of a schizophrenic genotype. Schizotypy is a clinical condition that can manifest with cognitive symptoms, alterations in perception, disorganization of behavior, and alterations in interpersonal functioning or present with positive and negative psychotic symptoms. For years, international classifications have differed in their classification of *schizotypal personality disorder* (SPD): in the International Classification for Diseases-11 (ICD-11) (WHO, 2020), it is referred to as schizotypal disorder and is listed under schizophrenia spectrum disorders, while in the Diagnostic and Statistical Manual of Mental Disorders-5 (DSM-5) (APA, 2013), it is classified as a personality disorder. In DSM-5, SPD is characterized by a pervasive pattern of intense distress and reduced capacity for close relationships, alterations in thinking and perceptions, and eccentric behavior. In ICD-11, schizotypal disorder is characterized by an enduring pattern (over a period of at least several years) of eccentricity in behavior, appearance, and language, accompanied by cognitive and perceptual distortions, unusual beliefs, and distress with reduced capacity for interpersonal relationships. Both ICD-11 and DSM-5 emphasize the possible presence of strange beliefs, magical thinking, bizarre behavior and language, social anxiety, and psychotic symptoms. The latter may include delusional thought content disorders, hallucinations, and

D. Catania · R. Popolo (✉)
Centro di Terapia Metacognitiva Interpersonale, Rome, Italy

DSM ASL Roma 1, Rome, Italy

G. Dimaggio
Centro di Terapia Metacognitiva Interpersonale, Rome, Italy

S. Cheli, P. H. Lysaker (eds.), *A Dimensional Approach to Schizotypy*, https://doi.org/10.1007/978-3-031-41788-7_16

affective flattening, of insufficient duration and intensity to meet the diagnostic criteria for schizophrenia.

The relationship between SPD and schizophrenia has been investigated at both the genetic and neurobiological levels. Genetic studies have documented a familial correlation between SPD and schizophrenia, to the point of hypothesizing that the two conditions represent different clinical manifestations of the same psychotic vulnerability. Imaging studies have found some similar patterns between schizophrenia and SPD, with differences appearing to show more attenuated alterations in SPD (Hazlett et al., 2012). These data lead to two possible conclusions: (1) SPD can be included among schizophrenia spectrum disorders and (2) patients with SPD present with attenuated psychotic symptoms affecting thinking, emotion expression, and behavior.

Although a recent review on SPD (Kirchner et al., 2018) concluded that it is not possible to make evidence-based recommendations for the treatment of this disorder. Metacognitive interpersonal therapy (MIT; Dimaggio et al., 2015, 2020), either alone or in combination with other modalities, has been shown to be effective in these cases with high rates of remission and good adherence to treatment with no dropouts (Cheli, 2020; Cheli et al., 2019, 2023). In this chapter, we will illustrate MIT as applied to a case of a patient with.

Forms and Content of the Schizotypal Experience

SPD patients have several problematic aspects similar to schizophrenia, albeit with less intensity frequency.

Alterations in Intersubjectivity Disorders that fall on the schizophrenic spectrum manifest alterations in intersubjectivity, that is, a difficulty in effortlessly understanding the communicative intention of the other; it is not a semantic or syntactic inability as much as a difficulty in intuitive, immediate, and pragmatic understanding of the other. Mario, a 56-year-old schizotypal patient, often shows great difficulty in grasping the other person's real intentions in his words: "*I used to tell my sister that I often go out and forget the lights on, once even the gas. And she with a smile tells me that maybe I need the 24-hour caregiver…that time I really got angry…I can't understand what she meant…does she think I'm demented? Or does she want to call social services to send me somewhere? I couldn't tell if she was joking or serious, and in the end we had a big argument and I kicked her out of the house.*"

What does not work properly is the immediate and intuitive understanding of the other's intention; this ability is a complex operation consisting of a *socio-cognitive component*, based on reasoning and prior knowledge, and a *socio-perceptual component* that is nonepistemic, prereflective, and implicit (Mitchell et al., 2006). The socio-cognitive component corresponds to the theory of mind (Frith, 2004) and acts through reasoning about mental states and context data. The socio-perceptual component corresponds to the capacity that Stanghellini (2010) defined as *prereflective function*. The deficit in prereflective function finds its fullest expression in schizophrenia and is also present in a less pervasive form in schizotypal disorder. This prereflexive tuning would be based on both an immediate perception of being similar to the other and an internal simulation of the other's finalized actions.

Schizophrenic patients, and to a lesser extent, SPD patients also exhibit impairment of the socio-cognitive component related to the ability to construct reasoning about the other's mind, to attribute mental states to others that may be different from one's own. The socio-cognitive component corresponds to *understanding others' mind*, a metacognitive skill that can be variously impaired, the malfunctioning of which generates what has been termed *contextual maladherence* (Salvatore et al., 2007, 2009, 2012). An old friend proceeding down the street toward us smiles at us and pointing his finger at us apostrophizes us with a phrase like "*You old rogue! What goes around comes around!*" What is his intention? Is he joking, or did he really think we were dead? Nonadherence to context often results in strangeness, eccentricity, or "oddity," which are characteristic and indispensable elements for posing a diagnosis of SPD.

Alterations in Narrative Functions Autobiographical memories are the best vehicle of the patient's subjective lived experience; patients with SPD may have a poor ability to relate specific narrative or tell stories that are disorganized. *Narrative poverty* is the difficulty in recalling detailed autobiographical memories that describe the cognitive, emotional, and somatic aspects of the subjective experience. Some SPD patients, as well as many schizophrenic patients, construct "prenarratives" (Holma & Aaltonen, 1998) that do not reach the minimum level of complexity because they are unable to convey information about the narrator's internal experience. Typical is the example of the patient who sits in front of the therapist and remains silent or responds monosyllabically or in a stereotyped manner. Other times, narrative poverty takes the form of "pseudo-narratives," that is, even very detailed accounts completely devoid of personal relevance; for example, a patient who describes in detail a program he or she watched the day before on television without being able to recognize the emotions associated with that viewing.

Narrative disorganization is a disjointed, unintegrated flow of words, the result of disorganized thinking. It can normally be observed in the presence of very intense negative emotions where stories lack internal coherence and structure. Marina, a patient with SPD, when questioned about what she was feeling at that moment in the session, replied "*I feel strange... strange to be here or yesterday with that heat I started... I don't always have to give sometimes even take... a decision once for all those who have never understood me (laughs)... I even happen to be stateless.*"

Maladaptive Interpersonal Patterns The interpersonal schema is a subjective representation of the fate our desires will meet in the course of our relationships with others. The schema derives from numerous early or recent learning experiences where a person's needs have been repeatedly frustrated; such experiences, experienced constantly over time, have been generalized. The schema is both a memory of how our desires were received by others in the past and an internalized expectation that has all the character of prediction. Think of an adolescent with temperamentally based emotional hypersensitivity who, starting high school, enters a peer group where he becomes the object of constant teasing. The adolescent's need to belong finds an aversive response in the environment that helps structure, along with the temperamental predisposition, a perception of self as vulnerable and/or weak. This perception may form the basis of future psychopathology.

Maladaptive interpersonal patterns are underlain by a negative self-image that generates suffering. In SPD, this image may be of a vulnerable, worthless, inadequate self or of a special self with talents not recognized by the other person that make him or her unique. In situations where a vulnerable representation emerges and the need for safety is felt, the image of others as hostile activates a feeling of danger; a flight response and avoidance of the relationship may ensue. The same coping strategy can be used to avoid the pain of being in relationship with other people when they represent themselves as worthless and inadequate. In such cases, they may experience a feeling of detachment from others, whom they see as different and distancing, or they may imagine the interlocutor as critical and judgmental. Even when the self-image is that of being special, a need to be recognized by the other is activated with the certainty, in reality that the other will remain distant or will even be judgmental. Patterns lead to bias in the interpretation of reality and decrease the likelihood of enacting adaptive behaviors; patients go through life guided by negative predictions, enacting dysfunctional coping, not implementing actions aimed at achieving their goals and desires.

Dysfunctional Interpersonal Cycles Pathogenic interpersonal patterns, when expressed in the relationship with the other, activate dysfunctional interpersonal cycles (Safran & Muran, 2000). A dysfunctional interpersonal cycle is a relational process in which one of the people involved, moved by negative expectations about the relationship, enacts coping strategies that induce aversive responses in the other, almost always confirming the initial negative expectations.

Michael, a patient with SPD with the idea that he had high value, in the presence of his peers closed himself off from dialogue by assuming an attitude of haughty detachment; if others spoke to him, he would respond steadily or assume an expression of condescension, convinced that others were unable to recognize this value. Faced with this attitude, others became irritated and distanced themselves; Michael perceived these behaviors as confirmation that the others were judging him negatively.

Metacognitive Dysfunctions By the term "metacognition," we mean the complex of skills that enable a person to make sense of his or her own experience, to access a representation of his or her own and others' internal states in order to pursue his or her own goals and purposes (Lysaker & Dimaggio, 2014). Along the lines of Semerari et al. (2003), metacognition is made of three different aspects:

Self-reflexivity is a function that enables a person to access a clear representation of his or her own internal states and make sense of subjective experience in order to define and pursue personal goals. *Understanding of others' mind* allows one to make truthful assumptions about the emotions, thoughts, and purposes that guide the other's action, perceiving, for example, that the other is sad based on a certain facial expression. *Decentering* is a subfunction of understanding another's mind and expresses the ability to describe the other's mental functioning independently of one's own perspective and involvement in the relationship. Then, we have *mastery*, which is the ability to use psychological knowledge intentionally and in full awareness to make decisions and formulate strategies to resolve interpersonal conflicts.

Metacognitive functions have the characteristic of being flexible; that is, they allow the construction of representations that change as external and internal elements change. For example, observing the emotional change in the other allows the person to modify the representation he had constructed of his intentionality in that specific situation. Many studies have confirmed metacognitive malfunctions in patients with schizophrenic spectrum disorders (Hasson-Ohayon et al., 2015; Lysaker et al., 2014) also present in SPD patients, with difficulty recognizing and distinguishing their own and others' thoughts.

MIT Procedures

Patients with SPD describe symptoms vaguely and tend to attribute their discomfort to external reasons, providing general theories or intellectualizations that others would hinder goals and desires. In MIT, the therapist does not seek abstract causal attributions about suffering, rather focuses on the ways in which the patient thinks and feels about something and how this is at the root of suffering and behaviors that hinder his or her well-being and relational stability.

MIT is (Dimaggio et al., 2007, 2015, 2019) is a third-wave approach that follows a series of formalized steps. A first goal is to form, jointly with the patient, a formulation of the latter's functioning (Dimaggio et al., 2015, 2020). Then, once the formulation is shared and agreed upon, the goal is to promote change at cognitive, affective, and behavioral levels. The first phase of treatment is shared case formulation; during this phase the therapist collects autobiographical episodes which are the place wheret to seek for the details of subjective experience. Collecting associated memories leads to the awareness that patients' actions, problems, and suffering stems from typical recurrent and crystalized ideas about self and others, namely maladaptive interpersonal schemas. In its more recent formulation (Dimaggio et al., 2020), MIT adopts experiential techniques early on in therapy for the sake of increasing access to subjective experiences. More in general, MIT uses experiential techniques in order to target interpersonal difficulties and other symptoms associated with any personality disorder. These techniques include guided imagery, chair work, role-play, bodily exercises, and behavioral experiments. Of note, growing evidence has shown that experiential techniques are both safe and effective (Dimaggio et al., 2020).

When therapy is focused on promoting change, the goals are to reduce symptoms and suffering, forming new and more benevolent ideas of self and others and using them as a ground for plan new and healthier behaviors in everyday life, so that social action becomes more adaptive (Dimaggio et al., 2013).

During the different steps, MIT is guided by the level of metacognition the patient displays in the moment. As the patient progresses to more advanced stages of treatment, interventions will indeed require more sophisticated metacognitive skills on the part of the patient. The aim will be to foster a progressive increase in the patient's metacognitive functioning and to use them in order to see interpersonal challenges more flexibly, restrain from problematic behaviors, and adopt healthier ones.

When working with SPD, there is the need to return many times working on the same problems. The patient may, for example, come to understand the connection between the appearance of persecutory ideas and schema activation in particular situations; he or she may also begin to place the schema in a critical spotlight by questioning it. However, under everyday life triggers, distrust and suspiciousness may emerge again in the session. In the course of therapy, therefore, a problem that appeared resolved may reoccur; in this case, the therapist will go over the parts of the procedure that have already been covered, as in a "physiotherapy" of metacognitive functions (Lysaker & Buck, 2010).

The therapist must maintain a constant focus on the therapeutic relationship. If relational problems emerge, the focus of the conversation shifts from attempting to understand and resolve the problem presented by the patient to assessing the reasons for the breakdown and attempting to repair them. It will return to the psychopathology after a good relationship has been restored.

When describing how MIT works with SPD, we will divide the interventions into three areas:

1. Relationship interventions
2. Shared formulation of functioning
3. Promotion of change

We now describe the MIT treatment of Luke, a 29-year-old male social worker who lives at home with his parents. He underwent individual psychotherapy after being admitted to a psychiatric ward for attacking his father from bizarre ideas, false recognition, and interpretive cues. In adolescence, he had few friends, tended to be isolated, fearful of others' judgment; gradually, his thinking became suspicious, with a state of alarm experienced mainly as physical activation and progressive detachment from others. At the time of hospitalization, Luke appeared perplexed, gloomy, and distrustful in relationship; only later, in the course of treatment, would he speak of his fear of having a demonic "presence" within him.

Interventions on the Relationship

In MIT, the focus on the therapeutic relationship is continuous (Dimaggio et al., 2013); the therapist must repair ruptures in the alliance and create a cooperative atmosphere in which to better reflect on one's mental states. Patients with SPD tend to construct the image of the therapist based on expectations derived from their own interpersonal schema: They ask for help but expect that the therapist will be disinterested, dismissive, dominant, or incapable. Relational problems are, then, enhanced by metacognitive dysfunction. If the patient has difficulty describing what he is feeling and thinking, the therapist will have trouble tuning in to him; the malfunction in understanding the mind of others makes it difficult for the patient to listen constructively to the therapist, who will, for example, feel frustrated or annoyed.

Interventions on the relationship involve operations that should be implemented whenever there is a threat of a rupture in the therapeutic alliance. First, the therapist should follow the patient *agenda* (Lysaker & Buck, 2010), that is, address the issues that the patient considers most urgent at that time while maintaining good interpersonal attunement. The patient should feel that the therapist's room is a welcoming and safe place, where one can enter without the risk of being hurt, rejected, or judged. This will be achievable by fostering in the patient's mind a representation of the other that is not opaque or negative, but as welcoming, caring, or validating as possible.

During one of the first sessions with Luke, the therapist was exploring the scene that had later led to his admission; at one point, he questioned the quality of the relationship by observing the patient's suspicious expression. The therapist felt evaluated by him as if he had to prove that he was not dangerous; he recognized his own internal state and handled it thinking that it could be complementary to that of the patient, who did not trust the interlocutor not understanding his intentions. He then interrupts the exploration to intervene in the relationship.

T: While we were talking about the reason for admission, I saw that you changed your expression, you became dark in the face, you seemed unnerved…

P: I don't know…

T: I was saying…maybe it's my impression, you seemed almost annoyed to talk about these things. If that's the case, I'm sorry, go ahead and tell me. I don't want to reconstruct how things went and then say what was wrong. What I want is to know you better and to understand how you feel even in relation to what happened to you; that's why, I ask you all these questions. I will always ask you how you feel, what you thought at a certain time, precisely because I am interested in that.

P: Yeah, okay…let's see.

The therapist makes his intentions explicit by assuming a transparent attitude, careful not to leave anything ambiguous in the exchange, given a certain disadherence to the patient's context. The effect achieved is to temporarily ease the climate of threat that seemed to characterize these first moments. Very important for preserving the relationship is to recognize the patient's disadherence with the therapist and to treat it as a priority. The disadherence represents, sometimes, a difficulty in the intersubjective functioning of the schizotypal patient; while in schizophrenic patients it is a trait-dependent condition, that is, always active and present, in patients with SPD it is activated mainly in the presence of the pathogenic interpersonal patterns. This also manifests itself in the encounter with the therapist, threatening the relationship throughout each session. The therapist is required, then, to carry out a series of internal discipline operations aimed at recognizing and regulating the negative emotional impact that the patient's disadherence causes on him (feeling of confusion and sense of ineffectiveness in communicating).

Shared Formulation of Functioning

In the first sessions, we accompany the patient in recognizing current unpleasant feelings and emotions and then link them back to past significant events. The narrative episode allows to explore the patient's experience; this episode allows the patient to return "into the thick of it," reliving the mental states experienced. Episodes involving interpersonal situations are experienced with suffering by the patient, where clinical aspects such as persecutory ideations or real delusional cues emerge.

The patient may narrate episodes spontaneously; if the patient shows difficulty in this, the therapist must assess the presence of possible problems in the relationship and put the focus on it. If not, go looking for what cause may be related to that difficulty. In SPD, the occurrence of positive symptoms is infrequent; if it does occur, it is necessary to calm the patient and help patients shift attention from the symptom to the suffering they cause. Therapists need to avoid challenging delusional belief. The goal is to focus on underlying emotional suffering associated with symptoms and jointly plan a series of behavioral strategies aimed at coping with that suffering. In the meantime, it is important to help patients become more aware of their inner experience; in some cases patients have a major impairment of this ability such that they are unable to recognize that they are masters of their thoughts, thinking they are inserted from outer forces.

To stimulate narrative capacity, the therapist may propose homework by inviting the patient to pay attention to emotionally activating situations; the emotional quality experienced is not important; the patient should observe the ongoing situation by dwelling on the thoughts and emotions emerging in his or her mind. The purpose is to train the patient to "feel" and place these emotional feelings in small stories that would otherwise have gone unnoticed. In the case of pseudo-narratives, without making judgments, the therapist should catch any flickers of vitality in the patient to bring the discourse to the source of vitality and work on positive modulation.

It may happen to counteract tendencies to intellectualizing and instead ask for specific autobiographical memories: "*Can you give me an example? Can you tell me about a time when someone made you feel exactly as you were telling me?*"

Luke had difficulty accessing emotionally marked memories. The therapist invited him to recount episodes, for example, that caused him pain, but he remained silent for a few moments. He would like to talk about the hospitalization, but appears conflicted; the therapist reiterates that he does not want to force him to talk about something if he does not want to, but to use the hospitalization as a temporal reference point to explore his internal states before and after.

P: Hospitalization was a tremendous experience. I was with so many people who were sick. I don't know what the others thought. I never bothered anyone, and yet I was hospitalized…I still don't understand why…

T: I see, that's exactly what I want to talk to you about; how you experienced this period…

P: I didn't understand what I was doing there. I was seeing everyone so strange, I was always by myself… I kept quiet, because otherwise they would punish me…

T: Okay…let me understand…so you were always on the alert and controlled?

P: No, I'm not saying that. It's just that I was lonely there, because everyone else had all their own problems. Then, I didn't want to see anybody. Some friends or relatives wanted me to visit, but I was ashamed to be seen locked up like a madman.

Having focused attention on a specific emotionally marked episode makes it easier, for the patient, to access his own internal states even if vague in detail. The patient refers, superficially, to three possible patterns: initially a sense of threat emerges where the other, moved by intentions unknown to him, may be dangerous; then, a state of interpersonal diversity/distance is observed, and then, the agonistic one related to the judgment theme is observed. The therapist catches, in particular, the latter pattern by fearing that he too may be seen as a potential judgmental other, thus always maintaining a validating attitude. Speaking of the fear of being criticized and excluded by others, Luke recalls, spontaneously, situations in which he felt judged in college and, even earlier, in a neighborhood group of friends.

Often SPD patients are unable to describe the content of their experience; in these cases, the patient must be helped to identify his or her own thoughts and emotions. This work should be done first of all from the traces that emerge in the session, in the patient's verbal and/or nonverbal content, from bodily aspects or in the therapeutic relationship. Experiential techniques such as guided imagery, body focusing, and role-playing are very effective in this respect.

In one session, the therapist invites Luke to focus on the body state, the way through which he most easily expresses his emotions.

P: At home, I kept having those strange physical sensations, once after an argument with my father … the feeling of having a presence inside me.

T: What do you mean by presence? Explain further.

P: Well… I don't think I'm possessed by the devil; it's like there's a presence inside me.
T: Can you describe this presence a little bit?
P: I don't know…when I feel this presence, I feel confused, I can't concentrate.
T: Where do you feel this presence?
P: In the chest, it's like a weight inside (puts hand on chest).
T: Stay with your hand on your chest, try to feel it now, how do you feel it?
P: It pushes inside my chest, I feel weak, tired…
T: Earlier you also said confused, do you feel the presence from other parts of the body?
P: I don't know (he continues to keep his hand on his chest), a little in the head… it's still a diffuse feeling…
T: Try to describe this presence.
P: It's not a person or an entity…I don't know, like demon…anyway it's not clear because I feel it in the body, as if I don't have control of the body in those moments.

The therapist invited the patient to feel the painful physical states, an expression of "embodied" sensations and patterns to try to grasp possible related emotions. The patient pauses to describe *bizarre thoughts* and *beliefs* related to religion from *unusual perceptions* not well defined. Luke still appears confused about this, does not have a clear theory about what is happening to him, and senses a presence "inside him" that is not well defined and which he experiences as threatening because of this. Physical sensations emerge more easily in situations of emotional stress throughout the days.

Once autobiographical memories are obtained, it will be possible to reconstruct the cause-and-effect links between events, thoughts, and actions; inviting the patient to relive such scenes in session, even using imaginative techniques, can facilitate the reconstruction of the connection between the different event cognition–self-perception–emotion variables. Helping the patient reconstruct these connections is the most important step that will lead him or her to reconstruct the pathogenic patterns.

P: Yesterday I felt the presence inside me again. I am not convinced that it is a possession, it is a presence.
T: How do you feel now as you tell me about it?
P: Good! (smiles)
T: I'm glad you talk about it smiling; it seems to me, however, that you think about this presence a lot. Would you like to tell how things went yesterday when you heard it?
P: Yes, it was evening when I had come home and I felt that sensation.
T: Let's see then what happened yesterday. Let's try to reconstruct what happened, as if we were there right now.
P: Nothing, I was back from work yesterday…
T: Look, try talking in present time, as if you were reliving the scene. I came home…

P: Alright. So…I finished all my rounds in the houses where I go to work, I come home and say hello to Dad.
T: How are you feeling right now?
P: Fine, physically tired…I had a little argument with one person, but nothing important.
T: Wait, are you tired emotionally?
P: Emotionally I'm a little nervous because of the discussion earlier…
T: So you're tired and a little nervous. You see your father, you say hello to him…describe what you are thinking right now.
P: That I'd like to go take a shower! So, I can relax a little bit.
T: Well…and what happens now?
P: My father calls me to tell me if I had done the shopping.
T: How do you feel when Dad tells you that?
P: I immediately got nervous because I had forgotten to do the shopping.
T: You forgot to go grocery shopping, let's stay in the scene. Try to feel what you feel inside… Dad tells you that you didn't do the grocery shopping.
P: That it's true, that I forgot…I made a mistake, I should have remembered…however, I've been working all day. I've been going around the houses. I make a mistake and immediately he takes me back; he never understands me, that sometimes I can be tired.
T: Nervous. Something like anger, it seems to me.
P: Yes…and right now I feel those strange feelings inside me.
T: The feeling of tiredness now how is it?
P: That's always there, but I feel again that strange weight on my chest, I don't know…
T: A weight on the chest…
P: Yes I can't breathe well, freely, like I have an obstacle… It's an unpleasant feeling, I look around…
T: Dad where is he right now.
P: He′s standing there, but I don't care. I have this physical feeling that worries me. I have to go to my room.

In proposing the experiential technique to explore the scene and reconstruct the patterns, the therapist feels that inviting the patient to close his eyes would not allow him to let go completely; he decides, then, to reconstruct the scene while keeping his eyes open. He invites Luke to dwell on the details of the scene while maintaining a welcoming and validating tone, not pressing but interested in what was being said; he invites him to pause in the individual states, to describe them as clearly as possible, not suggesting interpretations or causal links between the individual representations. The patient used to describe right away that feeling of presence that he experienced as inexplicable and perturbing; now, guided in the telling and "restrained" by the therapist to stay in the individual moments of the episode, he was able to describe and "discover" representations and sensations that most of the time were fleeting, and that did not attract his attention. Luke thus discovered that, just before he felt the sensation of a presence, he had physically felt a fatigue that had followed an overworked morning.

Once patient and therapist have reconstructed the relationships between variables during the narrative episode, the therapy moves toward the understanding that these processes are not only related to the event just narrated, but also represent stable modes of meaning attribution, that is, patterns that are repeated: The therapist will then request associated memories on the basis of thematic relevance to the state of suffering and the scene just described. Having collected a number of memories, it is possible to reconstruct the interpersonal pattern by observing that there are affinities or recursiveness in the different narrated events.

Let us look at Luke's patterns together. At the moment when he experiences unclear physical sensations, a vulnerable self-image emerges, causing him to enter a state of alarm. The safety system is activated, where the other is not seen as protective and supportive, but in turn threatening and hindering: the coping adopted is protective isolation such that he hides his vulnerability from others, as well as brooding to try to find an explanation for unexplained perceptions. The moment he perceives an altered bodily state, he feels different from others; a pattern of estrangement/detachment is activated where others are seen as people who have nothing in common with him; he would like to relate to others to share how he feels, but he feels he is having a unique experience, different from others. So, he avoids talking to them, certain that no one would understand him, locking himself in a withdrawal that accentuates the condition of interpersonal distance. In other situations, Luke also appears to be driven by a competitive interpersonal pattern. Luke would like to prove his worth, but fearful of receiving criticism from the other (as was the case in college); he avoids relationships so as not to expose himself to judgment, or he resorts to perfectionism or overwork to avoid negative judgment.

Having reconstructed the patterns together by observing that there are recurring relational modes, the patient may say, "Then it is I who tend to see these things all the time." This marks the beginning of the change promotion phase.

Promotion of Change

At the end of the previous phase, the therapist had invited Luke to recall autobiographical memories pertaining to the problematic episodes, in order to be able to grasp how some relational modes are repeated the same over time and in different situations; this is to get to the point of constructing new modes of thought and action that lead toward adaptation. The patient must now be helped to *differentiate*, because a desire for change arises only after experiencing and perceiving interpersonal patterns as egodystonic.

To gradually foster a critical distance from the schemas, the therapist invites the patient to revise the way he or she imagines the course of the relationship ("I will surely be misjudged") from a more effective self-image previously reconstructed ("I remember when the lady told me I was good"); in this way, the certainty of receiving a negative judgment becomes less firm. In other cases, the therapist showed Luke how certain relational modes ("I feel strange, different, and that's why others will definitely not want to deal with me") are repeated equally under certain circumstances ("every time I feel physically strange I feel that others experience a different reality and that's why they will stay away from me"): the therapist shows the patient that if a mode of reading events remains the same over time, it may be related to the way of interpreting events rather than to the situations themselves.

Parallel to the work on differentiation, there is also an attempt to encourage access to the healthy parts, to show the patient that he or she is capable of feeling trust or comfortable with the other. It is necessary, then, for the therapist to pay attention to nonverbal signals, to the contents of narratives in which the patient shows signs of positive states and tells himself in a way that is discrepant from pathogenic patterns. These moments should be pointed out to the patient and carefully explored to thus activate adaptive modes of functioning.

Having reached a critical distance from the schemas and from positive representations of self, the patient's behavioral change is designed in therapy. Having realized that the patient is being guided into action by pathogenic schemas, the therapeutic contract is reformulated, pointing out to the patient that well-being increasingly depends on actions taken outside the sessions: the patient must take the new structured beliefs outside the therapeutic setting, put them to the test of actual exchanges in the world. It is explained, for example, that without leaving home and meeting others, the sense of alienation will not go away; if autonomy is not experienced, the feeling of fragility will not diminish. Instead, we can be satisfied and experience well-being if we pursue goals and desires that we feel are ours and that we believe in.

The therapist proposes going over the course of the week to check the activation of the various patterns and how they are progressing without enacting the usual protective coping (e.g., avoidance of situations, resorting to perfectionism in performance, falling into brooding, or control). He then invites him to try to expose himself to conditions usually activating the patient's schemas (e.g., in Luke's case, the subject of judgment), always starting with those with less emotional load, to see how it is possible to stay in the feared scenes without being overwhelmed by the emotional reaction. Exposures build new memories where relationships are not guided by schemas; these accumulate by going to depower a rigid procedural mode such as schema-related. Exposures bring out the healthy parts of the patient together with a greater sense of agency; Luke tells how he dealt with criticism at work or difficulties with his father, experiencing a sense of efficacy in dealing with interpersonal issues: he now feels able to take charge of his life independently.

Final therapy steps with Luke included the following: (a) Starting from a greater awareness of his own schemata, the therapist stimulates Luke's ability to understand the other's inner states. In the session, after showing his tendency to automatically read the interlocutor's intentions, he invites him to imagine what other thoughts and images might be present in his mind, in order to make his representation flexible. He then reproduces relational exchanges using role-play; the role-reversal in the exercise allows the patient to put himself in the other person's shoes and thus have a different reading of his mind. The therapist then invites Luke to stay in real relationships and try to read the other's intentionality starting from his attitude and mimicry, his behavior, and his way of speaking, ignoring for a moment his usual interpretation. (b) Starting from a better understanding of the other's mind, the therapist helps the patient to recognize the interpersonal cycles that are activated within relationships starting from the behaviors that Luke enacts guided by his own schemes, to understand the role he plays in the genesis and maintenance of these interpersonal dynamics. For example, in the course of a role-play, the therapist invites Luke to adopt different relational modalities from his usual ones; in the discussion that follows, the relationship's progress is assessed together and which of the modalities proved to be more adaptive to the situation represented, (c) helping Luke realize when he is driven again by schema-related negative views about himself and learn to see himself from a more benevolent stance.

In order to consolidate understanding and distancing from one's maladaptive schemas, the therapist tries to catch moments in the patient's experience when the schema still seems to appear, even if less pervasive and disabling. For example, when thinking about "presence," Luke tended to see himself as strange or "crazy" as he realized that this idea was an irrational reading of his own physical states; thinking himself "crazy" still brought out the inadequate and different self-image from others, with lowered mood and consequent tendency to closure. The therapist shows the patient how certain stimuli still question his value by activating a sense of diversity; he reminds how these internal states are the expression of known patterns that have been structured and maintained over time. Already in the session, she invites him to interrupt his brooding, making him experience a sense of agency over his own internal state; this consolidates the healthy self-image that contrasts the powerless one that has always accompanied him. Starting from this effective self-representation, from the re-evocation of recent exposures that have seen Luke confronted with difficult relational situations, the therapist invites Luke to reevaluate that sense of inadequacy previously experienced in order to affirm, in this way, a different, more adaptive self-image.

Conclusions

After 2 years of psychotherapy treatment, the patient presented a significant improvement in symptoms, a reduction and discontinuation of psychopharmacological therapy, and no relapse such that further hospitalizations were necessary. Luke at the end of the therapy feels less sense of helplessness and constraint, has greater ability to describe his internal world, experiences greater sense of agency, and is aware that his ideas of being vulnerable to others perceived as threatening are not necessarily true. These changes allow the patient to access ideas of himself as more effective and adequate and of others as less critical, distant, and hostile. Luke thanks to MIT now possesses a more articulate and realistic map of the world, enabling him to realize his desires in the domain of interpersonal relationships.

In conclusion, the evolution of Luke's therapeutic journey shows how MIT allows for the formulation of procedures that can be successfully applied to schizotypal personality disorder. The results obtained cannot be generalized since this is a single case study, but they certainly encourage further study in this direction.

References

American Psychiatric Association. (2013). *Diagnostic and statistical manual of mental disorders* (5th ed.). American Psychiatric Publishing, 2013. Trad. it. Manuale diagnostico e statistico dei disturbi mentali. Raffaello Cortina, 2014.

Cheli, S. (2020). Assessment and treatment planning for schizotypal personality disorder: A metacognitively oriented point of view. *Psychiatric Rehabilitation Journal, 43*(4), 335–343. https://doi.org/10.1037/prj0000429

Cheli, S., Lysaker, P. H., & Dimaggio, G. (2019). Metacognitively oriented psychotherapy for schizotypal personality disorder: A two-case series. *Personality and Mental Health, 13*(3), 155–167. https://doi.org/10.1002/pmh.1447

Cheli, S., Cavalletti, V., Lysaker, P. H., Dimaggio, G., Petrocchi, N., Chiarello, F., Enzo, C., Velicogna, F., Mancini, F., & Goldzweig, G. (2023). A pilot randomized controlled trial comparing a novel compassion and metacognition approach for schizotypal personality disorder with a combination of cognitive therapy and psychopharmacological treatment. *BMC Psychiatry, 23*, 113. https://doi.org/10.1186/s12888-023-04610-5

Dimaggio, G., Semerari, A., Carcione, A., Nicolò, G., & Procacci, M. (2007). *Psychotherapy of personality disorders: Metacognition, states of mind and interpersonal cycles*. Routledge.

Dimaggio, G., Montano, A., Popolo, R., & Salvatore G. (2013). *Terapia metacognitiva interpersonale dei disturbi di personalità*. Raffaello Cortina Editore.

Dimaggio, G., Montano, A., Popolo, R., & Salvatore, G. (2015). *Metacognitive interpersonal therapy for personality disorders: A treatment manual*. Routledge.

Dimaggio, G., Ottavi, P., Popolo, R., & Salvatore, G. (2019). *Corpo, immaginazione e cambiamento*. Raffaello Cortina Editore.

Dimaggio, G., Ottavi, P., Popolo, R., & Salvatore, G. (2020). *Metacognitive interpersonal therapy body, imagery and change*. Routledge.

Frith, C. D. (2004). Schizophrenia and theory of mind. *Psychological Medicine, 34*(3), 385–389.

Hasson-Ohayon, I., Avidan-Msika, M., Mashiach-Eizenberg, M., Kravetz, S., Rozencwaig, S., Shalev, H., & Lysaker, P. H. (2015). Metacognitive and social cognition approaches to understanding the impact of schizophrenia on social quality of life. *Schizophrenia Research, 161*(2–3), 386–391.

Hazlett, E. A., Collazo, T., Zelmanova, Y., Entis, J. J., Chu, K. W., Goldstein, K. E., Roussos, P., Haznedar, M. M., Koenigsberg, H. W., New, A. S., Buchsbaum, M. S., Hershowitz, J. P., Siever, L. J., & Byne, W. (2012). Anterior limb of the internal capsule in schizotypal personality disorder: Fiber-tract counting, volume, and anisotropy. *Schizophrenia Research, 141*, 119–127.

Holma, J., & Aaltonen, J. (1998). Narrative understanding in acute psychosis. *Contemporary Family Therapy: An International Journal, 20*(3), 253–263.

Kirchner, S. K., Roeh, A., Noldenand, J., & Hasan, A. (2018). Diagnosis and treatment of schizotypal personality disorder: Evidence from a systematic review. *NPJ Schizophrenia, 4*, 20.

Lysaker, P. H., & Buck, K. D. (2010). Metacognitive capacity as a focus of individual psychotherapy in schizophrenia. In G. Dimaggio & P. H. Lysaker (Eds.), *Metacognition and severe adult mental disorders: From research to treatment* (pp. 217–232). Routledge/Taylor & Francis Group.

Lysaker, P. H., & Dimaggio, G. (2014). Metacognitive capacities for reflection in schizophrenia: Implications for developing treatments. *Schizophrenia Bulletin, 40*(3), 487–491.

Lysaker, P. H., Leonhardt, B. L., Brüne, M., Buck, K. D., James, A., Vohs, J., Francis, M., Hamm, J. A., Salvatore, G., Ringer, J. M., & Dimaggio, G. (2014). Capacities for theory of mind,

metacognition, and neurocognitive function are independently related to emotional recognition in schizophrenia. *Psychiatry Research, 219*(1), 79–85.
Mitchell, J. P., Macrae, C. N., & Banaji, M. R. (2006). Dissociable medial prefrontal contributions to judgments of similar and dissimilar others. *Neuron, 50*(4), 655–663.
Rado, S. (1953). Dynamics and classification of disordered behavior. *American Journal of Psychiatry, 110*, 406–416.
Safran, J. D., & Muran, J. C. (2000). *Negotiating the therapeutic alliance: A relational treatment guide*. Guilford Press.
Salvatore, G., Dimaggio, G., & Lysaker, P. H. (2007). An intersubjective perspective on negative symptoms of schizophrenia: Implications of simulation theory. *Cognitive Neuropsychiatry, 12*(2), 144–164.
Salvatore, G., Procacci, M., Popolo, R., Nicolò, G., Carcione, A., Semerari, A., & Dimaggio, G. (2009). Adapted metacognitive interpersonal therapy for improving adherence to intersubjective contexts in a person with schizophrenia. *Clinical Case Studies, 8*(6), 473–488.
Salvatore, G., Lysaker, P. H., Gumley, A., Popolo, R., Mari, J., & Dimaggio, G. (2012). Out of illness experience: Metacognition-oriented therapy for promoting self-awareness in individuals with psychosis. *American Journal of Psychotherapy, 66*(1), 85–106.
Stanghellini, G. (2010). Common sense, disembodiment and schizophrenic delusions. In G. Dimaggio & P. H. Lysaker (Eds.), *Metacognition and sever adult mental disorders: From research to treatment* (pp. 134–149). Routledge.
World Health Organizational. International Classification of Diseases – 11th version. Disponibile su: https://bit.ly/37gJdRO [ultimo accesso 30 novembre 2020].

Chapter 17
Evolutionary Systems Therapy for Schizotypy: An Integrated Look at Attachment, Compassion and Metacognition

Simone Cheli

Introduction

Schizotypy is an enigma for the clinician. Hundreds of theoretical studies have been published about this construct; however, no treatment guidelines have ever been formulated for treating schizotypal traits. Schizotypy, as a continuum of diverse conditions, ranging from sub-clinical or even healthy states to severe disorders (Kwapil & Barrantes-Vidal, 2015), is possibly one of the first psychopathological dimensions ever formulated and studied. Since the very first attempts of Eugen Bleuler (1911) to define traits recurring between patients diagnosed with schizophrenia and their siblings and between premorbid and clinical states, the main assumption was that certain personality features expose individuals to a heightened risk for psychopathology. As Paul Meehl (1962) later suggested, this would imply the possibility of locating specific markers of this schizotypal vulnerability and therefore of predicting the risk for severe disorders such as schizophrenia. Although the original formulation by Meehl has been revised by Gordon Claridge (Claridge & Broks, 1984) and others in terms of a full continuum from adaptive to maladaptive states rather than a taxon of pathological clusters (Cicero et al., 2019), schizotypy can be considered an early attempt to overcome a categorical and normative approach to psychopathology that is traced back one century ago. The wide range of experiences of those presenting schizotypal traits is usually understood in respect to three sets of features, including: positive (e.g., magical thinking), negative (e.g., anhedonia), and disorganized (e.g., odd behaviors) features (see Kwapil & Barrantes-Vidal, Chap. 6, this book).

S. Cheli (✉)
Department of Psychology, St. John's University, Rome, Italy

Center for Psychology and Health, Tages Charity, Florence, Italy
e-mail: chelis@stjohns.edu

S. Cheli, P. H. Lysaker (eds.), *A Dimensional Approach to Schizotypy*,
https://doi.org/10.1007/978-3-031-41788-7_17

Unfortunately, this long history was primarily shaped by the search for specific biomarkers to detect schizotypal vulnerability taking resources away from trying to develop trait-specific therapeutic interventions. A recent systematic review on schizotypal personality disorder (SPD) – which is probably the most representative clinical manifestation of schizotypy and the more prevalent together with brief psychotic disorder (BPD) – confirmed this trend: only a few studies on the feasibility of antipsychotic medications and just three studies on talk therapy or multimodal interventions were found (Kirchner et al., 2018). Similarly, the Cluster A of personality disorders has received limited attention. Schizoid personality disorder (SZPD) is discussed only in terms of anecdotal experiences (Hopwood & Thomas, 2012) and just a few studies included the diagnosis of paranoid personality disorder (PPD) as an inclusion criterion (Triebwasser et al., 2013). It is noteworthy how all the studies recruiting persons diagnosed with SPD, PPD, and SZPD did not clearly formulate a model of the intervention specific for schizotypal traits. The most interesting attempt is possibly a large randomized controlled trial (RCT) on the effectiveness of Schema Therapy (Bamelis et al., 2014). Authors included a few persons diagnosed with PPD ($N = 14$), but presented a general model of personality disorders (PDs) fitting with all the possible disorders.

The rise of dimensional and hierarchical models has fostered a look at psychopathology that is transdiagnostic, but at the same time informed by specific traits or spectra. The Five Factor Model (FFM), the Alternative Model of Personality Disorders (AMPD), and the Hierarchical Taxonomy of Psychopathology (HiTOP) have converged on two pivotal assumptions (Cicero et al., 2019; Gurrera et al., 2005; Kwapil & Barrantes-Vidal, 2022): (i) a general level of functioning or severity can better support the clinician in understanding the presenting problem than categorical diagnoses and (ii) the traits and facets are practical and trans-theoretical tools in anticipating the patient's trajectory and defining effective therapeutic strategies. Although these dimensional models have dominated the scientific debate for 15 years, we are once again without therapeutic guidelines for traits such as schizotypal traits characterized by a heightened severity. It has been suggested that thought disorders – as clinical manifestations of schizotypy – would represent the final psychopathological end of either externalizing or internalizing trajectories along a broad developmental continuum (Sharp, 2020).

Indeed, schizotypal traits may be associated with different and highly prevalent forms of severe impairment in psychosocial functioning. If we exclude a Norwegian sample as a possible outlier (prevalence = 0.6%), two American studies suggest a prevalence of SPD in the general population ranging between 3.9% and 4.6% (American Psychiatric Association, 2013). The course of the disorder is supposed to be stable with a possible risk for transitioning to schizophrenia (prevalence in population = 1%; APA, 2013) and psychotic experiences (prevalence in population = 5.8%; McGrath et al., 2015). Studies on course of impairment in psychosocial functioning report mixed outcomes: one out of four would later develop schizophrenia spectrum disorders, and paranoid ideation and unusual experience would be stable over time whereas oddity was more changeable (Kirchner et al., 2018). The relevance of SPD along the schizotypal continuum is even higher if we consider this diagnosis from the AMPD viewpoint. Indeed, AMPD includes SPD in the six (out of ten) remaining mixed categorical-dimensional diagnoses in the DSM-5. This diagnosis comprises two main domains (i.e., psychoticism and detachment) that can be used – either through a pure dimensional or a mixed approach – to assess what was previously defined as Cluster A of PDs (PPD; SZPD; SPD). Therefore, schizotypal traits would refer to a personality functioning that is highly prevalent, possibly leading to severe manifestations.

That said, when it comes to the issue on how to treat persons with prominent schizotypal traits, therapeutic options were in the past and are still today scarce. The aim of this chapter is to describe a recently implemented form of therapy – namely, Evolutionary Systems Therapy for Schizotypy (ESTS) – that is supposed to be feasible in targeting schizotypal traits (Cheli et al., 2023a). Its theoretical background is based on evolutionary theory and complex systems theory (Cheli, 2018, 2023). In the following pages, I describe the rationale of ESTS and how this supports a shared conceptualization with the patient, and then the structure of the manualized protocol and evidence supporting its clinical utility. I conclude by summarizing recent trends and future directions of research on ESTS.

ESTS can be possibly considered the first attempt to outline and test a psychotherapy tailored to schizotypal traits. It is informed by existing theoretical and experimental studies on schizotypy, but it is primarily oriented toward clinical practice. It has been designed to target schizotypal traits along the continuum of clinical manifestations: from early psychosocial distress in the general population (where the prevalence of schizotypy is almost 10%) to rigid and maladaptive traits as in SPD (prevalence ranging between 3.9% and 4.6%).

Roots and Background

During 2018, we started at the Center for Psychology and Health, Tages Charity (Tages Onlus) in Florence with a project aimed to test possible interventions for SPD. As a mental health center focused on a recovery-oriented approach, we were experiencing an increasing demand for support for those presenting in states at risk for psychosis and, concurrently, hesitant or even oppositive attitudes with respect to standard treatments. Since there were no guidelines to rely upon, we opted for an intervention based on a highly transdiagnostic target that has been shown to be predictive of psychosocial functioning in both PDs and schizophrenia spectrum disorders: metacognition (see Lysaker and Wiesepape, Chap. 8, this book). Metacognition refers to the integrated and nuanced ability to understand one's own mental states and the mental states of others (Lysaker et al., 2018). It is similar in this respect to well-established constructs such as mentalizing and social cognition; however, it is also reputed to offer an architectural look at self-organizing functions through which persons make sense of their subjective and intersubjective experience (Lysaker et al., 2021). It comprises four sub-functions: self-reflectivity (i.e., understanding one's own mental states), awareness of the other's mind (i.e., understanding the mental states of others), decentration (i.e., awareness that others have their own valuable view of the world), and mastery (i.e., the ability to use metacognitive functions to cope with daily psychosocial challenges). By considering how metacognition is capable of predicting psychosocial functioning in severe mental disorders and how specific treatments based on it were effective in treating schizophrenia and PDs (Lysaker et al., 2020; Semerari et al., 2014), we tested two different forms of Metacognitively Oriented Psychotherapy (MOP): Metacognitive Reflection and Insight Therapy (MERIT; Lysaker & Klion, 2017) and Metacognitive Interpersonal Therapy (MIT; Dimaggio et al., 2020). In two cases conducted in collaboration with Paul H. Lysaker (Indiana University) and Giancarlo Dimaggio (Center for MIT), we showed how a 6-month MOP may be a feasible intervention for those diagnosed with SPD (Cheli et al., 2019). Both patients remitted from diagnosis and reported reliable changes in symptomatology. During a post-hoc analysis, we noticed that the case successfully treated with MERIT had higher proneness to schizophrenia and possibly a higher vulnerability (i.e., early detached temperament and a family history of psychiatric disorders), whereas the one successfully treated with MIT had several developmental stressors (i.e., a personal history of traumas) and comorbid traits related to other personality disorders (i.e., dysregulated and antagonistic traits). In a second larger cases series ($N = 12$; Cheli, 2020), we tested a modular intervention where MERIT was used for the early phases (being reputed more feasible for severer symptoms) and MIT for the advanced phases (being reputed more feasible for targeting complex interpersonal schemas). This one-year intervention was effective even if the patients were reporting a limited acceptability of the experiential interventions proposed during the later phases of MOP. It is noteworthy how in this latter cases series the SPD diagnosis was made using the AMPD, rather than the categorical diagnosis as in the first two-cases series.

In the meanwhile, we tested alternative interventions aimed to reduce the criticisms we experienced during the first studies. As previously discussed, experiential techniques were not fully perceived as safe and viable by the patients. Second, during the early shared conceptualization phase we experienced two diametrically opposite problems. A fully non-stigmatizing approach to schizotypy based on metacognitive functioning without referring to a categorical diagnosis was well accepted at the beginning, but then perceived as limited (i.e., people did not feel fully understood in their longstanding difficulties). In contrast, an early presentation of the SPD diagnosis was perceived as stigmatizing and generated several significant ruptures in the therapeutic alliance. Thus, we explored the feasibility of alternatives.

In a few single cases and cases series, we tested the feasibility of experiential techniques that were integrated with the evolutionary psychoeducation of Compassion Focused Therapy (CFT; Gilbert, 2009). Indeed, CFT is an evolutionarily informed therapy that posits how self-soothing, a mammalian effect regulation system normally triggered by cues of social safeness, is impaired by criticisms about self and others leading to a counteracting activation of the threat detection and response system (Gilbert, 2020; Petrocchi & Cheli, 2019). This model offers an extremely valuable approach to understand proximate and evolutionary factors involved in a specific trait (see Cheli & Brüne, Chap. 2, this book). Criticism about the self and others would be shaped by the phylogenetic history of our species (e.g., shame and self-criticism had a pivotal role in a hyper-affiliative species such as humans) and triggered by early stressors within relationships with attachment figures and peers (Bucci et al., 2017; Gumley et al., 2014). This is consistent with the transdiagnostic role of self-criticism, early attachment experiences, and interpersonal criticism among different mental health disorders (See Berry et al., Chap. 10, this book; Gilbert, Chap. 11, this book; Asan et al., Chap. 12, this book). From a neurodevelopmental point of view, early experiences in the form of attachment relationships are fundamental in generating interpersonal schemas (or internal working models according to attachment theory) about how we perceive ourselves and the others during interactions (Antonucci et al., 2018; Luyten & Fonagy, 2015). Moreover, distressful or even traumatic experiences may generate or foster a vulnerability for psychopathology that has been reported in both patients diagnosed with psychosis and healthy subjects with prominent schizotypal traits (Varese et al., 2012; Velikonja et al., 2015). The same patterns (i.e., interpersonal schemas, interpersonal cycle, internal working models, etc.) that in adults are associated with critical beliefs about self and others are rooted in early developmental experiences and have progressively become more rigid and inflexible.

In collaboration with the Italian association of CFT (Compassionate Mind Italia), we explored the viability of compassion-focused psychoeducation and experiential techniques to schizotypy through two cases series (Cheli et al., 2020, 2021b). Then, in a large sample of healthy young adults ($N = 2065$), we confirmed how the protective factor of metacognition in respect to delusional ideation may fail when people experience severe forms of self-criticism (Cheli et al., 2021a, b).

Finally, I integrated existing knowledge about schizotypy with the data we have collected during these preliminary studies (Cheli, 2023). This model was the foundation of the shared conceptualization in ESTS.

The Early Shared Conceptualization

A growing body of evidence suggests that personality traits are better understood as a continuum from adaptive to maladaptive experiences consistent with a between-persons perspective, whereas from a within-person point of view, a trait can evolve into diverse clinical manifestations related to a specific spectrum (Kotov et al., 2021). Schizotypy primarily refers to facets of openness to experience and introversion, plus facets of neuroticism (Edmundson & Kwapil, 2013). This pattern parallels the conceptualization of schizotypal personality proposed by the AMPD as defined by psychoticism and several facets of detachment (Kwapil & Barrantes-Vidal, 2022), and similarly by the HiTOP as a super-spectrum of psychosis (Kotov et al., 2020). Thus, it is reasonable that odd behaviors, emotions, cognitions, and emotional and social detachment may evolve during development from prominent openness and introversion.

In ESTS, this data is presented through an evolutionary framework (Cheli, 2023). The phylogenetic rise of the social brain is linked with the rise of schizotypy, suggesting how the complexity of our metacognition and social life is linked to both advantages and disadvantages (Burns, 2007; Dunbar, 2009). Similarly, the neurodevelopment of the human social brain is so complex that humans are exposed to extreme vulnerability when dealing with threatening social experiences, from childhood maltreatment to difficulties in peer-to-peer relationships (Teicher et al., 2022). From the ESTS point of view, the clinical manifestations of schizotypy would represent a failure in socializing one's own openness to experience and introversion, finally leading to odd and distorted beliefs (i.e., psychoticism) and severe social withdrawal (i.e., detachment). Since human adaptation always happens within a social context, schizotypal traits would expose a person to a vicious cycle (see Fig. 17.1). The more a person perceives a threat in socializing, the more they foster defensive patterns in the form of unique-maximizing (i.e., crystallizing one's own subjective beliefs) and risk-minimizing (i.e., reducing social and emotional expression) strategies. This would lead to increasing levels of psychoticism and detachment, and the more these maladaptive traits are rigid, inflexible, and recurrent, the more the person experiences a threat maintaining this vicious cycle. A pivotal role is played by critical beliefs about self and others in the forms of self-criticism and

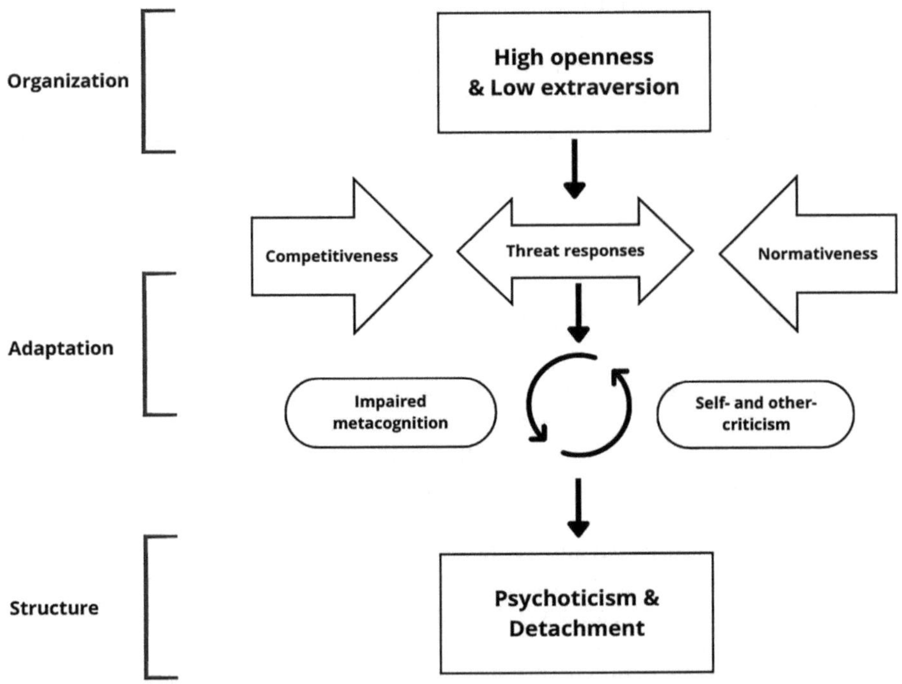

Fig. 17.1 An evolutionary model of schizotypy. (Modified from *New Ideas in Psychology*, 68, 100993, Simone Cheli, An evolutionary look at oddity and schizotypy: How the rise of social brain informs clinical practice, Copyright Elsevier (2023))

suspiciousness that, through a vagally mediated neurophysiological cascade, impairs metacognitive functioning (Cheli et al., 2020; Wood & Irons, 2016). When under stress, the vagus nerve may mediate a hypo-activation of the prefrontal cortex (a brain region directly involved in metacognition) with consequences on a variety of regulatory functions. And obviously, the more metacognitive functioning is impaired, the more likely defensive strategies based on our temperamental dispositions and our learned automatisms will be. Figure 17.1 is indicative of these patterns, suggesting a distinction between a bio-temperamental tendency (organization as high openness and introversion) and a resulting personality structure (high psychoticism and detachment) through subjective and intersubjective forms of adaptation (see Maturana & Varela, 1984). It is noteworthy how a trait, such as openness, that can be considered valuable and socially reinforced may incur in an evolutionary paradox: social pressure may force the persons to compete for innovation and creative solutions, while the same community may sanction those who are diverging from societal norms and standards. Therefore, either a limited capacity to socialize ones' own ideas or an extremely judgmental attitude of the environment may trigger and maintain the previously described vicious cycle.

This evolutionary model is presented and discussed with the patient avoiding scientific jargon. While collecting information about the presenting problem, the therapist tries to validate emotional distress and the difficulty in finding a way out from this distress. Special attention is paid to threatening experiences in the forms of attachment relationships, self-criticism, and interpersonal criticism, before introducing the first element of psychoeducation. The neurophysiological cycle previously described is explained through simple metaphors. For example, the therapist may say: "If It – the Stephen King character – enters into the room holding an axe, what do you do? Do you remain seated in your chair, or do you try to defend yourself, fleeing or attacking? Obviously, the latter! And that's healthy, that's adaptive!". Then, this defensive mechanism is detailed and generalized, trying to connect the threatening experiences reported by the patient and this neurophysiological vicious cycle. Second, the therapist aims to progressively explore the life history of the patient. Different techniques can be used in a structured way (e.g., asking the patient to write as a homework a brief summary of past life) or during the flow of therapeutic dialogue. When discussing the elements emerging during this phase, it is important that the therapist explores early temperament. The goal is to share an integrated view of early personality organization and the series of negative experiences that are relevant for the patient. Consistent with the ESTS model and existing literature, those with schizotypal traits usually report prominent openness to experience and varying degrees of introversion and other traits. They also describe several turning points (they are clearly aware of some of them and become aware of others during the dialogue) that have negatively conditioned their life in the form of automatizing defensive strategies.

This shared conceptualization is often crucial during therapy, and our recent post-hoc analysis of past interventions has confirmed this. Patients describe this conceptualization as validating and usually not judgmental. They also see a pattern in their past behaviors that is an attempt – albeit maladaptive – to take care of themselves and live decently. Moreover, this first step supports the therapist in formulating and sharing a therapeutic plan: the goal is not to change the personality or restructure their identity, but rather to value their core traits implementing new and more adaptive strategies in socializing their experience.

The Four-Module Structure of the Therapy

ESTS is an individual therapy. It has been tested in either 6-month (RCT on SPD; Cheli et al., 2023a) or 10-month (cases series on SZPD; Cheli et al., 2022) format, ranging between 24 and 40 weekly sessions. The length is not strictly determined, but rather is supposed to be consistent with the specific needs and goals discussed with the patient. In clinical practice, we usually include a final follow-up phase with biweekly or monthly sessions.

ESTS comprises four modules (see Table 17.1): (1) sharing, (2) subjective systems, (3) intersubjective systems, and (4) consolidation. These labels were chosen

Table 17.1 The structure of evolutionary systems therapy for schizotypy

Module	Primary goal	Main steps	Therapeutic alliance
First – sharing	Sharing treatment goals and conceptualization	(a) Sharing evolutionary conceptualization (b) Introducing psycho-education (c) Defining preliminary goals	The therapist may be perceived as threatening and their compassion as something to defend from. A destigmatizing approach is pivotal
Second – subjective systems	Experiencing mind-body awareness of subjective experience	(a) Exploring early schemas (b) Understanding present schemas (c) Linking past and present	The exploration of the past may be distressful, but it is important to discuss and confirm recurring schemas and mechanisms to prevent future ruptures of alliance
Third – intersubjective systems	Experiencing mind-body awareness of intersubjective experience	(a) Exploring interpersonal cycles (b) Exploring socialization (c) Exploring communication	The tendency to intellectualize can take the focus away from experiential work on relationships. The therapist must not be conniving with this mechanism
Fourth – consolidation	Managing and consolidating changes	(a) Reflecting on changes (b) Reflecting on error friendliness (c) Consolidating adaptive strategies	The two biggest risks to the alliance are: patients may downplay the changes and therapists may avoid confirming the processes that facilitated those changes

Note. Evolutionary Systems Therapy for Schizotypy comprises four modules or phases, partially overlapping each other. Each module ranges between 4 and 8 sessions. Primary goals of the single module, main therapeutic steps, and a few tips about therapeutic alliance are presented to refer to two main theoretical roots. First, as I discussed in the previous paragraph, the early goal is to share a conceptualization that is based on an evolutionary view of human suffering, generally speaking, and, specifically, schizotypal traits. Consistent with evolutionary psychopathology, I hypothesize that a trait is not pathological per se. Even severe disorders – such as in schizotypy – are the maladaptive manifestations of complex evolutionary trade-offs and direct advantages related to human traits. A diagnosis such as SPD would be the final result of a failure in socializing one's own openness to experience and introversion (see Fig. 17.1).

Second, from an epistemological point of view, persons are considered complex systems whose experience is shaped by the continuousness of and contiguousness between subjective and intersubjective systems (Cheli, 2018). Therefore, the intervention should take into account this complexity, progressively moving back and forth from an increase of metacognitive self-reflectivity to a nuanced understanding of the other's mind and fallibility of any individual perspective. Complex systems theory informs the epistemological stance of the ESTS therapist, by valuing the unique meaning-making of any person and acknowledging how a tight distinction between personal and interpersonal experience is a convention rather than a matter of fact. This epistemology is consistent with several therapeutic approaches such as the not-knowing stance in Mentalization-Based Treatment (see Salaminios & Debannè, Chap. 9, this book), the recovery-oriented framework of Metacognitively Oriented Psychotherapy (see Lysaker & Wiesepape, Chap. 8, this book), and an interpersonal look at personality disorders (see Asan et al., Chap. 12, this book). Together, these models suggest the need for a non-stigmatizing approach to conceptualization and a therapy practically oriented toward the social life of our species. Moreover, this epistemological stance is related to specific focus on the therapeutic relationship and alliance. Those with prominent schizotypal traits – especially if they are under any psychosocial threat – will present specific patterns in negotiating goals, tasks, and bond. The human need for a safe social space will be hindered by defensive mechanisms in the form of fueling oddity and detachment to distance the other even at the cost of getting worst. Critical beliefs about self and others will manifest themselves in extreme ways (e.g., self-hatred, paranoia, terrifying fear of other's compassion, etc.), maintaining a vicious cycle that is the main and primary obstacle to therapy. The therapist should be aware of that and directly use the therapeutic relationship to explore these cyclical patterns and how the patient makes sense of them. As Lorna Benjamin (1993) would say, any form of suffering is a gift of love, that is an attempt – albeit a maladaptive one – to maintain or look for human relationships. This fine-grained understanding may support the therapist in understanding their countertransference in the recurrent maladaptive forms of either a fearful/anxious sense of unpredictability (triggered by odd or disorganized narratives) or a worried/annoyed frustration (when dealing with a constant fluctuation of symptoms and mentalizing).

Finally, consolidation (the 4th module) is considered a flexible phase aimed to stabilize and consolidate changes through a sort of experimental approach. This is reputed to be consistent with evolutionary conceptualization and systemic epistemology, and so with the need to implement new strategies in being in the world. The flexibility refers to both a variable length of sessions and different strategies in accordance with person's needs, whereas the experimental approach refers to a therapeutic way of promoting curiosity and error-friendliness in facing daily psychological challenges. Consistent with experiential approaches to psychotherapy, the therapist invites the patient to experience rather than talk about change.

In Table 17.2, I present a brief summary of the case of Abigail (fictional name), a 21-year-old patient I worked with. The therapy is discussed in relation to the four modules of ESTS, highlighting how, on the one hand, there is an ideal sequence of narrative and experiential techniques, and on the other hand, the therapist is supported in tailoring the intervention to the specific personality styles of the patient and their actual needs. Indeed, the predominance of schizotypal traits does not imply a tight definition of patient's personality. Each person has their own uniqueness in terms of specific schizotypal patterns (e.g., prominent positive or negative features) and concomitant traits (e.g., more internalizing or externalizing features). This subjective complexity, together with the complexity of the intersubjective world we live in, generates infinite possibilities and trajectories, and makes our profession so fascinating.

Supporting Evidence and Future Research

ESTS is a novel form of psychotherapy that has collected preliminary evidence. It cannot be considered a treatment of choice for SPD, but together with a good psychiatric management tested in Danmark (Nordentoft et al., 2006), it is one of the few available treatments specifically tailored to schizotypal traits and then tested through RCTs (see Kirchner et al., 2018).

Indeed, we recently concluded an RCT reporting promising evidence about the feasibility and effectiveness of ESTS (Cheli et al., 2023a). We compared this new form of therapy (without drugs) with a combination of Cognitive Behavioral Therapy (CBT) for PDs (Beck et al., 2015) and tailored psychopharmacological treatment for SPD. The study was a pilot non-inferiority trial, and we randomized (on a 1:1 ratio) 24 patients diagnosed with SPD. At the end of the 6-month intervention (24 weekly sessions), the primary outcome – reduction of personality pathology as assessed monthly over time – confirmed the non-inferiority of experimental treatment. Moreover, ESTS showed a larger reduction of general symptomatology ($\eta^2 = .558$) and a larger increase in metacognition ($\eta^2 = .734$) than control group. It is noteworthy that two other scores suggested a possible inferiority of the combination of CBT and drugs. First, at certain phases of treatment (i.e., second month of intervention, final, and at 1-month follow-up assessment), ESTS reported greater reduction in personality pathology, such that there was a greater gain in respect to control group. Second, even though we did not find significant differences, remission rates in ESTS were more than double those in control group (9 vs. 4), and dropout rates were one-third (1 vs. 3). All these changes were maintained at 1-month follow-up.

Table 17.2 The case of Abigail

Presenting problem	Abigail was a 21-year-old patient who identified herself as female. Her presenting problem was a growing sense of lack of control in her daily life and a perduring psychosocial distress in the form of anxious and depressive symptoms and social withdrawal. She was a first year student at a social science university. Her father abandoned the family when she was 5 years old, and she always lived with her mother who was a high school teacher. Her mother was described as a very judgmental person with high perfectionism (both self-oriented and other-oriented). Abigail had always described herself as introverted and imaginative, even though her shy attitude was constantly criticized by her mother and triggered bullying behaviors by her peers. She presented prominent positive and disorganized schizotypal symptoms together with recurring self-criticism, socially prescribed perfectionism, suspiciousness, and emotional dysregulation. During the first sessions, she reported how she dropped out of university since she experienced increasing levels of paranoid ideation about staying in class and meeting other students
Module 1: Sharing	Abigail had an oppositive and paranoid attitude during the first sessions. She constantly criticized the therapy and the therapist, taking for granted that the latter was either not sincerely interested in helping her or not capable of understanding her view of the world. This pattern was considered a test of relational safeness by the therapist and managed through a validating approach to negative feelings and compassionate curiosity about personal meaning and life history. As the therapy moved on, Abigail felt more safe and her narratives become more detailed and open to therapist feedback. An early conceptualization was shared that was consistent with the ESTS model and with a specific – albeit frequent among patients with schizotypal traits – mechanism: Abigail was frightened by compassion from others. In her experience, the others had always been judgmental if not abusive and her highly critical self-image was consistent with this narrative
Module 2: Subjective systems	During Module 2, this early conceptualization was deepened and discussed in relation to several narrative episodes. Abigail felt safe enough to share her personal diaries where she wrote fictional stories about her inner world. Although enriched by the patient's vivid fantasy, this fictional world followed the same dramatic rules as her life. She had creative representations of a few fantasy creatures (e.g. a necromant resembling an inner critic) who were constantly and severely judging her behaviors and thoughts. Abigail reported to have had experiences of hearing voices. And these voices hated her as much as she hated herself. The therapist introduced a few basic experiential techniques (i.e., grounding; soothing breathing) that during Module 1 were rejected by the patient. Indeed, for Abigail, it was not easy to feel safe enough to close her eyes in front of the therapist and try some mindfulness practices. Progressively, she recognized how the oppositive, suspicious, and even aggressive behaviors were the effect rather than the cause of her distress. She was simply trying to protect herself in the only way she had. A guided imagery (realities of life meditation) was then introduced to envision how she was trying to do her best to live decently. And it was not her fault to have experienced negative events or have been born with her temperament

(continued)

Table 17.2 (continued)

Module 3: Intersubjective systems	Through a validating stance, the therapist introduced the usefulness of exploring interpersonal cycles during Module 3. That is, the previously described schemas were contextualized into lived relational experiences, understanding how defensive automatisms may have shaped and channelized the mutual understanding. The therapist recalled the evolutionary conceptualization shared during the early sessions, and helped Abigail recognize how a threatening view of the other always led her to distancing, paranoid, or aggressive patterns. To the extent that the therapeutic relationship was perceived as safe, Abigail felt free to explore her deep need for socialization and compassion, and progressively acknowledge her authentic interest in others. She also became aware about several maladaptive interpersonal cycles. The patient and the therapist worked on these cycles using diverse forms of role-playing: primarily chairwork and theatrical techniques. Then, behavioral experiments were discussed, planned, applied, and evaluated. Moreover, emerging changes were consolidated using imagery with rescripting about past traumatic interpersonal experiences
Module 4: Consolidating	The last module aimed at consolidating the changes and preventing relapses. The frequency of therapy changed from weekly to biweekly. In addition to reviewing the relationship experiments, the therapist invited Abigail to write a brief history of the therapy. The goal was to identify critical points and stages of change. The therapist invited the patient to consolidate the ability to recognize adaptive and maladaptive strategies and the early indicators of the latter. Finally, follow-ups were scheduled (at 3 and 6 months) and the therapy ended. During the final stage, Abigail had resumed attending university and taking exams. She felt that she had learned to value her own characteristics (e.g., imagination) rather than hide and consider them a risk in her relationship with others

These results are in line with a few pilot cases series and a post-hoc analysis of this RCT. During follow-up interviews, patients recruited for the RCT reported two important elements. Those in the experimental group were seemingly experiencing a greater flourishing and purpose of life after the intervention. They reported how the therapy was useful in valuing their own personal identity and supported them in experimenting with new strategies. This narrative was consistent with the viability of an evolutionarily oriented conceptualization, as in contrast with a categorical diagnosis or more normative conceptualization usually presented during CBT. Interviewed patients suggested how this element was pivotal in either supporting a flourishing (ESTS) or fueling internal stigma (control group). That said, collected findings may have been biased by several limitations. Indeed, the limited sample size does not allow for a generalizability of results. The promising outcomes I have reported may be due to subjective differences among either patients or therapists. More importantly, the mandatory use of psychopharmacological treatment was possibly associated with a higher level of internalized stigma in the patients of the control group. Therefore, a new RCT has been registered and will compare ESTS with CBT without any mandatory pharmacotherapy (National Library of Medicine, NCT05710926).

Another criticism is under consideration. The ESTS model is primarily focused on psychoticism and so on positive and disorganized symptoms. Further evidence is needed to confirm that it would be effective in targeting schizotypal persons with prominent detached traits (and so negative symptoms). At this early stage, we concluded a cases series that may support this claim. Two patients diagnosed with SZPD reported a remission from diagnosis and reliable changes in several measures through a 10-month intervention (Cheli et al., 2022). These initial findings would support the need for confirmatory studies about the effectiveness of ESTS for severe forms of emotional and social detachment.

Finally, it is important to explore the feasibility of ESTS in two specific contexts. First, early manifestations of schizotypal traits during adolescence may benefit from the integrated and destigmatizing approach of ESTS. An evolutionary conceptualization of the presenting problems may help adolescent patients to value their identity rather than feeling judged by a normative approach to their distress. In a pilot five cases series, we recruited adolescents with prominent schizotypal traits and reported promising results (Cheli et al., 2023b). All the participants showed reliable changes in personality pathology and distress at the end of the intervention. Four out of five remitted from diagnosis after the scheduled 6-month ESTS, and one after an additional 2-month intervention. Second, I hypothesize that ESTS would be beneficial for acute conditions or at high-risk states for psychosis in those with prominent schizotypal traits, but I do not have any evidence to support this claim. Further research is needed.

Conclusion

ESTS is a form of psychotherapy tailored to schizotypal traits. It is based on a four-module intervention integrating an evolutionary conceptualization shared with the patient, and relational, narrative and experiential techniques aimed to recover metacognition and the capacity to soothe one's own suffering. Despite its recent development, it has collected promising evidence. A few cases series suggested its feasibility, and a pilot RCT reported an effectiveness at least equal to a good psychiatric management comprising CBT and psychopharmacological treatment. Further research is needed to confirm the clinical utility of ESTS.

Importantly, ESTS may be considered an emerging form of psychotherapy that is both specifically tailored on schizotypal traits and explicitly aimed at a full recovery. A few interventions tailored either to personality disorders, broadly speaking, or schizophrenia have been tested on a few cases of SPD, where treatment as usual was tested to reduce the risk of transitioning to psychosis. On the contrary, ESTS has been developed, since its earliest formulation, to target schizotypal traits and consistently with a dimensional look at schizotypy and personality pathology. Since the very first sessions, the presenting problem is discussed with the patient in terms of a maladaptive pattern in socializing one's own openness to experience and introversion. Along a continuum from healthy states to severe manifestations of schizotypy, schizotypal traits may lead to rigid, inflexible, and painful strategies. This evolutionary and dimensional approach to conceptualization aspires to support the person in valuing their own identity and looking for adaptive strategies. Although collected evidence is limited, the pilot RCT reported drop-out rates below 10% and SPD remission rates of 75%. These results would be consistent with the effectiveness of ESTS in targeting psychoticism, and so positive and disorganized features of schizotypy. Moreover, a cases series on SZPD seemingly suggests the feasibility of ESTS in treating severe forms of detachment and so of negative symptoms of schizotypy.

I suggest considering these promising – albeit preliminary – findings as the result of two main characteristics of ESTS: (i) a constant integration of relational, narrative, and experiential techniques in accordance with the here-and-now levels of metacognitive functioning and perceived threat, and (ii) a full consideration of subjective and intersubjective experience as an attempt to make sense of one's own world, rather than a cue of any sort of madness.

References

American Psychiatric Association. (2013). *Diagnostic and statistical manual of mental disorders: DSM-5™* (5th ed.). American Psychiatric Publishing. https://doi.org/10.1176/appi.books.9780890425596

Antonucci, L. A., Taurisano, P., Coppola, G., & Cassibba, R. (2018). Attachment style: The neurobiological substrate, interaction with genetics and role in neurodevelopmental disorders risk pathways. *Neuroscience and Biobehavioral Reviews, 95*, 515–527. https://doi.org/10.1016/j.neubiorev.2018.11.002

Bamelis, L. L., Evers, S. M., Spinhoven, P., & Arntz, A. (2014). Results of a multicenter randomized controlled trial of the clinical effectiveness of schema therapy for personality disorders. *The American Journal of Psychiatry, 171*(3), 305–322. https://doi.org/10.1176/appi.ajp.2013.12040518

Beck, A. T., Davis, D. D., & Freeman, A. (2015). *Cognitive therapy for personality disorders* (3rd ed.). The Guilford Press.

Benjamin, L. (1993). Every psychopathology is a gift of love. *Psychotherapy Research, 3*(1), 1–24. https://doi.org/10.1080/10503309312331333629

Bleuler, E. (1911). *Dementia praecox oder die Gruppe der Schizophrenien*. Deutike.

Bucci, S., Emsley, R., & Berry, K. (2017). Attachment in psychosis: A latent profile analysis of attachment styles and association with symptoms in a large psychosis cohort. *Psychiatry Research, 247*, 243–249. https://doi.org/10.1016/j.psychres.2016.11.036

Burns, J. (2007). *The descent of madness: Evolutionary origins of psychosis and the social brain*. Routledge/Taylor & Francis Group.

Cheli, S. (2018). On the Eigenform and viability of human complex systems: A view to epistemologically ground current psychotherapy. *Systems Research and Behavioral Science, 35*, 505–519. https://doi.org/10.1002/sres.2559

Cheli, S. (2020). Assessment and treatment planning for schizotypal personality disorder: A metacognitively oriented point of view. *Psychiatric Rehabilitation Journal, 43*(4), 335–343. https://doi.org/10.1037/prj0000429

Cheli, S. (2023). An evolutionary look at oddity and schizotypy: How the rise of social brain informs clinical practice. *New Ideas in Psychology, 68*. Advance online publication. https://doi.org/10.1016/j.newideapsych.2022.100993

Cheli, S., Lysaker, P. H., & Dimaggio, G. (2019). Metacognitively oriented psychotherapy for schizotypal personality disorder: A two-case series. *Personality and Mental Health, 13*(3), 155–167. https://doi.org/10.1002/pmh.1447

Cheli, S., Cavalletti, V., & Petrocchi, N. (2020). An online compassion-focused crisis intervention during COVID-19 lockdown: A cases series on patients at high risk for psychosis. *Psychosis: Psychological, Social and Integrative Approaches, 12*(4), 359–362. https://doi.org/10.1080/17522439.2020.1786148

Cheli, S., Cavalletti, V., Mancini, F., & Goldzweig, G. (2021a). What if metacognition is not enough? Its association with delusion may be moderated by self-criticism. *Current Psychology*. Advance online publication. https://doi.org/10.1007/s12144-021-02451-7

Cheli, S., Petrocchi, N., & Cavalletti, V. (2021b). Hearing divine voices: A qualitative enquiry about criticism, connectedness, and compassion. *Psychosis: Psychological, Social and Integrative Approaches, 15*, 100. https://doi.org/10.1080/17522439.2021.2011387

Cheli, S., Chiarello, F., & Cavalletti, V. (2022). A psychotherapy oriented by compassion and metacognition for schizoid personality disorder: A two cases series. *Journal of Contemporary Psychotherapy*. Advance Online Publication. https://doi.org/10.1007/s10879-022-09566-3

Cheli, S., Cavalletti, V., Lysaker, P. H., Dimaggio, D., Petrocchi, N., Chiarello, F., Enzo, C., Velicogna, F., Mancini, F., & Goldzweig, G. (2023a). A pilot randomized controlled trial comparing a novel compassion and metacognition approach for schizotypal personality disorder with a combination of cognitive therapy and psychopharmacological treatment. *BMC Psychiatry, 23*, 113. https://doi.org/10.1186/s12888-023-04610-5

Cheli, S., Goldzweig, G., Lysaker, P. H., Chiarello, F., Wiesepape, C., & Cavalletti, V. (2023b). An evolutionarily informed therapy for adolescents with prominent schizotypal traits: A pilot five case series. *Psychosis*, 1. https://doi.org/10.1080/17522439.2023.2199325

Cicero, D. C., Jonas, K. G., Li, K., Perlman, G., & Kotov, R. (2019). Common taxonomy of traits and symptoms: Linking schizophrenia symptoms, schizotypy, and normal personality. *Schizophrenia Bulletin, 45*(6), 1336–1348. https://doi.org/10.1093/schbul/sbz005

Claridge, G., & Broks, P. (1984). Schizotypy and hemisphere function-I. Theoretical considerations and the measurement of schizotypy. *Personality and Individual Differences, 5*(6), 633–648. https://doi.org/10.1016/0191-8869(84)90111-9

Dimaggio, G., Ottavi, P., Popolo, R., & Salvatore, G. (2020). *Metacognitive interpersonal therapy. Body, image and change*. Routledge.

Dunbar, R. I. (2009). The social brain hypothesis and its implications for social evolution. *Annals of Human Biology, 36*(5), 562–572. https://doi.org/10.1080/03014460902960289

Edmundson, M., & Kwapil, T. R. (2013). A five-factor model perspective of schizotypal personality disorder. In *Personality disorders and the five-factor model of personality* (3rd ed., pp. 147–161). American Psychological Association. https://doi.org/10.1037/13939-010

Gilbert, P. (2009). *The compassionate mind: A new approach to the challenge of life*. Constable & Robinson.

Gilbert, P. (2020). Compassion: From its evolution to a psychotherapy. *Frontiers in Psychology, 11*, 586161. https://doi.org/10.3389/fpsyg.2020.586161

Gumley, A. I., Taylor, H. E., Schwannauer, M., & MacBeth, A. (2014). A systematic review of attachment and psychosis: Measurement, construct validity and outcomes. *Acta Psychiatrica Scandinavica, 129*(4), 257–274. https://doi.org/10.1111/acps.12172

Gurrera, R. J., Dickey, C. C., Niznikiewicz, M. A., Voglmaier, M. M., Shenton, M. E., & McCarley, R. W. (2005). The five-factor model in schizotypal personality disorder. *Schizophrenia Research, 80*(2–3), 243–251. https://doi.org/10.1016/j.schres.2005.08.002

Hopwood, C. J., & Thomas, K. M. (2012). Paranoid and schizoid personality disorders. In T. A. Widiger (Ed.), *The Oxford handbook of personality disorders* (pp. 582–602). Oxford University Press. https://doi.org/10.1093/oxfordhb/9780199735013.013.0027

Kirchner, S. K., Roeh, A., Nolden, J., & Hasan, A. (2018). Diagnosis and treatment of schizotypal personality disorder: Evidence from a systematic review. *NPJ Schizophrenia, 4*(1), 20. https://doi.org/10.1038/s41537-018-0062-8

Kotov, R., Jonas, K. G., Carpenter, W. T., Dretsch, M. N., Eaton, N. R., Forbes, M. K., Forbush, K. T., Hobbs, K., Reininghaus, U., Slade, T., South, S. C., Sunderland, M., Waszczuk, M. A., Widiger, T. A., Wright, A., Zald, D. H., Krueger, R. F., Watson, D., & HiTOP Utility Workgroup. (2020). Validity and utility of Hierarchical Taxonomy of Psychopathology (HiTOP): I. Psychosis superspectrum. *World Psychiatry: Official Journal of the World Psychiatric Association (WPA), 19*(2), 151–172. https://doi.org/10.1002/wps.20730

Kotov, R., Krueger, R. F., Watson, D., Cicero, D. C., Conway, C. C., DeYoung, C. G., Eaton, N. R., Forbes, M. K., Hallquist, M. N., Latzman, R. D., Mullins-Sweatt, S. N., Ruggero, C. J., Simms, L. J., Waldman, I. D., Waszczuk, M. A., & Wright, A. G. C. (2021). The Hierarchical Taxonomy of Psychopathology (HiTOP): A quantitative nosology based on consensus of evidence. *Annual Review of Clinical Psychology, 17*, 83–108. https://doi.org/10.1146/annurev-clinpsy-081219-093304

Kwapil, T. R., & Barrantes-Vidal, N. (2015). Schizotypy: Looking back and moving forward. *Schizophrenia Bulletin, 41*(Suppl 2), S366–S373. https://doi.org/10.1093/schbul/sbu186

Kwapil, T. R., & Barrantes-Vidal, N. (2022). Schizotypal personality disorder in the alternative model for personality disorders. *Personality Disorders, 13*(4), 392–396. https://doi.org/10.1037/per0000538

Luyten, P., & Fonagy, P. (2015). The neurobiology of mentalizing. *Personality Disorders: Theory, Research, and Treatment, 6*(4), 366–379. https://doi.org/10.1037/per0000117

Lysaker, P. H., & Klion, R. E. (2017). *Recovery, meaning-making, and severe mental illness: A comprehensive guide to metacognitive reflection and insight therapy*. Routledge.

Lysaker, P. H., Hamm, J. A., Hasson-Ohayon, I., Pattison, M. L., & Leonhardt, B. L. (2018). Promoting recovery from severe mental illness: Implications from research on metacognition and metacognitive reflection and insight therapy. *World Journal of Psychiatry, 8*(1), 1–11. https://doi.org/10.5498/wjp.v8.i1.1

Lysaker, P. H., Kukla, M., Leonhardt, B. L., Hamm, J. A., Schnakenberg Martin, A., Zalzala, A. B., Gagen, E. C., & Hasson-Ohayon, I. (2020). Meaning, integration, and the self in serious mental illness: Implications of research in metacognition for psychiatric rehabilitation. *Psychiatric Rehabilitation Journal, 43*(4), 275–283. https://doi.org/10.1037/prj0000436

Lysaker, P. H., Cheli, S., Dimaggio, G., Buck, B., Bonfils, K. A., Huling, K., Wiesepape, C., & Lysaker, J. T. (2021). Metacognition, social cognition, and mentalizing in psychosis: Are these distinct constructs when it comes to subjective experience or are we just splitting hairs? *BMC Psychiatry, 21*(1), 329. https://doi.org/10.1186/s12888-021-03338-4

Maturana, H., & Varela, F. G. (1984). *El arbol del conocimiento*. Editorial Universitari.

McGrath, J. J., Saha, S., Al-Hamzawi, A., Alonso, J., Bromet, E. J., Bruffaerts, R., Caldas-de-Almeida, J. M., Chiu, W. T., de Jonge, P., Fayyad, J., Florescu, S., Gureje, O., Haro, J. M., Hu, C., Kovess-Masfety, V., Lepine, J. P., Lim, C. C., Mora, M. E., Navarro-Mateu, F., Ochoa, S., et al. (2015). Psychotic experiences in the general population: A cross-national analysis based on 31,261 respondents from 18 countries. *JAMA Psychiatry, 72*(7), 697–705. https://doi.org/10.1001/jamapsychiatry.2015.0575

Meehl, P. E. (1962). Schizotaxia, schizotypy, schizophrenia. *American Psychologist, 17*(12), 827–838. https://doi.org/10.1037/h0041029

National Library of Medicine (U.S.). (2023, February–). *Evolutionary systems therapy for schizotypy (ESTS)*. Identifier NCT05710926. https://clinicaltrials.gov/ct2/show/NCT05710926

Nordentoft, M., Thorup, A., Petersen, L., Ohlenschlaeger, J., Melau, M., Christensen, T. Ø., Krarup, G., Jørgensen, P., & Jeppesen, P. (2006). Transition rates from schizotypal disorder to psychotic disorder for first-contact patients included in the OPUS trial. A randomized clinical trial of integrated treatment and standard treatment. *Schizophrenia Research, 83*(1), 29–40. https://doi.org/10.1016/j.schres.2006.01.002

Petrocchi, N., & Cheli, S. (2019). The social brain and heart rate variability: Implications for psychotherapy. *Psychology and Psychotherapy, 92*(2), 208–223. https://doi.org/10.1111/papt.12224

Semerari, A., Colle, L., Pellecchia, G., Buccione, I., Carcione, A., Dimaggio, G., Nicolò, G., Procacci, M., & Pedone, R. (2014). Metacognitive dysfunctions in personality disorders: Correlations with disorder severity and personality styles. *Journal of Personality Disorders, 28*(6), 751–766. https://doi.org/10.1521/pedi_2014_28_137

Sharp, C. (2020). Adolescent personality pathology and the alternative model for personality disorders: Self development as nexus. *Psychopathology, 53*(3–4), 198–204. https://doi.org/10.1159/000507588

Teicher, M. H., Gordon, J. B., & Nemeroff, C. B. (2022). Recognizing the importance of childhood maltreatment as a critical factor in psychiatric diagnoses, treatment, research, prevention, and education. *Molecular Psychiatry, 27*, 1331–1338. https://doi.org/10.1038/s41380-021-01367-9

Triebwasser, J., Chemerinski, E., Roussos, P., & Siever, L. J. (2013). Paranoid personality disorder. *Journal of Personality Disorders, 27*(6), 795–805. https://doi.org/10.1521/pedi_2012_26_055

Varese, F., Smeets, F., Drukker, M., Lieverse, R., Lataster, T., Viechtbauer, W., Read, J., van Os, J., & Bentall, R. P. (2012). Childhood adversities increase the risk of psychosis: a meta-analysis of patient-control, prospective- and cross-sectional cohort studies. *Schizophrenia Bulletin, 38*(4), 661–671. https://doi.org/10.1093/schbul/sbs050

Velikonja, T., Fisher, H. L., Mason, O., & Johnson, S. (2015). Childhood trauma and schizotypy: A systematic literature review. *Psychological Medicine, 45*(5), 947–963. https://doi.org/10.1017/S0033291714002086

Wood, L., & Irons, C. (2016). Exploring the associations between social rank and external shame with experiences of psychosis. *Behavioural and Cognitive Psychotherapy, 44*(5), 527–538. https://doi.org/10.1017/S1352465815000570

Chapter 18
Mentalization-Based Treatment for Schizotypal Personality

Jeremy M. Ridenour, Daniel P. C. Knauss, and Alice Pozzi

Over the past decade, mentalization-based treatment (MBT) has been increasingly applied to persons experiencing psychosis (Brent, 2009, 2015; Debbané et al., 2016; Ridenour et al., 2019, 2021) to address the underlying social cognitive deficits and impairments in monitoring self and other mental states that give rise to symptoms (Knauss et al., 2018). Despite this rich emerging literature, much less has been written about how to apply MBT for individuals experiencing schizotypal personality disorder (SPD), even though persons with SPD display mentalizing deficits (Cheli, 2020). In contrast to schizophrenia, persons with SPD experience subthreshold psychotic symptoms, such as magical thinking, bodily illusions, or suspiciousness. They might also experience brief psychotic episodes that do not last as long and are not as severe compared to persons with schizophrenia (APA, 2013).

In the schizotypy literature (Kemp et al., 2021), schizotypal symptoms have been divided into three categories: positive schizotypy (magical ideation, perceptual illusions, suspiciousness, and ideas of reference), disorganized schizotypy (odd thinking and peculiar behavior), and negative schizotypy (constricted affect and lack of close friends). For this chapter, we will argue that these elements of schizotypy can be best conceptualized in a developmental framework (Debbané & Barrantes-Vidal, 2015). First, we will describe some of the developmental research on trauma and schizotypy to contextualize the symptoms of SPD. Next, we will explore the emotional deficits of people with SPD and their impact on mentalization capacities. After reviewing the research, we will outline how an MBT approach can strengthen underlying emotional and mentalization capacities through the therapeutic

J. M. Ridenour (✉) · D. P. C. Knauss · A. Pozzi
Austen Riggs Center, Erikson Institute for Education, Research, & Advocacy, Stockbridge, MA, USA
e-mail: jeremy.ridenour@austenriggs.net; daniel.knauss@austenriggs.net; alice.pozzi@austenriggs.net

S. Cheli, P. H. Lysaker (eds.), *A Dimensional Approach to Schizotypy*, https://doi.org/10.1007/978-3-031-41788-7_18

relationship. Specific treatment targets will be identified along with brief case vignettes to illustrate the intervention strategies.

Developmental Context

Recently, an effort has been made to conceptualize schizotypy from a developmental perspective and establish its relation to the spectrum of psychotic disorders (Debbané & Barrantes-Vidal, 2015; Snyder et al., Chap. 1, THIS BOOK). Several factors have been considered including epigenetic, social, and psychological factors contributing to the emergence of schizotypal phenomenon. One area of growing emphasis is on early childhood adversity. In a systematic review and meta-analysis of studies addressing early childhood adversity and schizotypy, Toutountzidis et al. (2022) found that all forms of childhood abuse and neglect were associated with schizotypy. However, the association between childhood emotional abuse and schizotypy was significantly stronger than other forms of adversity. Emotional abuse was associated with positive schizotypy such as hallucination-like experiences (e.g., perceptual illusions), aberrant salience, and ideas of reference. These findings are consistent with previous research by Quidé et al. (2018), who found that trauma-exposed individuals demonstrated higher levels of schizotypy, with marked elevations in suspiciousness and concurrent social cognitive deficits. In conceptualizing the link between early adversity and later schizotypy, Weijers et al. (2018) have found that mentalizing impairments play a significant mediating role only in the emergence of negative symptoms, for those who experienced the most severe abuse and neglect.

According to a standard measure of childhood trauma (Bernstein et al., 1994), emotional abuse is defined as a parent or older adult in the household who frequently insulted, humiliated, or cursed the child, leaving the child scared and fearful of being harmed. The child might be regularly demeaned and may be anxious and wary of interacting with the abusive parent. In such a contentious household, the child likely struggles to develop a secure attachment in which they could learn how to make sense of their thoughts, emotions, and intentions as well as the mental states of the caregivers. For a child to form a model of their mind, they need to have a relationship with a caregiver who can help them understand their thoughts, emotions, and desires (Bateman & Fonagy, 2016), which requires a sense of interpersonal security and trust. However, if the child consistently experiences emotionally threatening and unpredictable behavior from their caregiver, they might defensively shut down their reflective capacity so as not to know the motivations of those inflicting harm on them (Brent, 2009). Without these reflective abilities, the child may have trouble drawing a clear boundary between their thoughts and the thoughts of others (i.e., ideas of reference), recognizing what factors are relevant to social interactions (i.e., aberrant salience), and forming benign interpretations of social interactions (i.e., suspiciousness). Although not all individuals who later develop SPD grow up in this social context, for those who experience such emotional turmoil, they likely struggle to modulate their emotions, reflect upon their thoughts, and identify the psychological states of others.

Consistent with this research, Pazar et al. (2022) investigated the link between the negative emotional environment in the relationship between children and their caregivers and the development of schizotypy. Their findings showed that high expressed emotion, a construct that account for caregivers' level of criticism, hostility, and emotional overinvolvement, may positively correlate to the development of schizotypy later in life. Given the potential role of mentalization as a moderator between childhood trauma and psychopathology, the researchers investigated the impact of reflective functioning in the development of schizotypy. Findings indicated that reflective functioning was significantly negatively correlated to schizotypy, suggesting that mentalization is an important factor in predicting good mental health outcomes and explaining pathways that connect childhood adversity to schizotypy in individuals with severe trauma history.

Based on this brief review of the developmental literature on schizotypy, many adults who later display SPD traits likely did not have the necessary developmental experiences to help them learn how to contain and label their emotions, understand their mental states, and reflect upon the mental states of others, which could partially explain their poor social skills in childhood, isolation (Ridenour, 2016), and high degrees of introversion (Cheli, 2020). Without these necessary psychological capacities, they might be at risk of becoming confused and overwhelmed by social interactions that might result in unusual thinking and subsequent withdrawal.

Emotions

Previous studies have found that persons with SPD tended to pay more attention to their emotions than controls (Kerns, 2005) but have consistent difficulty labeling their feelings (Dmitryeva et al., 2021; Ridenour, 2016), leading to increased ruminations (Kerns, 2005). Berenbaum et al. (2006) have argued that heightened awareness of emotions, coupled with an inability to identify the sources of their emotions, could result in the misattribution of feelings to others and therefore provoke paranoia. Other studies have also found that individuals with SPD tend to display a high degree of neuroticism and emotional distress (Cheli, 2020). To manage these negative emotions, people with SPD might rely on defense mechanisms such as denial, avoidance, reaction formation, splitting, undoing, and projection (Ridenour, 2016). Although these defense mechanisms allow for the person to escape painful emotions, they also result in reality distortions that can lead to disorganization and poor mentalization.

In addition to a high degree of negative emotionality, case studies have noted that persons with SPD may have particular struggles managing aggressive and sexual impulses (Dmitryeva et al., 2021; Ridenour, 2016). Difficulties with anger could stem, in part, from exposure to emotional abuse, criticism, shame, and a high degree of expressed emotion in the family (Pazar et al., 2022). Bender et al. (2003) found that persons with SPD, compared to people with other personality disorders, reported having the most frequent aggressive and sexual thoughts about their therapist. These findings suggest that intense emotions and impulses might be particularly overstimulating for people with SPD and, if not properly contained, might result in disorganized thought or suspiciousness.

Mentalization

Mentalization impairments are evident in persons with SPD (Cheli, 2020; Salaminios & Debanné, Chap. 9, THIS BOOK). A couple of recent studies have investigated the relationship between different types of mentalization difficulties and facets of schizotypy. Wastler and Lenzwenger (2019) explored the relationship between mentalization errors in people with SPD. Mentalization errors can be divided into two categories: undermentalization (i.e., the tendency to make overly simplistic or incomplete mental state attributions) and hypermentalization (i.e., the proclivity to make excessive mental state attributions that extend beyond the social cues evident in the interaction). The researchers found that persons with schizotypy made significantly more hypermentalization errors compared to the negative affect and healthy control groups. These errors were correlated with referential thinking, aberrant salience, lack of close friends, social anxiety, and poor functional outcomes.

A more recent study by Salaminios et al. (2021) found that interpersonal schizotypal manifestations pertaining to social anxiety are associated with high mentalizing uncertainty for a community adolescent sample. In addition, SPD features of odd speech correlated with high mentalization uncertainty and reduced mentalizing certainty. The first finding is in line with previous data suggesting that mentalizing deficits are linked with social withdrawal in patient samples (e.g., Weijers et al., 2018), highlighting a bidirectional relationship between social anxiety and mentalizing dysfunction. As in the case of social anxiety, odd speech impedes effective interpersonal communication, potentially disrupting the developmental elaboration of complex meta-representations of experience (Salaminios et al., 2021). Furthermore, high mentalization uncertainty suggests that people with schizotypy have difficulty discerning their own thoughts and making sense of the minds of others.

Linking these findings to developmental literature, this inability to read the mind of others could be influenced by a chaotic home environment in which the mind of the caregiver was potentially threatening and dangerous, causing the child to withdraw into their own mind (Brent, 2009). Without being able read and access the other's mind, the child is then left alone with their own imagination to try to sort out what is going on in a social interaction. Based on the study by Wastler and Lenzwenger (2019), it appears that people with schizotypy are likely to read too much meaning into a given social interaction, which can result in a confusing and distorted interpretation, potentially leading to magical thinking, ideas of reference, suspiciousness, and odd ideas.

One concept from the mentalization literature that can help contextualize these findings is the relevance of non-mentalizing modes of thought, a form of early cognition that precedes the development of mentalization. As outlined by Bateman and Fonagy (2016), there are three non-mentalizing modes of thoughts: psychic equivalence (i.e., the assumption that a mental state is a direct representation of reality), teleological mode (i.e., the belief that the minds of others can only be known through their actions and not their words), and pretend mode (i.e., a mode of thought in which the internal world of the mind is decoupled from reality). Pretend mode emerges in early childhood when the child creates an imaginative world in which they can exert control by disconnecting from external reality and largely focus on their mental representations (Freeman, 2016). Bateman and Fonagy (2006) argue that pretend mode is evident in adults who often intellectualize in therapy or speak at length about their experiences with little genuine connection to their sense of self, emotions, or bodily sensations (Muller & Midgley, 2020). In this type of mindset, the individual is mostly lost in their fantasies and idiosyncratic interpretations of what might be going in the mind of the other with little capacity to realistically reflect on a given social interaction. This pretend mode of thought is potentially linked to the hypermentalization errors that are commonly exhibited by persons with SPD (Wastler & Lenzwenger, 2019).

Psychic equivalence may also occupy a unique position in relation to SPD (Ridenour et al., 2019). Specifically, the sort of odd, idiosyncratic, or unusual thinking typical of the personality type can manifest as an entrenched style of perceiving the world. On the more extreme end, the individual with SPD may become convinced that their internal experience is a direct representation of the external world. This sort of difficulty can lead to difficulties in their social interactions with others, including basic confusion regarding the underlying mental states behind others' behavior. In the case examples to follow, we hope to illustrate how these two non-mentalizing modes of thought might appear during the course of treatment.

Treatment Targets

Before introducing MBT principles, we want to briefly summarize some relevant treatment targets based on the schizotypy literature. First, given the high rates of childhood trauma (particularly emotional abuse), the therapist should assess for a history of trauma for a patient with SPD. If trauma is reported, the therapist should hold this in mind, especially as it might pertain to disorganized thought, dissociation, paranoia, or interpersonal sensitivity. Second, people with SPD have significant difficulties labeling and regulating their emotional reactions and bodily sensations. Therapists should be especially aware of the impact that anger and sexual impulses can have on the person's thinking and mentalization of the mind of the therapist. Helping the patient identify emotional arousal and locating its source might be useful to reduce confusion. Finally, the research on mentalization errors for schizotypy has shown that hypermentalization errors and mentalization uncertainty are common in this population and likely result in magical ideation and self-referential thinking. Working with the patient to notice moments when their thinking becomes more emotionally disconnected and unconventional and the contexts that lead to breakdown in rational thought could help boost mentalization and self-awareness.

Therapists should also be aware of moments when the patient's thinking begins to feel unreal or pretend, as this might signify that the patient is primarily lost in fantasy, with little to no realistic connection to their sense of self or the mind of the other. Finally, people with SPD often exhibit high degrees of social anxiety and struggle with intimate relationships (APA, 2013). Despite their introverted presentation, research by Bender et al. (2003) suggests that people with SPD are quite invested in the therapeutic relationship and are easily overstimulated by their thoughts and feelings about the therapist. The therapist should hold this sensitivity in mind and be attentive to the therapeutic relationships and any ruptures that might result in interpersonal withdrawal or affective and cognitive disorganization. In summary, the treatment targets include the following: (1) Assessment of trauma; (2) Promote awareness of emotions and bodily sensations (especially anger); (3) Notice breakdowns in mentalizations and the potential factors that lead to unusual thinking; (4) Attend to the therapeutic relationship and consider how changes in the relationship might impact the patient's mentalization capacity.

MBT for SPD

The central goal for MBT is for the therapist to facilitate mentalization and attempt to keep the patient's mind "in mind" to promote reflection and curiosity. What distinguishes MBT from other treatments that focus on social cognition (see Ridenour et al., 2019 for more detail) is a particular sensitivity to how disruptions in attachment relationships lead to breakdowns in mentalization. Therefore, the therapist is continuously monitoring the relationship with the patient and assessing possible ruptures or misunderstandings that could lead to heightened confusion or lapses into non-mentalizing modes of thoughts (Ridenour et al., 2021). For instance, if following a therapist's comment about the patient's anxiety, the patient begins to suddenly monologue about a science fiction novel that has seemingly no relevance to the previous discussion, the therapist might wonder if their comment might have upset the patient, driving them to withdraw into a self-enclosed narrative. Although patients with SPD can sometimes present as withdrawn or flat, research indicates that they are quite sensitive to the therapist and think about their therapist often (Bender et al., 2003).

To accomplish these aims, the therapist adheres to a couple of principles. First, the therapist adopts a "not knowing stance" in which they embody a curious attitude toward their mind and to the patient's mind (Ridenour et al., 2019). To model this openness, the therapist asks questions to try to understand the patient's perspective while also holding their own opinions lightly, willing to change their mind based on emerging evidence. Underlying this stance is a belief in the opacity of the mind (Brent, 2009), a recognition that mental states can never be known with absolute certainty. The therapist offers their mind as a model to illustrate mentalization, attempting to describe their mental states while spelling out the underlying reasons for their thoughts, as best as they understand them (Ridenour et al., 2021).

Second, interventions are grounded in the present and especially attuned to the patient's feelings and bodily sensation, as they evolve over the course of a session (Weijers et al., 2020). Keeping an eye on the emergence and escalation of emotion can help the therapist and patient collaboratively assess how feelings affect the patient's thinking and experience of the therapeutic relationship. The therapist works with the patient to downregulate emotions that are unbearable and interfere with the capacity to reflect on their experiences.

Third, the therapeutic relationship is a central focus of the conversation and dialogue. Attending to shifts in the relationship and their subsequent impact on the patient's (and therapist's) capacity to mentalize can deepen the patient's learning and self-awareness. Furthermore, reflecting upon the relationship provides an opportunity to compare different perspectives on shared experiences (Ridenour et al., 2019). During the session, both therapist and patient might be vulnerable to having breakdowns in mentalization. In these moments, the therapist can "stop and rewind" the process with the patient to try to pinpoint the causes for these lapses in mentalization (e.g., the patient felt too vulnerable talking about a painful memory and therefore shifted into a more disconnected, intellectual monologue). With these principles in mind, we will now highlight some relevant practice points when working with people with SPD.

MBT for psychosis is a treatment that is 18 months long and includes weekly group therapy and half-hour individual sessions once per two weeks that is offered in an outpatient setting (Weijers et al., 2020). The intensity of the individual and group therapy sessions is usually attenuated to avoid overwhelming the patients with mentalization interventions. Given that MBT has not been specifically applied to persons with SPD, it is not clear what kind of treatment package would be best suited to address their specific needs and challenges. The following cases examples are pulled from naturalistic settings, including a residential treatment center and outpatient setting.

Practice Point 1: Promote Awareness of Emotions and Bodily Sensations

The following clinical example is of Max, a 23-year-old, single, cisgender man who was in residential treatment, where he attended four-time weekly mentalization-informed psychodynamic individual psychotherapy for about four months along with psychopharmacology and daily group therapy (both skills-based and process groups). Max had been to several other treatment centers in his young adult life due to depression, dissociative symptoms, suicidality, perceptual disturbances, post-traumatic symptoms, interpersonal problems, and non-suicidal self-harm. Abandoned at birth, Max spent the first few months of his life in an orphanage before being adopted. Max did not have a good relationship with either of his adoptive parents, and, following the loss of his adoptive mother who left the family abruptly, he was left to be raised by his father, who was generally misattuned and, at times, emotionally and physically abusive. Max's two main presentations in sessions were a state of sustained reverie in his fantasies, and a transference-filled state in which he directly engaged with his therapist about his fear of being abandoned. For this example, we will describe Max's reveries. Many of Max's fantasies were grandiose and driven by a wish for omnipotence. Some of the fantasies were also malevolent and retaliatory. The latter usually came up when Max felt threatened or angry.

The following clinical example illustrate Max's use of fantasies to flee unbearable emotions.

During this session, Max was talking about feeling lonely and shared his desire to go on a trip to his home state, where he could visit old friends. Though Max was identifying feeling homesick, the initial tone of the session was upbeat, as he excitedly talked about his plan to spend time with people he loved. Suddenly, Max's expression shifted when he explained that his father had told him that he would like Max to also visit him while on this trip.

Max: I can't believe he is demanding that. I will kill myself if I have to spend a day with my father!

Therapist: It really upset you that he asked you to spend time with him. You don't imagine making it out of that encounter alive.

Max: I cannot. I won't.

Therapist: What are you worried will happen?

Max: My dad knows better than to attack me. I would destroy him. I have claws and sharp teeth, I'm not a bunny – I might be small, but I am no bunny. I am a fucking honey badger. I have the strength of hundreds-year old animals that live inside of me. They have seen it all and will never die.

Therapist: What happened there? You were talking about not wanting to visit your father and, as I asked you to explain what you're worried about, you seemed to have gone away.

Max sits quietly for a while, his breathing is fast, and he looks agitated.

Therapist: You seem frightened, and maybe quite angry at the same time?

Max: I guess…I don't want to be thinking about the times I had to hide in the shower in the basement, so he wouldn't find me.

Therapist: What happens when you're forced to remember those times? What do you feel?

Max: I feel weak, I never want to feel that way again – weak and small.

Therapist: It makes sense that you'd want to conjure the strength of ancient immortal animals to help you through this helplessness.

Max: Yes, when I do that, I am not alone. I can count on them, and no one will ever hurt me again.

In this exchange, the therapist attempted to help Max to identify what feelings and thoughts led to a momentary break with reality. By paying attention to the shifts in emotional tone, nonverbal cues, and verbal content, the therapist paused the state of fantasy to understand the cognitive and emotional sequence of Max's retreat into fantasy. In this case, Max became overwhelmed with fear and feelings of helplessness and regressed to pretend mode of thought. By clinging to fantasied omnipotence, Max managed to no longer feel like a weak, abused orphan, by adopting a strong, powerful stance. By encouraging him to identify his emotional experience preceding the escape into fantasy, the therapist helped Max to access and explore relevant memories and reach a more mentalized understanding of his defensive adaptations.

Practice Point 2: Notice Breakdowns in Mentalization and the Underlying Causes

Kyle is a 32-year-old, bi-racial, cisgender, single, asexual man who sought outpatient therapy within the context of extreme social anxiety and difficulty launching an independent life following the completion of college. Although he was highly trained and gifted engineer, he persistently struggled to sustain employment as he would become intensely preoccupied and worried about how his co-workers were experiencing him, often resigning preemptively when he feared he was disliked. Furthermore, he had been unable to sustain friendships outside of several online groups focused on niche interests in South Korean culture. He has been in once-weekly psychodynamic therapy for six months, largely processing his difficulty in his newest job which he started one month into treatment. Recently, he has become concerned that his co-workers negatively received the wording in one of his emails. The following exchange comes from a session in which Kyle is lamenting the expected impact of an email he sent to his team at work. Of note, his affect appears flat, and he seems to have little awareness that his steady stream of a narrative has left the therapist bored, confused, and disconnected.

Kyle: I know they could not read my tone of voice in the email. I sent it too quickly. I also know that I didn't edit it for grammar and afterwards I caught a misspelling and a misplaced comma. At lunch, I saw my supervisor and she was turned away from me in an unusual way during the lunch line. It seemed clear that she had caught on to me. She must know I am awkward and terrible with people. She even said much less to me when we crossed paths coming back from our lunches that she usually does. This happens at each job, I can't help but mess up in a particular way and then everyone else catches on. She probably is wondering what is wrong with me.

Therapist: How do you feel about that?

Kyle: Well, when she wrote me an email later in the day she didn't sign off in any particular way. She didn't say "warmly" or "sincerely" or "thanks"… just wrote her name at the end. When this happens there is a way that you can know the other person is off. She must have spent the afternoon thinking about my message and how it wasn't adequate and that I was a very awkward person. It's like there are alarms going off for everyone else in the office about me and now they know. I keep track of how she ends her emails, and it is often predictable what mood she is in by the language she chooses…

Therapist: I'm sorry I find myself a bit confused. I was wondering how you felt about the idea that others might think something was wrong with you? It was hard for me to tell if you were answering that in some way that I missed?

Kyle: Oh… no I guess I hadn't answered it. Um… I feel shitty. I feel awful. [Kyle begins to tear up]

Therapist: It really feels bad.

Kyle: Yes. I want to be liked and have good relationships with my co-workers, but I feel so different. I spend so much time trying to figure out how to fit in.

Therapist: I see. Kind of like paying such close attention to your co-workers' language in her email? You feel like you've outed yourself as being awkward and then look very carefully for signs that this might be true in what others say? All the while it makes you feel like rubbish?

In this example, the therapist noticed their own feeling of disconnection from the engagement, signaling something off in the degree of mentalization. The boredom and confusion they felt were taken to be a possible sign of pretend mode or hypermentalization, which they then attended to in Kyle's narrative. As Kyle fled from his own emotional experience into a hypermentalizaed examination of his co-workers' intentions, the therapist tried to attend to this process and re-engage Kyle emotionally while trying to contextualize his desperate attempts to discern his co-workers' intentions. At the same time, Kyle was at risk of becoming entrenched in certainty that his internal experience was representative of external reality (i.e., psychic equivalence).

Practice Point 3: Attend to the Therapeutic Relationship

Bella is a 24-year-old, single, bi-sexual, cisgender woman in outpatient treatment with her therapist whom she has been seeing for two years at a frequency of twice a week. She initially sought treatment in relation to intrusive sexual thoughts about a family member that left her feeling increasingly isolated, paranoid and on guard. She described feeling "porous" and easily intruded on by others, yet desperate to form intimate friendships. More importantly, she hoped to establish a sexual and romantic connection with a partner that might blossom into a more serious, long-term relationship. As treatment unfolded, it became clear that Bella would become easily overwhelmed by the experience of sexual desire and then profoundly confused about where to locate and understand her feelings. Often, she would become frightened and overwhelmed by the sense that others were attracted to her and looking at her body lustfully. Even more distressing, she could quickly become worried that others wanted to rape her or take control her body in ways that were frightening. In response to her confusion, Bella would often retreat into fantasy, isolate from others, and deny her longing for actual interpersonal engagement. In her mind, she would play out intricate scenarios in which others would present themselves to her with their longing which she could cautiously join.

The following example illustrates the ways that Bella's desire could quickly bring about confusion, eliciting anxiety about safety and security of the therapeutic relationship and precipitating flight into fantasy (i.e., pretend mode). The therapist's engagement was directed toward helping Bella identify the antecedents to her retreat as a means of re-establishing a mentalizing stance. Although there were clear, rich transference implications, more traditional forms of interpretation were not utilized as the emphasis was on restoring mentalizing in the therapeutic dyad. Prior to this appointment, the therapist had been away for a brief vacation and Bella had struggled with a sense of abandonment, longing for reconnection with her therapist, and building confusion regarding what her longing meant.

At the beginning of the hour, Bella spoke about the time she spent alone working on art projects the week prior during the missed appointments. She stated that she had not noticed many feelings about the time apart and was hesitant to explore what it had been like for her to not have therapy. Following a prolonged period of quiet and stillness in the middle of the session, Bella's eyes begin to dart around the room, and she appears to the therapist to be anxiously distressed.

Therapist: Something seems to have just changed a moment ago. You were quite still but that has shifted.

Bella: I was lost in thought. I was starting to imagine if you had ever had sex with someone who was intoxicated. I don't think you'd be the type, but I was playing it out in my mind.

Therapist: How did you come to that thought?

Bella: I don't know. It makes me feel gross. I'm not sure if you are a safe person. I know in my mind you are, but when I started imagining you taking advantage of someone, I feel this bad sensation in my body. I know logically you wouldn't, but I can't get out of this feeling.

Therapist: Can you describe it? Does it feel like you could translate it to an emotion?

Bella: Creeped out. I feel creeped out. The idea that you would have to force yourself on someone when they might not really want it. Not quite as transgressive as rape, but creepy. Maybe disgust? Or something intrusive about it.

Therapist: If we try and rewind to the silence, we had been talking about how you occupied your time during my vacation and then something played out in your mind that led to a frightening fantasy about me which left you feeling creeped out, disgusted, and intruded upon.

Bella: Well, the thought in between was about missing you. Ugh, I felt it there… the creepy feeling.

Therapist: You felt that gross feeling when you thought about having missed me?

Bella: I was worried that if you knew I missed you, you would feel intruded on. Like it was something you wouldn't want, and I remember feeling really anxious that you'd know I was missing you and then wouldn't want to see me after your vacation.

Therapist: I see, you were worried I'd be disgusted and wouldn't tolerate your having missed me? Like I'd want to get rid of you?

Bella: Yeah. I feel anxious about it and worried that you wouldn't accept it. Then I got worried about sharing my fantasy that you would take advantage of someone, and you would want to get rid of me for having that thought.

In this exchange, the therapist has focused on trying to ascertain what thoughts, feelings, and experiences precipitated a retreat into fantasy that was both distressing (in its content) for Bella, but also apparently a means of projecting her own conflict over desire and longing. The focus was not on the transference explicitly, nor interpreting unconscious determinants of the symptom. Rather, the therapist attempted to make sense of the overwhelm and confusion of the experience with Bella by adopting an accepting, curious stance in relation to her internal experience and what it might indicate about the relationship in that moment. Given Bella's anxiety about the stability and safety of the relationship, acceptance remained a key factor in addressing what felt like disturbing and transgressive fantasies. This is consistent with Cheli's (2020) report that patients noted acceptance as a key factor for the therapists to embody in such clinical encounter.

Conclusion

MBT is specifically designed to help people develop a greater awareness of their mental states and the mental states of others. The MBT therapist aims to promote curiosity and reflection while also attending to ruptures in the therapeutic relationship that may result in breakdowns in mentalization in both the therapist and patient. MBT seems particularly relevant for persons with schizotypy given that they have difficulties identifying their emotions and often hypermentalize, which can lead to distorted interpretations of interpersonal interactions and subsequent withdrawal. Three brief case vignettes were offered to help illustrate how therapists can understand breakdowns in mentalization during session and respond thoughtfully and sensitively to try to restore reflectivity while also attending to the therapeutic relationship. Key practice points also include the importance of helping people with schizotypy recognize their emotions and bodily sensations and notice breakdowns in their capacity for mentalization and possibly underlying causes. While MBT for psychosis is an emerging treatment, MBT has not specifically been applied to people exhibiting schizotypy; therefore, more research is needed to develop a comprehensive treatment package that can provide effective and timely interventions.

References

American Psychiatric Association. (2013). *Diagnostic and statistical manual of mental disorders* (5th ed.). American Psychiatric Publishing.

Bateman, A., & Fonagy, P. (2006). *Mentalization-based treatment for borderline personality disorder: A practical guide*. Oxford University Press.

Bateman, A., & Fonagy, P. (2016). *Mentalization-based treatment for personality disorders*. Oxford University Press.

Bender, D. S., Farber, B. A., Sanislow, C. A., Dyck, I. R., Geller, J. D., & Skodol, A. E. (2003). Representations of therapists by patients with personality disorders. *American Journal of Psychotherapy, 57*(2), 219–236.

Berenbaum, H., Boden, M. T., Baker, J. P., Dizen, M., Thompson, R. J., & Abramowitz, A. (2006). Emotional correlates of the different dimension of schizotypal personality disorder. *Journal of Abnormal Psychology, 115*(2), 359–368.

Bernstein, D. P., Fink, L., Handelsman, L., Foote, J., Lovejoy, M., Wenzel, K., Sapareto, E., & Ruggiero, J. (1994). Initial reliability and validity of a new retrospective measure of child abuse and neglect. *American Journal of Psychiatry, 151*(8), 1132–1136.

Brent, B. (2009). Mentalization-based psychodynamic psychotherapy for psychosis. *Journal of Clinical Psychology, 65*(8), 803–814.

Brent, B. K. (2015). A mentalization-based approach to the development of the therapeutic alliance in the treatment of schizophrenia. *Journal of Clinical Psychology, 71*(2), 146–156.

Cheli, S. (2020). Assessment and treatment planning for schizotypal personality disorder: A metacognitively oriented point of view. *Psychiatric Rehabilitation Journal, 43*(4), 335–343.

Debbané, M., & Barrantes-Vidal, N. (2015). Schizotypy from a developmental perspective. *Schizophrenia Bulletin, 41*(2), S386–S395.

Debbané, M., Benmiloud, J., Salaminios, G., Solida-Tozzi, A., Armando, M., Fonagy, P., & Bateman, A. (2016). Mentalization-based treatment in clinical high-risk for psychosis: A rationale and clinical illustration. *Journal of Contemporary Psychotherapy, 46*(4), 217–225.

Dmitryeva, N., Chernov, N., Kostyuk, G., & Lysaker, P. H. (2021). Utilizing MERIT to promote recovery in schizotypal personality disorder: An illustrative case study. *Journal of Clinical Psychology, 77*(8), 1798–1806.

Freeman, C. (2016). What is mentalizing? An overview. *British Journal of Psychotherapy, 32*(2), 189–201.

Kemp, K. C., Bathery, A. J., Barrantes-Vidal, N., & Kwapil, T. R. (2021). Positive, negative, and disorganized schizotypy predict differential patterns of interview-rated schizophrenia-spectrum symptoms and impairment. *Assessment, 28*(1), 141–152.

Kerns, J. G. (2005). Positive schizotypy and emotion processing. *Journal of Abnormal Psychology, 114*(3), 392–401.

Knauss, D., Ridenour, J., & Hamm, J. A. (2018). Emerging psychotherapies for psychosis. *Journal of Psychiatric Practice, 24*(5), 348–353.

Muller, N., & Midgley, N. (2020). The clinical challenge of Mentalization-based therapy with children who are in "pretend mode". *Journal of Infant, Child, and Adolescent Psychotherapy, 19*(1), 16–24.

Pazar, Ö., Steele, H., & Todman, M. (2022). Expressed emotion and reflective functioning across the schizotypy spectrum: Developmental experiential factors. *Psychoanalytic Psychology, 39*(3), 266–276.

Quidé, Y., Cohen-Woods, S., O'Reilly, N., Carr, V. J., Elzinga, B. M., & Green, M. J. (2018). Schizotypal personality traits and social cognition are associated with childhood trauma exposure. *British Journal of Clinical Psychology, 57*(4), 397–419.

Ridenour, J. M. (2016). Psychodynamic model and treatment of schizotypal personality disorder. *Psychoanalytic Psychology, 33*(1), 129–146.

Ridenour, J., Knauss, D., & Hamm, J. A. (2019). Comparing metacognition and mentalization and their implications for psychotherapy for individuals with psychosis. *Journal of Contemporary Psychotherapy, 49*(2), 79–85.

Ridenour, J. M., Knauss, D., & Neal, D. W. (2021). Promoting an integrating recovery style: A mentalization-informed approach. *Journal of Clinical Psychology, 77*(8), 1786–1797.

Salaminios, G., Morosan, L., Toffel, E., Tanzer, M., Eliez, S., Badoud, D., et al. (2021). Associations between schizotypal personality features, mentalizing difficulties and thought problems in a sample of community adolescents. *Early Intervention in Psychiatry, 15*(3), 705–715.

Toutountzidis, D., Gale, T. M., Irvine, K., Sharma, S., & Laws, K. R. (2022). Childhood trauma and schizotypy in non-clinical samples: A systematic review and meta-analysis. *PLoS One, 17*(6), e0270494.

Wastler, H. M., & Lenzenweger, M. F. (2019). Self-referential hypermentalization in schizotypy. *Personality Disorders: Theory, Research, and Treatment, 10*(6), 536–544.

Weijers, J., Fonagy, P., Eurelings-Bontekoe, E., Termorshuizen, F., Viechtbauer, W., & Selten, J. P. (2018). Mentalizing impairment as a mediator between reported childhood abuse and outcome in nonaffective psychotic disorder. *Psychiatry Research, 259*, 463–469.

Weijers, J. G., Ten Kate, C., Debbané, M., Bateman, A. W., De Jong, S., Selten, J. P., & Eurelings-Bontekoe, E. H. M. (2020). Mentalization and psychosis: A rationale for the use of mentalization theory to understand and treat non-affective psychotic disorder. *Journal of Contemporary Psychotherapy, 50*(3), 223–232.

Chapter 19
A View on the Treatment of Schizotypy in Terms of Psychoanalysis

Ondrej Pec and Vaclava Probstova

Introduction

The concept of schizotypy has a long and varied history in psychopathology and the diagnosis of mental disorders. In this development, psychoanalysis provided useful conceptions in addition to diagnostics, psychometrics, and genetic or neurobiological hypotheses. The classic work on schizotypy by Paul E. Meehl "Schizotaxia, schizotypy, schizophrenia" of 1962 already postulated schizotaxia as a genetically inborn neural integrative defect that transforms into a personality organisation called schizotypy, with four basic types of behaviour (interpersonal aversiveness, cognitive slippage, anhedonia, and ambivalence). These were later more precisely identified and defined (Barrantes-Vidal & Kwapil, Chap. 6, THIS BOOK; Kirchner et al., 2018; Reynolds et al., 2000; Su & Cicero, Chap. 3, THIS BOOK). According to Meehl, interpersonal development in the interaction between mother and child, especially maternal ambivalence and aversive stimuli towards the child, should have an effect on this transformation. The question of the intensity of this effect should be whether an individual develops schizophrenia, schizotypal personality disorder, or only subtle signs of the disorder that do not reach clinical significance (Meehl, 1962). These ideas were part of the view that also shaped the stress diathesis (vulnerability–stress) model in the following decades (Lenzenweger, 2006, 2018).

O. Pec (✉)
Center for Neuropsychiatric Research of Traumatic Stress, Department of Psychiatry and UHSL, First Faculty of Medicine, and Department of Psychiatry, Faculty of Medicine Pilsen, Charles University, Prague, Czech Republic

ESET, Psychotherapeutic and Psychosomatic Clinic, Prague, Czech Republic
e-mail: ondrej.pec@1lf.cuni.cz

V. Probstova
Department of Social Work, Faculty of Arts, Charles University, Prague, Czech Republic
e-mail: probstova@volny.cz

S. Cheli, P. H. Lysaker (eds.), *A Dimensional Approach to Schizotypy*,
https://doi.org/10.1007/978-3-031-41788-7_19

It is the understanding of the circumstances of early intrapsychic and interpersonal development together that could lead to the manifestations of schizophrenic psychosis, which has been the focus of psychoanalysis for many decades. The guide for this understanding was the practice of interpersonal experience in the psychotherapeutic treatment of patients with schizophrenic illness or with personality disorders of the schizotypal spectrum (especially schizotypal and schizoid) and observational studies of early mother–child interactions. These experiences were formulated into clinical theories and used in the treatment of patients.

In the same way that there is a wide and relatively continuous scale in the psychopathology of schizotypy (Su & Cicero, Chap. 3, THIS BOOK), one can observe a clinical-theoretical focus in psychoanalysis on pathological mental processes that describe psychic disintegration or mental fragmentation and loss of psychic differentiation, with an emphasis on their presence in schizophrenic psychoses up to dissociative events in schizoid mechanisms, covering the entire spectrum of schizotypy from personality disorders to psychotic illnesses.

Theoretical Concepts

The disintegration of mental experience in schizophrenia was formerly described by Freud (1914/1953, 1915/1953) as the primary process of thinking, and by Bleuler as autistic thinking (Bleuler, 1913). This form of thinking comprises several characteristics: the absence of contradiction, negation of time, forming of substitution and condensation of mental products, wish-fulfilment ignoring obstacles, immediate discharge of psychic energy, fragmentation, and concreteness in thinking. Recently, we can find new re-formulations of Freud's primary process (Modell, 2014; Robbins, 2018). Very close to this concept is also the hypothesis of damaged emotional unconsciousness, which is conceived as a state in which a person is unable intuitively to perceive emotional nonverbal signs and communications, to respond to emotions, to construct a sense of personal identity, to make self-observations, and to be aware of her/his mental and emotional processes (Rosenfeld, 1947; De Masi, 2016, 2017).

The description of the lack of psychic differentiation between inner and outer experience was derived from Freud's model of decathexis, when the ego, after strong emotional pressure, gives up emotional bonds to external objects or to mental representations of the objects and renews the primitive narcissistic state (secondary narcissism). The absence of any difference between outer and inner simultaneously refills the vacant psychic space with delusions and hallucinations (Freud, 1914/1953, 1915/1953). As a result, ordinary terms lose their content, which is given by the relationship to the surrounding world, they lack their internal and mutual logical connection and are the basis of schizophrenic disintegrated thinking (Freud, 1914/1953, 1923/1953). Bodily sensations, feelings, and emotions are also poorly differentiated (Lombardi, 2003). The concept of deficit differentiation was later further developed by a number of followers (Bleger, 1974; Caparros, 1999; Kernberg,

1982; Grotstein, 1990; Robbins, 1993, 2011). A lack of differentiation in principle leads to disruption of the formation of mental representations of outer and inner objects and of self. Where there is this lack, emotional bonds are missing, even at the cost of the absence of bonds based on severe projections. Simultaneously, attraction from external objects is disabled. Therefore, this state is connected with bland affect and passivity (Ogden, 2018). This type of disintegrative process in schizophrenia was also pointed out by Bleger (1974), who characterised it as a special symbiotic type of relationship in which a person does not psychologically distinguish between his own space and that of other people. In this situation, the mechanism of psychic splitting and projection is also limited. Bleger considered that "schizophrenia results from a pathological splitting with inability to build up the schizoid content of the paranoid-schizoid position" (Bleger, 1974, p. 24). He described these deficient and undeveloped mental states [glyschro-caryc position, from Greek γλίσχροσ – sticky and καρυο – nucleus] and supposed that this mental state precedes the paranoid-schizoid position described by Klein (1946) in the development. Ogden (1989) similarly characterized such an early developmental position (autistic contiguous position) and concluded that early experiences from this undifferentiated state belong to bodily touches on the skin surface, rhythmicity, and regularity of sucking.

In this context, we can therefore say that, prior to the paranoid position as described by Melanie Klein, there is a more primitive position, characteristic defences of which are abnormal splitting, immobilisation, and fragmentation (what Bleuler (1911/1950) called 'Zerspaltung'), which gives rise to confusional rather than persecutory anxiety, and in which, instead of real object relations, there are various "ego nuclei" together with the objects to which they correspond. These nuclei exist psychologically, but in an undifferentiated state because the splitting (Bleuler's 'Spaltung'), which later will characterise the paranoid-schizoid position, has not yet occurred. This more primitive position – Bleger terms it the glyschro-caryc position – and the residue of its relational structure persists throughout normal and pathological development as an "agglutinated nucleus", which he equates with what Bion (1957) called the psychotic part of the personality. Throughout life, the agglutinated nucleus remains ready to form symbiotic relationships, characterised by massive projective identifications. It is this nucleus that is deposited in the setting and remains hidden there, unanalysed, until a disruption to the setting causes it to become manifest (Churcher, 2023). The discovery of these early persistent states had an impact on Bleger's thinking about the so-called frame (setting). Bleger (1967, pp. 513–514) wrote: "In psychotic transference, affection is not transferred but 'a total situation, the whole of a development' (Lagache); it would be better to state: 'the whole of a non-development'. For Melanie Klein, transference repeats the primitive object relationships, but I think that what is still most primitive (the non-differentiation) repeats itself in the frame."

Another psychoanalyst who contributed to the considerations about early undifferentiated states was Tustin (1988), who defined them as autistic shapes (e.g., gentle touches) or autistic objects (that cause hard pressure against the infant's skin). According to Anzieu (1993), the cause of a deficient differentiation from mother–child symbiosis is probably linked to the missing bonds between mother and child (a negative attachment), which were later connected with a fantasy of "…an area of skin common to both mother and infant" (Anzieu, 1993, p.46). In accordance with this fantasy, they can communicate through this area, they have the same feelings and sensations and may mutually "…read the thoughts". The self is fragmented into an incoherent collection of pieces that create internal undifferentiated "*black holes*" of separateness, in which actual representations of otherness are missing (Anzieu, 1974, 1993).

Disintegration and loss of differentiation between the internal and external world can have a common origin in the effects of the very early traumatic factors that do not allow differentiation of primarily undifferentiated self-object representation through the interrelated processes of exteroception and interoception (Kernberg, 1982). Impaired mother containing functioning during early mother–child relationships was considered as the traumatic factor. This means that an infant cannot use a primary object – the mother as a 'container' (Bion's term) – for endangering unthinkable emotional experiences that can then be processed and passed back to the child in an acceptable form. Because, in a favourable case, the child can identify with this containing function as a basis for his/her mental processing (Bion, 1984; Mawson 2017).

The existence of this form of dysfunctional attachment was further supported by observational studies of early child–mother interactions. The period between the second and seventh months of life has been assumed as being critical for a predisposition to schizophrenia when many important capacities are established from these interactions: the sense of authorship of one's actions, being non-fragmented as a physical whole, and continuity in time. The creation of these capacities is very closely linked to further abilities, such as the ability to distinguish between self and non-self as an agent of internal experience. Their absence can predispose the person to paranoid symptoms, mental fragmentation, affective indifference, or distorted perception of time (Michels, 2017; Stern, 1985). These concepts now have a lively response in the research that is being focused on the immediate sense of mine-ness, a disturbance of "minimal self" (Ameller et al., 2015; Henriksen et al., 2019; Madeira et al., 2019), comprising neural models (Taylor, 2011) and describing the experience of agency in schizophrenia (Synofzik et al., 2013).

While disintegration and loss of psychic differentiation are the domain of mental processes primarily in schizophrenia, schizoid mechanisms as a defense covers the entire range of schizotypy. This concept was used for the first time by Fairbairn (1952), and elaborated on by Melanie Klein and her successors. Klein's theories were inspired by her clinical work with severely disturbed adults and with children. She described the mechanism of psychic splitting as a result of early exposure to intense intrapsychic and relational stress, which slows down the integrative processes in psychic maturation. As a result, during psychic splitting, the individual keeps the negative and positive parts of the representation of himself and other relational persons divided, and places them in close people (paranoid-schizoid position). The more stressful the relationship and the more intense the corresponding emotional burden, and the earlier it occurs, the more probable it is that the psychic splitting has the nature of disintegration (Klein, 1940, 1945, 1946). Such disintegrative forms of splitting, which are mainly found in patients with schizophrenic psychosis, were discussed by Bion (1959) and characterised as "splitting attacks". In these, a person splits internal mental objects or functions and identifies them with real objects or persons, enabling his/her own mental states to be sensed and experienced as a part of the external world. For example, various bizarre objects or events, such as a "listening chair", "sight" of inanimate objects, and others, based on a projective mechanism in which a split [unconscious] seeing or other sensations may be transferred to other persons or things (Bion, 1959). Splitting can be viewed as a disturbance or disconnection between two (or more) mental states or thoughts, preventing conscious awareness of unbearable negative emotions. A consequence of these "attacks on the link" is an inability to bring together two disconnected thoughts and to form a new mental object and related emotional experience (Bion, 1957, 1959).

Following Klein and Bion, Matte-Blanco (1988) also contributed significantly to the understanding of mental states in a continuous spectrum of schizotypy, from schizophrenia to personality disorders. For the area of the unconscious and the primary process, he defined what was called the "principle of symmetry", which states that if A has some relation to B, then B must also have the same relation to A. The opposite is asymmetric relationships, which are part of our ordinary logic. On the principle of symmetry, it is possible to explain a number of properties belonging to the unconscious system and the primary process (Freud, 1915/1953). It is usual for a symmetric relationship to be "nested" into an asymmetric relationship, whereby a dual relationship is created, which is called "bi-logic". Matte-Blanco assumes that the human mind is more than three-dimensional, which is especially true for its unconscious part. Therefore, what takes place in the unconscious mind, we can perceive consciously only in three-dimensional space-time. A space, which has more dimensions than three, is converted into three-dimensional space (tridimensionalisation). Tridimensionalisation is important for understanding phenomena such as displacement, condensation, and projective identification. The same psychic contents can exist separately internally and externally (seen three-dimensionally) and, at the same time, without distinction between inside and outside (seen more than three-dimensionally). Matte-Blanco (1988) developed a theory of five layers of the human mind, according to the ability to distinguish phenomena and classify them into classes or categories and according to the degree of involvement of asymmetrical or symmetrical relationships. The first layer belongs to conscious perception, to the limited perception of individual phenomena. Asymmetric relationships prevail here. The second layer is still conscious and includes the differentiation of specific objects into individual classes or categories. This layer also includes emotions, where symmetrisation can already enter, albeit in a limited way. The third layer discussed by him roughly corresponds to the mental state of schizoid mechanisms. All elements in a certain category are identical, their parts are equal to the whole, the succession of phenomena disappears. For psychotic states, the fourth layer is the most relevant. The symmetrisation here affects wider classes (e.g. man = woman = child). People with schizophrenia see as identical what belongs to different subgroups of some broader class. The fifth layer is the deepest. Thinking that requires a certain amount of asymmetry is no longer practically possible. Symmetrisation has already progressed in such a way that anything is experienced as anything else, an infinite number of things tend to be a single thing. This layer belongs to the deeper layers of the unconscious. The meaning of therapeutic work is the journey from symmetrisation to asymmetrisation (Lombardi, 2003). There are many psychoanalytical contributions to an understanding of schizotypy. Due to limited space, we present only some of these. They provide access to a psychological understanding of symptoms and their occurrence in time. Clinical work with patients with schizotypy has taken place mainly in psychoanalytic therapeutic practices, or in clinical outpatient and inpatient settings, inspired by and using psychodynamic understanding.

Empirical Findings in Clinical Practice

Evaluation of clinical effectiveness, which is already beginning to be seen in other psychosocial approaches (Nordentoft et al., 2006), has so far been very sparse (Dixon-Gordon et al., 2011; Kirchner et al., 2018). Karterud et al. (1992) evaluated a sample of 97 patients with various diagnoses of personality disorders, treated in a daily psychotherapy programme, using individual and group psychodynamic psychotherapy in combination with other approaches. In schizotypal patients, of whom there were only 13 in the entire sample, he noted only a statistically insignificant improvement after 6 months of treatment in the area of symptoms of the disorder. Later published data from a subsample of 26 schizotypal patients being treated in a psychodynamic day programme showed similar results (Karterud et al., 2003). On the other hand, patients with schizotypal personality disorder in a similar daily psychodynamic programme in a prospective follow-up of 3–6 years showed moderate symptom reduction, but still with problematic global functioning (Mehlum et al., 1991).

Patients with borderline personality disorder appear to show faster and greater progress in psychoanalytically focused therapy than patients with schizotypal disorder. Stone (1983) compared a group of 21 borderline-affective patients with a group of 27 schizotypal patients (borderline schizophrenic patients), in terms of clinical effect after several months of psychoanalytic treatment. He found that in the group of patients with borderline disorder, the majority made significant progress, whereas in the group with schizotypal disorder, some patients made progress, some stagnated, and some even showed deterioration. He observed that a greater representation of anhedonia and social withdrawal, the predominance of the autistic type of attachment over the symbiotic type, and the absence of signs from the area of affective symptoms in patients could be predictors of stagnation in therapy. More recent studies regarding the therapeutic effectiveness of psychodynamic psychotherapy can be found in the treatment of patients with schizophrenia. Here we may mention, for example, the Danish schizophrenia project demonstrating the additive effect of supportive psychodynamic psychotherapy to conventional treatment in the area of symptoms and social functioning (Rosenbaum et al., 2012; Rosenbaum, 2015). Although more systematic empirical research on psychodynamic treatment in the field of schizotypy is still lacking, psychoanalytic treatment had and still has an important influence in the field of case studies, conceptual and theoretical works, in which we can trace a long-standing tradition and influence on other psychotherapeutic approaches.

Practical Recommendations for Therapy

In the following discussion of the psychoanalytic treatment of patients, we rather concentrate on the broader spectrum of schizotypy, because this kind of psychotherapy has been practised on patients classified as schizoid, pseudoneurotic schizophrenic (Hoch & Polatin, 1949), schizoaffective (Kasanin, 1994), "borderline" non-delusional schizophrenic (Knight, 1953), and later on schizotypal patients (Rado, 1953). From today's point of view, it is difficult to retrospectively determine their exact diagnostic classification according to current standards. In the treatment, the psychodynamic approach mainly tried to respect some of the above-mentioned characteristics of the mental organisation of patients with schizotypy, such as the permeability of ego boundaries, intensely expressed splitting mechanisms with a strong involvement of projective mechanisms and the related important role of countertransference or a stronger representation of the primary process or symmetrical relationships in thinking.

Psychodynamic characteristics of patients with schizotypy are important for some specificity of psychotherapeutic work with them.

To mention several topics in this regard – these are mainly questions of therapeutic alliance and stance, therapeutic setting, the therapeutic relationship in general, a question of interpretations and progress in treatment.

The establishment of a therapeutic alliance is the cornerstone of the success of psychotherapeutic treatment of patients with schizotypy. Empirical studies have shown us the high drop-out of schizotypal patients from treatment, reaching several tens of percent (Kirchner et al., 2018). In patients with schizophrenia, a similar problem prompted the search for more flexible forms of individual psychotherapy (Fenton, 2000) and the development of tools that would be able to evaluate the quality of the therapeutic alliance before starting the therapy (Valbak et al., 2003). The relationship with objects, including the therapist, seems to be paradoxical in people with the schizotypal spectrum: a great need and fear of it simultaneously. On the one hand, we observe significant social withdrawal in these people, due to paranoid alertness and a fear of the unpredictability of the other person's reactions. On the other hand, when we get to know the patient more closely, we discover a desire for an intense bond with the other person. This contradiction corresponds, for example, to how schizotypal patients represent the person of the therapist. For example, Bender et al. (2003) found that schizotypal patients, compared to other personality disorders, are more concerned with the relationship with the therapist outside of the session and are far more sensitive to treatment interruptions, wishing to establish a personal friendship with him/her. Their motivation for therapy may therefore be influenced by the desire not to be alone, even in the form of a “hired friendship” (Stone, 1985). However, such intense embedding in the person of the therapist is complicated by the permeability of ego boundaries, which we can detect, for example, by the presence of transitivistic phenomena during the session, e.g. that the therapist can know what the patient is thinking (Stone, 1985). In order to maintain a quality therapeutic alliance, it is therefore important to take measures that limit intermingling as much as possible, i.e. firm boundaries and a structured therapeutic frame (Ridenour, 2016). Another aspect in schizotypal patients that can complicate the therapeutic alliance is strong anhedonia. Every interpersonal relationship is very painful, including a therapeutic relationship, and is balanced slightly by the pleasant experiences that also result from the relationship. It then requires considerable patience from the therapist (Stone, 1983). To summarise, we can state that building a therapeutic alliance is a long-term process, in which it is very important to be able to stay with the patient’s inner chaos, to give a message that one is able to stay with it, and to avoid giving premature interpretations (countertransferential tendency to defend himself from projective identifications by forcing them back to the patient).

Regarding the therapeutic setting, there is no consensus on the use of a couch or face-to-face session. On the one hand, the patient needs not to be disturbed too much by the therapist’s visible gestures, and on the other hand, he also needs visual contact for greater support (Stone, 1985). Psychoanalytically oriented psychotherapy for patients with schizotypy is a long-term commitment. It can take several months, but we often encounter treatments that last several years. Improvement of anhedonia, reduction of paranoid ideation, and improved social inclusion are important markers for consideration of the termination of therapy. The frequency of sessions is 2–4 per week. The frequency depends to a large extent on the psychological fragility of the patient, i.e. to what extent it has been possible to establish a quality therapeutic alliance with the patient and if the patient is able to withstand the intensity of contact with the therapist without major psychological discomfort. A greater frequency of sessions is usually agreed upon with the patient later in the therapy, when the therapeutic alliance has improved (Ridenour, 2016; Stone, 1983).

In the technique of the psychodynamic approach to patients with schizotypy, we place much more emphasis on the function of the therapist as a container than as a bearer of interpretations. Psychodynamic therapy for these patients tends to be supportive rather than insight-oriented psychotherapy. This implies that the aim is rather to strengthen the repression of thoughts, feelings, and fantasies that provoke anxiety, and the task of the therapist is to be an auxiliary ego for the patient, supporting the patient’s ego functions (Ridenour, 2016).

Let us now bear in mind the heavily represented primary thought process in these patients and the large representation of projective processes. Therefore, as therapists, we should offer “narcissistic” identification in the relationship to maintain emotional contact (Stone, 1985), which, as a more primitive nucleus of the superego, is a precursor of object cathexis (Perdigão, 1985). The function of the container means that the analyst has the ability to tolerate the projections and interpret them in a way that creates the possibility that the hitherto isolated attributes of the psychic material are more tolerable and the patient can reintegrate them into his/her personality for the benefit of his/her enrichment (Bion, 1984). In this context, considerable attention needs to be paid to the choice and timing of interpretations of the content to the patient. The patient tends to be overwhelmed by a large number of fantasies that have incestuous, homosexual, or aggressive content. Direct interpretations confronting these contents can induce intense shame and, in some cases, a brief psychotic episode (Stone, 1985). More appropriate in these cases are the interpretations directed at the analyst as the bearer of the threat in the projective transference situation, which results from these fantasies. Steiner (1994) called this type of interpretation "analyst-centred interpretations" stating, for example, "You experience me as …" However, excessive use of these interpretations can lead the patient to becoming overly concerned with the person of the therapist, instead of with the patient himself. Patient-directed interpretations can rather be used later in therapy, at a stage when the patient better distinguishes the therapist as a real person from thoughts about the therapist (Carsky & Rand, 2018). In his extensive practice with schizotypal patients, Stone (1983) did not find many opportunities for directly interpreting the symbolic content of the patient's message. Instead, there are more opportunities for these patients to interpret resistance, such as: "I find it hard to understand what you're telling me today; I suspect there's something troubling you that you're more comfortable concealing than telling me straight out about." (Stone, 1983, p. 108).

From these considerations of containment and interpretation, it follows that transference analysis in schizotypal patients is not as much a primary goal of therapy as it is in other types of patients. Ridenour (2016), for example, recommends using transference interpretations only occasionally as a point of reference when the patient's relationship issues are discussed in therapy. On the other hand, in these patients, the goal comes to the fore, so that the patient can experience feelings and emotions more hand in hand with gaining a better understanding of the boundary between self and others, along with reducing the intensity of projective and introjective psychological mechanisms. As a vehicle for this development in therapy, for example, Benedetti (1980) mentions "identification", by which he means the mutual introjection between the patient and the therapist, when the therapist introjects the pathological parts of the patient's self and is able to transform them. In this context, he also talks about the "transitional subject", which arises on the basis of fusal transference, when the therapist takes the place of the self-object within the patient's fusion, having creative, progressive, and communicative functions. The transitional subject is gradually absorbed into the patient's incipient identity and has the role of a certain third person in the dyad. A new symptom may also appear that is still psychotic, but serves a communicative function. It is what is called "progressive psychopathology" (Benedetti & Peciccia, 1998). However, this mental inclusion of the patient's parts in the therapist also presents difficult aspects to the therapy. Unconscious "living in the object" prompts excessive control of the therapist, efforts not to be abandoned by him, including the painful experience of a break in therapy. Another peculiarity is also persecutory fears of the therapist, if there is an inner conviction that the patient's split and projected parts have the character of envious, greedy, and destructive impulses (Rey, 1994). In this context, other authors would rather talk about the role of countertransference and the containing function of the therapist, in which the therapist accepts and transforms the projected and split pathological aspects of the patient, integrates them and passes them back to the patient in a form more acceptable to him. At the same time, the patient identifies with the containing function of the therapist, which supports his mentally synthesising abilities (Mawson, 2017; Ogden, 1980).

Distinctive aspects of the therapy of patients with schizotypy include the use of language, which reflects a strong representation of the primary thought process and concreteness in thinking. Language use is therefore often idiosyncratic. Ridenour (2016) describes states of confusion in the therapist, when the patient could not find the correct expression for an affectively coloured word and had a magical premonition that the wrongly chosen word would forever change her relationship with the therapist. Finally, a suitable word helped to contain her anxiety stemming from the destructive and dangerous nature of giving voice to such feelings. Stone (1985) states that the therapist should first learn the patient's language. This is because language is also used for defensive purposes, and speech is used as an elaborate manoeuvre to conceal what is not to be said. The therapist is then in the role of a detective who reveals the real hidden person behind the said content (Stone, 1983).

Psychoanalytically focused individual psychotherapy for patients with schizotypy is very often a long-term process, lasting for many years if we want to achieve a favourable change. Therapists should not push for a quick therapeutic effect. Such pressure would lead to an unfavourably unsuccessful self-concept in therapy, both in the therapist and in the patient, and exacerbate his anhedonia. Small favourable changes should be considered a success by the therapist (Stone, 1983). Stone (1985) also emphasises that the therapist should not hesitate to provide advice, education, and clarification when needed. In patients with schizotypy, this is more appropriate than in other types of patients. The therapist serves as a "reality organ" for the patient (Stone, 1985, p.586). In this regard, it should be borne in mind that patients with schizotypy cover the entire range of disorders, from lower social functioning (schizophrenic patients and some patients with schizotypal disorder) to higher functioning (part of schizotypal patients and patients with schizophrenia, patients with schizoid personality disorder). The level of support should therefore reflect this functionality, ranging from community or rehabilitation services to psychotherapeutic support.

Conclusion

Our intention in this chapter was to describe the main psychological processes that underlie disorders in the diagnostic spectrum of schizotypy. We mentioned the psychological phenomena of disintegration, the blurring of boundaries between self and others, and schizoid mechanisms. The representation of these phenomena in individual patients corresponds to the severity of the disability, from schizophrenia to schizotypal disorder or schizoid personality disorder. Psychoanalytic treatment for these patients has a long tradition and uses the therapeutic relationship as the main tool for positive change. Individual treatment for these patients consists mainly of integration of the patient's fragmented internal psychic contents to alleviate the intensity of projective psychic mechanisms, and to strengthen the boundaries of the ego and the sense of self. This treatment also includes supportive interventions, which we use in this group more than in other types of patients.

The benefit of the psychoanalytic approach to the treatment of schizotypy can generally be seen in two directions. The first of these is psychoanalytically focused psychotherapy, which will be used by patients with schizotypy who have gone through a painful experience associated with that disorder and for whom there is a certain level of insight that their psychological problems are connected to their relationship experiences and that they are searching for a longer-term processing of these experiences in a therapeutic relationship. The second direction is the possibility of finding an understanding for the relationships of these patients, for their behaviour and problems, even outside the framework of the psychotherapeutic setting. In this regard, psychoanalytic concepts (e.g. projective identification, container) with their comprehension of interpersonal patterns (transference and countertransference phenomena with acting out/in, enactments) can play a significant role in the work of mental health workers outside of direct psychotherapeutic work, for example, in community care in relationships between social workers or nurses and patients.

References

Ameller, A., Dereux, A., Dubertret, C., Vaiva, G., Thomas, P., & Pins, D. (2015). What is more familiar than I? Self, other and familiarity in schizophrenia. *Schizophrenia Research, 161*(2–3), 501–505. https://doi.org/10.1016/j.schres.2014.12.007

Anzieu, D. (1974). A discussion of the paper by Gisela Pankow on "The body image in psychosis". *International Journal of Psychoanalysis, 55*, 415–416.

Anzieu, D. (1993). Autistic phenomena and the skin ego. *Psychoanalytic Inquiry, 13*, 42–48.

Bender, D. S., Farber, B. A., Sanislow, C. A., Dyck, I. R., Geller, J. D., & Skodol, A. E. (2003). Representations of therapists by patients with personality disorders. *American Journal of Psychotherapy, 57*(2), 219–236. https://doi.org/10.1176/appi.psychotherapy.2003.57.2.219

Benedetti, G. (1980). Individual psychotherapy of schizophrenia. *Schizophrenia Bulletin, 6*(4), 633–638. https://doi-org.ezproxy.is.cuni.cz/10.1093/schbul/6.4.633

Benedetti, G., & Peciccia, M. (1998). The ego structure and the self-identity of the schizophrenic human and the task of psychoanalysis. *International Forum of Psychoanalysis, 7*, 169–174.

Bion, W. R. (1957). Differentiation of the psychotic from the non-psychotic personalities. *International Journal of Psychoanalysis, 38*, 266–275.

Bion, W. R. (1959). Attacks on linking. *International Journal of Psychoanalysis, 40*, 308–315.

Bion, W. R. (1984). *Elements of psycho-analysis*. Karnac.

Bleger, J. (1967). Psycho-analysis of the psycho-analytic frame. *International Journal of Psychoanalysis, 48*(4), 511–519.

Bleger, J. (1974). Schizophrenia, autisms, and symbiosis. *Contemporary Psychoanalysis, 10*, 19–25.
Bleuler, E. (1911/1950). *Dementia praecox or the group of schizophrenias* (J. Zinkin, Trans.). International Universities Press.
Bleuler, E. (1913). Autistic thinking. In D. Rapaport (Ed.), *Organization and pathology of thought, selected sources* (pp. 399–437). Columbia University Press.
Caparrós, N. (1999). Splitting and disavowal in group psychotherapy of psychosis. In V. L. Schermer & M. Pines (Eds.), *Group psychotherapy of the psychoses* (pp. 83–96). Jessica Kingsley Publishers.
Carsky, M., & Rand, S. N. (2018). Conflict between fantasy and reality: A patient and therapist talk about psychotherapy and schizophrenia. *Psychoanalytic Psychology, 35*(4), 401–409. https://doi.org/10.1037/pap0000178
Churcher, J. (2023). The psychoanalytic setting, embodiment and presence: Exploring José Bleger's concept of encuadre. In C. Moguillansky & H. B. Levine (Eds.), *Psychoanalysis of the psychoanalytic frame revisited. A new look at José Bleger's classic work* (pp. 38–56). Routledge. https://doi.org/10.4324/9781003252252
De Masi, F. (2016). Herbert Rosenfeld in Italy, 1978–1985. *International Forum of Psychoanalysis, 25*(4), 241–248. https://doi.org/10.1080/0803706X.2015.1127423
De Masi, F. (2017). Some paths towards psychotic alienation. *American Journal of Psychoanalysis, 77*(4), 347–358. https://doi.org/10.1057/s11231-017-9111-8
Dixon-Gordon, K. L., Turner, B. J., & Chapman, A. L. (2011). Psychotherapy for personality disorders. *International review of psychiatry (Abingdon, England), 23*(3), 282–302. https://doi-org.ezproxy.is.cuni.cz/10.3109/09540261.2011.586992
Fairbairn, W. D. (1952). Chapter I. Schizoid factors in the personality (1940). *Psychoanalytic Studies of the Personality, 7*, 1–27.
Fenton, W. S. (2000). Evolving perspectives on individual psychotherapy for schizophrenia. *Schizophrenia Bulletin, 26*(1), 47–72. https://doi-org.ezproxy.is.cuni.cz/10.1093/oxfordjournals.schbul.a033445
Freud, S. (1914/1953). On narcissism: An introduction. In J. Strachey, A. Freud, A. Richards, & C. L. Rothgeb (Eds.), *The standard edition of the complete psychological works of Sigmund Freud* (Vol. 14, pp. 67–102). Hogarth Press and the Institute of Psycho-Analysis.
Freud, S. (1915/1953). The unconscious. In J. Strachey, A. Freud, A. Richards, & C. L. Rothgeb (Eds.), *The standard edition of the complete psychological works of Sigmund Freud* (Vol. 14, pp. 159–215). Hogarth Press and the Institute of Psycho-Analysis.
Grotstein, J. S. (1990). Nothingness, meaninglessness, Chaos, and the "Black Hole" I – The importance of nothingness, meaninglessness, and Chaos in psychoanalysis. *Contemporary Psychoanalysis, 26*(2), 257–290. https://doi.org/10.1080/00107530.1990.10746658
Henriksen, M. G., Parnas, J., & Zahavi, D. (2019). Thought insertion and disturbed for-me-ness (minimal selfhood) in schizophrenia. *Consciousness and Cognition, 74*, 102770. https://doi-org.ezproxy.is.cuni.cz/10.1016/j.concog.2019.102770
Hoch, P., & Polatin, P. (1949). Pseudoneurotic forms of schizophrenia. *The Psychiatric Quarterly, 23*(2), 248–276. https://doi.org/10.1007/BF01563119
Karterud, S., Vaglum, S., Friis, S., Irion, T., Johns, S., & Vaglum, P. (1992). Day hospital therapeutic community treatment for patients with personality disorders. An empirical evaluation of the containment function. *The Journal of Nervous and Mental Disease, 180*(4), 238–243. https://doi-org.ezproxy.is.cuni.cz/10.1097/00005053-199204000-00005
Karterud, S., Pedersen, G., Bjordal, E., Brabrand, J., Friis, S., Haaseth, O., Haavaldsen, G., Irion, T., Leirvåg, H., Tørum, E., & Urnes, O. (2003). Day treatment of patients with personality disorders: Experiences from a Norwegian treatment research network. *Journal of Personality Disorders, 17*(3), 243–262. https://doi-org.ezproxy.is.cuni.cz/10.1521/pedi.17.3.243.22151
Kasanin, J. (1994). The acute schizoaffective psychoses. 1933. *The American Journal of Psychiatry, 151*(6 Suppl), 144–154. https://doi.org/10.1176/ajp.151.6.144

Kernberg, O. F. (1982). Self, ego, affects, and drives. *Journal of the American Psychoanalytic Association, 30*(4), 893–917. https://doi-org.ezproxy.is.cuni.cz/10.1177/000306518203000404

Kirchner, S. K., Roeh, A., Nolden, J., & Hasan, A. (2018). Diagnosis and treatment of schizotypal personality disorder: Evidence from a systematic review. *NPJ Schizophrenia, 4*(1), 20. https://doi-org.ezproxy.is.cuni.cz/10.1038/s41537-018-0062-8

Klein, M. (1940). Mourning and its relation to manic-depressive states. *International Journal of Psychoanalysis, 21*, 125–153.

Klein, M. (1945). The Oedipus complex in the light of early anxieties. *International Journal of Psychoanalysis, 26*, 11–33.

Klein, M. (1946). Notes on some schizoid mechanisms. *International Journal of Psycho-analysis, 27*(Pt 3–4), 99–110.

Knight, R. P. (1953). Borderline states. *Bulletin of the Menninger Clinic, 17*(1), 1–12.

Lenzenweger, M. F. (2006). Schizotaxia, schizotypy, and schizophrenia: Paul E. Meehl's blueprint for the experimental psychopathology and genetics of schizophrenia. *Journal of Abnormal Psychology, 115*(2), 195–200. https://doi-org.ezproxy.is.cuni.cz/10.1037/0021-843X.115.2.195

Lenzenweger, M. F. (2018). Schizotypy, schizotypic psychopathology and schizophrenia. *World Psychiatry: Official Journal of the World Psychiatric Association (WPA), 17*(1), 25–26. https://doi-org.ezproxy.is.cuni.cz/10.1002/wps.20479

Lombardi, R. (2003). Catalyzing the dialogue between the body and the mind in a psychotic analysand. *The Psychoanalytic Quarterly, 72*(4), 1017–1041. https://doi-org.ezproxy.is.cuni.cz/10.1002/j.2167-4086.2003.tb00148.x

Madeira, L., Pienkos, E., Filipe, T., Melo, M., Queiroz, G., Eira, J., Costa, C., Figueira, M. L., & Sass, L. (2019). Self and world experience in non-affective first episode of psychosis. *Schizophrenia Research, 211*, 69–78. https://doi-org.ezproxy.is.cuni.cz/10.1016/j.schres.2019.07.001

Matte-Blanco, I. (1988). *Thinking, feeling, and being: Clinical reflections on the fundamental antinomy of human beings and world.* Taylor & Frances/Routledge.

Mawson, C. (2017). Interpretation as Freud's specific action, and Bion's container-contained. *The International Journal of Psychoanalysis, 98*(6), 1519–1532. https://doi.org/10.1111/1745-8315.12668

Meehl, P. E. (1962). Schizotaxia, schizotypy, schizophrenia. *American Psychologist, 17*(12), 827–838. https://doi.org/10.1037/h0041029

Mehlum, L., Friis, S., Irion, T., Johns, S., Karterud, S., Vaglum, P., & Vaglum, S. (1991). Personality disorders 2-5 years after treatment: A prospective follow-up study. *Acta Psychiatrica Scandinavica, 84*(1), 72–77. https://doi-org.ezproxy.is.cuni.cz/10.1111/j.1600-0447.1991.tb01423.x

Michels, R. (2017). Stern on "Self". *Psychoanalytic Inquiry, 37*(4), 265–269. https://doi.org/10.1080/07351690.2017.1299502

Modell, A. H. (2014). The evolutionary significance of the primary process—The Freudian concept and its revision. *Psychoanalytic Inquiry, 34*(8), 810–816. https://doi.org/10.1080/07351690.2014.968023

Nordentoft, M., Thorup, A., Petersen, L., Ohlenschlaeger, J., Melau, M., Christensen, T. Ø., Krarup, G., Jørgensen, P., & Jeppesen, P. (2006). Transition rates from schizotypal disorder to psychotic disorder for first-contact patients included in the OPUS trial. A randomized clinical trial of integrated treatment and standard treatment. *Schizophrenia Research, 83*(1), 29–40. https://doi-org.ezproxy.is.cuni.cz/10.1016/j.schres.2006.01.002

Ogden, T. H. (1980). On the nature of schizophrenic conflict. *International Journal of Psychoanalysis, 61*, 513–533.

Ogden, T. H. (1989). On the concept of an autistic-contiguous position. *International Journal of Psychoanalysis, 70*, 127–140.

Perdigão, H. G. (1985). Revista De Psicoanálisis, XL. 1983: Roots of the Superego. Hugo Mayer. pp. 573-582. *Psychoanalytic Quarterly, 54*, 332–333.

Rado, S. (1953). Dynamics and classification of disordered behavior. *American Journal of Psychiatry, 110*(6), 406–416. https://doi.org/10.1176/ajp.110.6.406

Rey, H. (1994). The schizoid mode of being and the space-time continuum (before metaphor). In J. Magagna (Ed.), *Universals of psychoanalysis in the treatment of psychotic and borderline patients* (pp. 8–30). Free Associations.

Reynolds, C. A., Raine, A., Mellingen, K., Venables, P. H., & Mednick, S. A. (2000). Three-factor model of schizotypal personality: Invariance across culture, gender, religious affiliation, family adversity, and psychopathology. *Schizophrenia Bulletin, 26*(3), 603–618. https://doi-org.ezproxy.is.cuni.cz/10.1093/oxfordjournals.schbul.a033481

Ridenour, J. M. (2016). Psychodynamic model and treatment of schizotypal personality disorder. *Psychoanalytic Psychology, 33*(1), 129–146. https://doi.org/10.1037/a0035531

Robbins, M. (1993). *Experiences of schizophrenia. An integration of the personal, scientific, and therapeutic*. The Guilford Press.

Robbins, M. (2011). *The primordial mind in health and illness: A crosscultural perspective*. Routledge.

Robbins, M. (2018). The primary process: Freud's profound yet neglected contribution to the psychology of consciousness. *Psychoanalytic Inquiry, 38*(3), 186–197. https://doi.org/10.1080/07351690.2018.1430965

Rosenbaum, B. (2015). Psychodynamic psychotherapy for persons in states of psychosis: Some research perspectives. *British Journal of Psychotherapy, 31*(4), 476–491. https://doi.org/10.1111/bjp.12187

Rosenbaum, B., Harder, S., Knudsen, P., Køster, A., Lindhardt, A., Lajer, M., Valbak, K., & Winther, G. (2012). Supportive psychodynamic psychotherapy versus treatment as usual for first-episode psychosis: Two-year outcome. *Psychiatry, 75*(4), 331–341. https://doi-org.ezproxy.is.cuni.cz/10.1521/psyc.2012.75.4.331

Rosenfeld, H. (1947). Analysis of a schizophrenic state with depersonalization. *International Journal of Psychoanalysis, 28*, 130–139.

Steiner, J. (1994). Patient-centered and analyst-centered interpretations: Some implications of containment and countertransference. *Psychoanalytic Inquiry, 14*, 406–422.

Stern, D. N. (1985). *The interpersonal world of the infant: A view from psychoanalysis and development*. Basic Books.

Stone, M. H. (1983). Psychotherapy with schizotypal borderline patients. *The Journal of the American Academy of Psychoanalysis, 11*(1), 87–111. https://doi-org.ezproxy.is.cuni.cz/10.1521/jaap.1.1983.11.1.87

Stone, M. (1985). Schizotypal personality: Psychotherapeutic aspects. *Schizophrenia Bulletin, 11*(4), 576–589. https://doi-org.ezproxy.is.cuni.cz/10.1093/schbul/11.4.576

Synofzik, M., Vosgerau, G., & Voss, M. (2013). The experience of agency: An interplay between prediction and postdiction. *Frontiers in Psychology, 4*, 127. https://doi-org.ezproxy.is.cuni.cz/10.3389/fpsyg.2013.00127

Taylor, J. G. (2011). A neural model of the loss of self in schizophrenia. *Schizophrenia Bulletin, 37*(6), 1229–1247. https://doi-org.ezproxy.is.cuni.cz/10.1093/schbul/sbq033

Tustin, F. (1988). The "black hole": A significant element in autism. *Free Associations, 1*, 35–50.

Valbak, K., Køster, A., Larsen, K. A., Nielsen, J. R., Norrie, B., & Danish National Multicenter Schizophrenia Project. (2003). The Danish national multicenter schizophrenia project: Assessment of psychotic patients for dynamic psychotherapy (APPP). *Nordic Journal of Psychiatry, 57*(5), 333–338. https://doi-org.ezproxy.is.cuni.cz/10.1080/08039480310002651

Ogden, T. H. (2018). The nature of schizophrenic conflict. Projective Identification and Psychotherapeutic Technique (pp. 135–172). London: Routledge.

Chapter 20
Clinical Staging of Schizotypal Disorder: Preliminary Considerations and Treatment Implications

Kristina Ballestad Gundersen, Andrea Polari, Louise Birkedal Glenthøj, Nikolai Albert, Patrick D. McGorry, Andreas Rosén Rasmussen, and Barnaby Nelson

Introduction

Many conditions, both in general medicine and in psychiatry, have been approached from a clinical staging perspective – that is, defined according to stages of disorder severity and extension. However, this perspective has not yet been applied to

K. B. Gundersen (✉)
Copenhagen Research Center for Mental Health (CORE), Copenhagen, Denmark
e-mail: Kristina.ballestad.gundersen@regionh.dk

A. Polari
Centre for Youth Mental Health, The University of Melbourne, Melbourne, VIC, Australia

Orygen, Parkville, VIC, Australia

Orygen Specialist Program, Melbourne Health, Melbourne, VIC, Australia

L. B. Glenthøj
Copenhagen Research Center for Mental Health (CORE), Copenhagen, Denmark

Department of Psychology, University of Copenhagen, Copenhagen, Denmark

N. Albert
Copenhagen Research Center for Mental Health (CORE), Copenhagen, Denmark

Mental Health Center Amager, University of Copenhagen, Copenhagen, Denmark

P. D. McGorry · B. Nelson
Centre for Youth Mental Health, The University of Melbourne, Melbourne, VIC, Australia

Orygen, Parkville, VIC, Australia

A. R. Rasmussen
Centre for Youth Mental Health, The University of Melbourne, Melbourne, VIC, Australia

Mental Health Center Amager, University of Copenhagen, Copenhagen, Denmark

Faculty of Health and Medical Sciences, Department of Clinical Medicine, University of Copenhagen, Copenhagen, Denmark

S. Cheli, P. H. Lysaker (eds.), *A Dimensional Approach to Schizotypy*,
https://doi.org/10.1007/978-3-031-41788-7_20

schizotypy, possibly indicative of the fact that it has generally been viewed as a stable, trait-like condition. In this chapter, we consider schizotypy from a clinical staging perspective. This is not merely a diagnostic issue but also has treatment implications. We therefore conducted a systematic review of the literature regarding treatment of schizotypal disorder and considered whether different treatment indications may vary by stage of the illness.

The Clinical Phenotype and Trajectories of Schizotypal Disorder

The clinical diagnosis of schizotypal disorder[1] comprises patients with relatively mild schizophrenia-spectrum psychopathology such as an "odd" pattern of cognition and affectivity, mild formal thought disorder, inadequate interpersonal behavior or withdrawal, and/or transient or attenuated psychotic experiences. Before the DSM-III (1980), this phenotype was captured via several overlapping diagnostic categories such as latent schizophrenia, borderline schizophrenia, and pseudoneurotic schizophrenia (Parnas et al., 2005). Rado and Meehl argued for the notion of a schizophrenia spectrum (Meehl, 1962; Rado, 1953) as a continuum from compensated sub-clinical cases to clinical pseudoneurotic schizophrenia (i.e., schizotypal disorder) to schizophrenia proper with manifest psychosis. The schizophrenia-spectrum concept was subsequently empirically validated in numerous family studies (for a review, see Parnas et al., 2005). The spectrum model was considered compatible with a diathesis-stress model emphasizing an interplay between innate (genetic) and environmental influences (Tienari et al., 2002).

The diagnostic criteria are superficially presented in the DSM and ICD, and a proper clinical assessment of these presupposes knowledge of the wider psychopathological literature (see Parnas et al., 2005). Most DSM criteria address expressive features (odd thinking and speech; inappropriate or constricted affect; behavior or appearance that is odd, eccentric, or peculiar; lack of close friends or confidants other than first-degree relatives) and subtle psychotic-like phenomena (ideas of reference; odd beliefs or magical thinking; suspiciousness or paranoid ideation). However, only one criterion (unusual perceptual experiences, including bodily illusions), relates to the rich literature on subjective experiential anomalies in the schizophrenia-spectrum (Blankenburg, 1971; Jansson & Parnas, 2020; McGhie & Chapman, 1961), investigated in recent decades as basic symptoms (Schultze-Lutter, 2009) or disturbances of basic self (Henriksen et al., 2021). Moreover, anhedonia and ambivalence (central to pre-DSM prototypical diagnosis (Bleuler, 1911/1950)) are not mentioned. The same applies to disorganized interpersonal behavior that most clinicians today associate with borderline personality disorder

[1] In this chapter, we use the term "schizotypal disorder" to refer to both the ICD diagnosis of this name as well as the DSM diagnosis of schizotypal personality disorder.

(Zandersen et al., 2018). Finally, the so-called "pseudo-neurotic" symptoms are represented by one criterion in the DSM (excessive social anxiety that does not diminish with familiarity) and another criterion in ICD-10 (obsessive ruminations without inner resistance). The pseudoneurotic symptoms are non-psychotic symptoms (such as obsessive-compulsive, depression, or anxiety symptoms) with specific phenomenology that in foundational twentieth-century psychopathological literature were considered relatively closely associated with the schizophrenia-spectrum in spite of a superficial similarity with symptoms of other disorders (Rasmussen et al., 2022). These symptoms are often classified as comorbidity in current clinical practice.

While recognizing that some patients could present with pre-diagnostic symptoms, most researchers of the pre-DSM era considered the phenotype of schizotypal disorder to be relatively stable, and as such distinct from chronic schizophrenia (Lingiardi & Boldrini, 2019). This was linked with a therapeutically optimistic attitude emphasizing the relevance of a flexible, personalized approach involving long-term supportive psychotherapy combined with psychopharmacological treatment (Hoch et al., 1962; Vanggaard, 1979). Due to duration criteria of a minimum of two years of symptoms (ICD-10) or "an enduring pattern of symptoms that are relatively stable over time" (DSM-5) a certain persistence of the symptomatology is implicit in the diagnosis. More recently, studies have reported 25–35% transition rates of schizotypal disorder to schizophrenia-spectrum psychoses in young patients as well as a high diagnostic stability of non-transitioning patients (Albert et al., 2017; Nordentoft et al., 2006, 2017; Parnas et al., 2011).

Clinical Staging

Longitudinal psychiatric research indicates substantial heterotypic continuity in the evolution of mental disorders (Caspi et al., 2020; Plana-Ripoll et al., 2019). In other words, psychopathology often evolves from one form to another with a variable level of accumulating comorbidity over a person's lifetime. There is also now strong evidence that psychopathology exists on a continuum of severity with different levels of need for care. The transdiagnostic clinical staging approach aims to capture this dynamic natural history and continuous nature of psychopathology and link to pragmatic models successfully developed in other medical fields. While recognizing the dimensional nature of psychopathology, staging also proposes subcategories, the boundaries of which are defined by treatment needs and/or potentially by underlying neurobiological changes. It attempts to define, especially at first diagnosis, the position that an individual is located at a given point in time along a continuum of illness (Fig. 20.1) (McGorry et al., 2006, 2018; McGorry, 2007; McGorry & Hickie, 2019). In this way, clinical staging takes a quasi-dimensional approach to symptomatology, delineating step changes on top of continuous symptomatology to guide treatment decision-making, prediction, and etiological research. The transdiagnostic element of clinical staging is that it delineates illness stages *across* symptom domains and true (non-polythetic) syndromes (psychosis, mood, anxiety, etc.),

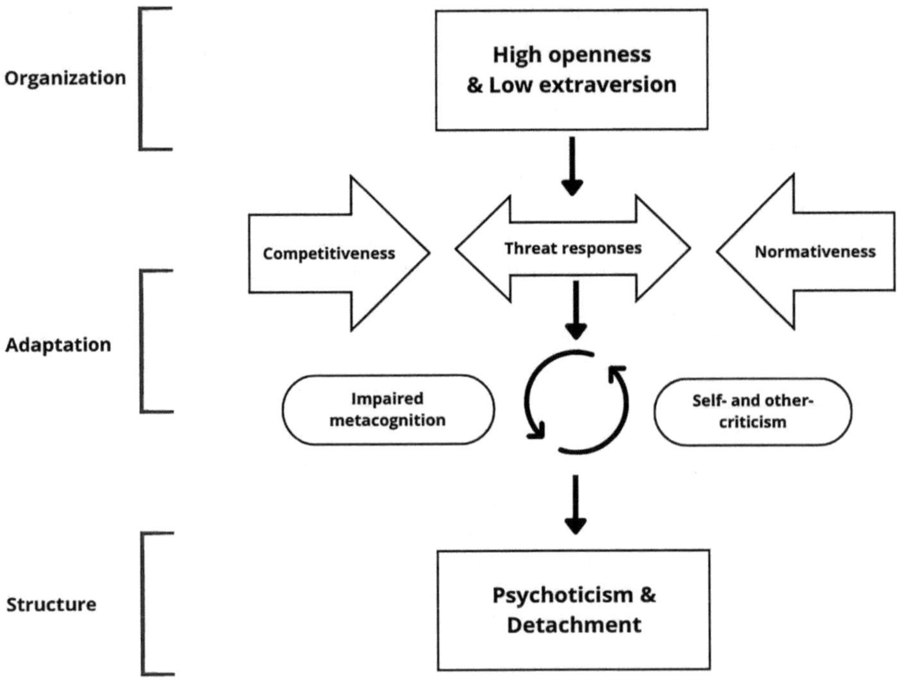

Fig. 20.1 Clinical staging model depicting the emergence of undifferentiated microphenotypes that may progress to macrophenotypes (e.g., psychosis, depression). (Reproduced from McGorry and Mei (2021) with permission)

rather than traditional disorders, which typically capture late-stage phenotypes, such as schizophrenia. This allows for a pluripotential mindset early in the course of disorder where fluid comorbidity is frequently present, as well as expecting the evolution of symptoms over time.

Current transdiagnostic models have proposed dimensional boundaries for progressive stages, signified by changes or increases in the severity of core clinical presentations. Specifically, stage 0 = asymptomatic; stage 1a = non-specific distress, generally anxiety and depressive symptomatology; stage 1b = distress with more complex but still attenuated symptoms; stage 2 = first episode of serious mental disorder; stage 3 = recurrent disorder; stage 4 = chronic/unremitting disorder (McGorry et al., 2010).

Clinical staging has utility in that it mandates early treatment of distress and functional impairment according to risk-benefit principles. This means that treatments used earlier should be established as safer, and also hold the promise of being more effective than late-stage treatments. Later stages justify more risk and potential adverse effects as the "clinical stakes" are higher. The evolution of clinical staging to clinicopathological staging, via the inclusion of pathophysiological biomarkers as in oncology, is a worthy ambition for psychiatry (McGorry & Hickie,

2019). Clinical staging allows changes in biomarkers to be studied and linked to (and potentially redefine) stage as well as syndrome (McGorry et al., 2014).

Schizotypal Disorder in the Clinical Staging Approach

Where does schizotypy fit in this framework? Because the clinical category of schizotypal disorder is closely linked with the concept of the schizophrenia-spectrum, a clinical staging approach addressing schizotypal disorder would address staging in the milder range of the schizophrenia-spectrum. However, we are not aware of any studies to date that have explicitly examined schizotypy according to the clinical staging model. It is possible that the ultra-high risk (UHR) for psychosis paradigm (stage 1b according to the clinical staging model), while immensely successful in promoting research into and clinical service delivery for early-stage psychosis and psychosis risk states, has inadvertently obscured the clinical/research view of schizotypy. That is, the UHR approach may have led to reduced recognition of and focus on schizotypy both in the clinic and in research study design. This may have occurred because, although schizotypal personality disorder is a formal component of the UHR criteria (in the Trait Vulnerability/Genetic Risk and Deterioration group), the UHR paradigm has promoted a particular focus on attenuated positive psychotic symptoms, with >80% of UHR samples consisting of those who meet this UHR sub-group (Fusar-Poli et al., 2020). Given that attenuated positive psychotic symptoms are part of the clinical phenotype of schizotypal disorder (e.g., magical thinking, ideas of reference, perceptual aberrations), individuals who might previously have been identified as suffering from schizotypal disorder may have come to be identified as belonging to the Attenuated Psychosis Symptom UHR sub-group instead. In some cases, insufficient awareness of other aspects of schizotypal disorder (e.g., odd speech, peculiar mannerisms, difficulty responding appropriately to social cues) and insufficient history taking (the longitudinal course of attenuated psychotic symptoms), particularly in clinical settings, may have contributed to this situation.

A related point concerns the increased interest in UHR research on attenuated psychotic symptoms that are still present at follow-up time points – referred to as "persistent" attenuated psychotic symptoms or UHR "non-remitters" – and the various clinical and biological predictors and correlates of this outcome (Beck et al., 2019; Cropley et al., 2016; Polari et al., 2018; Yung et al., 2007). It is of course possible that these persistent or non-remitting cases are in fact schizotypal disorder cases, as they show an enduring presence of attenuated positive psychotic symptoms and possibly a reduced clinical responsiveness to UHR-targeted treatments, perhaps indicating a more trait-like disturbance. This suggestion is worthy of further direct investigation and may indicate that the UHR paradigm is in fact functioning as an early identification approach for schizotypal disorder, as well as for first-episode psychosis.

Another area worthy of further research is that schizotypy may be misdiagnosed as Autism Spectrum Disorder, particularly when schizotypal signs/symptoms develop early in life (Tonge et al., 2020). Bleuler referred to "autistic" features (poor ability to enter into contact with others, withdrawal and inaccessibility, indifference, rigid attitudes and behaviors, unconventional hierarchy of values and goals, inappropriate behavior, idiosyncratic logic, and a propensity to delusional thinking) as a core feature of the schizophrenia-spectrum (Parnas, 2011). This characterization was later refined by Minkowsi (Minkowski, 1927). This phenotype can readily be misrecognized as symptoms of Autism Spectrum Disorder as currently defined in diagnostic manuals.

Schizotypy Symptom Development Across Clinical Stages

Although schizotypal disorder is usually diagnosed in young adulthood, symptoms and signs are often first apparent in childhood. Studies indicate that the condition can in fact be reliably and validly diagnosed in childhood aged 5–12 years (Tonge et al., 2020). Therefore, developing an adequate clinical staging perspective on schizotypal disorder will probably require longitudinal studies that track the developmental course of emerging signs and symptoms from childhood in order to identify clinical characteristics of early (stage 1a, 1b) stages of the disorder, biopsychosocial correlates, and associated risk/resilience factors. Given the low prevalence of schizotypal disorder and the frequent lack of help-seeking behavior, using enriched samples, such as those presenting to specialized childhood mental health services, subcultural groups with unusual beliefs, or family members of those diagnosed with psychotic disorders may be required.

Small longitudinal studies suggest that schizotypal symptoms persist and may develop into schizophrenia or other schizophrenia-spectrum disorders (Asarnow, 2005; Esterberg et al., 2010; Nagy & Szatmari, 1986; Olin et al., 1997; Parnas & Schulsinger, 1986; Robins, 1966; Roff, 1963; Wolff & Chick, 1980; Wolff et al., 1991). Although there is some evidence for the relative stability of schizotypal traits in children (Tonge et al., 2020), the dynamic nature of brain plasticity and psychosocial development in children suggests that longitudinal studies are required to determine whether schizotypal symptoms in childhood may resolve or morph into other phenotypes, consistent with the heterotypic continuity mentioned above. For example, it has been reported that brain structural connectivity abnormalities observed in siblings of those with childhood schizophrenia normalize by mid-adolescence (Zalesky et al., 2015). The study of these presentations in childhood is made possible by child-appropriate dimensional measures such as the Melbourne Assessment of Schizotypy in Kids (MASK) (Jones et al., 2015).

As noted above, the clinical phenotype of schizotypal disorder consists in a persistent, although possibly fluctuating, pattern of relatively mild schizophrenia-spectrum psychopathology. However, it is conceivable that detailed longitudinal research may indicate that *certain features* of schizotypal disorder may show more of a stage-based evolution than other features. The Hierarchical Taxonomy of

Psychopathology (HiTOP) makes a distinction between spectra, subfactors, syndromes, traits, and symptoms (DeYoung et al., 2022). Using this taxonomy, it is possible that certain *traits* remain relatively (although not completely) stable across stage progression and the *symptom* components in the HiTOP model become more severe as an individual progresses through stages. There is some support for this view from longitudinal research into "basic self-disturbance" in schizophrenia-spectrum disorders (see Chap. 1 The phenomenological perspective). The subjective anomalies indicative of basic self-disturbance are frequent in schizotypal disorder and predict transition to schizophrenia in high-risk samples (Henriksen et al., 2021). Moreover, longitudinal data indicate that basic self-disturbance remains reasonably stable from earlier stages in schizophrenia-spectrum disorder evolution (high-risk and first-episode cases) to later stages in these disorders, while the psychotic symptoms wax and wane in an episodic fashion and become more entrenched in more advanced stages (Henriksen et al., 2021; Nordgaard et al., 2018).

Similar patterns may be evident regarding other features of schizotypal disorder, with (for example) eccentricity, lack of social attunement, odd thinking/language being reasonably stable "background" features and attenuated psychotic symptoms showing a stage progression. Another example may be the relative balance of positive and negative schizotypal features across stages. In line with evidence from general population studies that attenuated positive psychotic symptoms ("psychotic-like symptoms") are most prominent in adolescence and young adulthood and decline with age, positive schizotypal features may be more characteristic of early clinical stages of schizotypal disorder and negative schizotypy of more advanced stages. Again, longitudinal studies are necessary to test these speculations.

Treatment of Schizotypal Disorder

Having considered a clinical staging approach to the phenomenology of schizotypal disorder and emphasized the need for further longitudinal research, we now turn to the issue of treatment. In order to determine whether treatment needs differ by stage of schizotypal disorder, we first need to review the existing evidence base for different treatments.

We performed a systematic review in order to take stock of the current state of the art for treating schizotypal disorder. We included studies on patients diagnosed with schizotypal personality disorder according to DSM-IV or DSM-III criteria or schizotypal disorder according to ICD-10 criteria that reported a targeted intervention for the disorder. The review is registered at PROSPERO (ID: CRD42022375001) and the protocol is in review (Gundersen et al., 2023a). Although this separate body of work is currently in preparation for a separate publication (Gundersen et al., 2023b), the preliminary findings are summarized below.

Psychotherapies and Integrated Treatments

A total of five studies were identified as having investigated the effect of psychotherapeutic- and integrated interventions for schizotypal disorder.

Two studies investigated the effect of metacognitively oriented psychotherapy (MOP) (Cheli, 2020; Cheli et al., 2019). A two-case series by Cheli et al. (2019) evaluated the effect of MOP in two different formats: metacognitive interpersonal therapy (MIT) and metacognitive reflection and insight therapy (MERIT). In both formats, patients received weekly individual psychotherapy over 6 months. Cheli (2020) investigated a metacognitively oriented individualized assessment and treatment plan based on multidisciplinary teamwork in a pilot mixed-methods study including 12 patients. Patients received individualized MOP once a week and received one of the following: MERIT or MIT alone, or a tailored sequence of MERIT (first) and MIT (second). The treatment program also included routine psychiatric evaluation and pharmacological treatments if needed, along with group therapy with different mindfulness-based cognitive therapy programs, and if necessary, a behavioral module targeting a single relevant problem (e.g., insomnia, tic management, medication management, etc.). The patients' families received interventions to reduce conflict and promote collaboration. All treatments were optional, and the participants could opt out of some components. Both studies found MOP to improve everyday functioning, to reduce disturbing and odd thoughts as well as reducing confusion about one's own and others' thoughts and feelings (Cheli, 2020; Cheli et al., 2019). Both studies also found MOP to promote recovery, defined as no longer fulfilling criteria for schizotypal disorder.

Abdul Salam et al. (2013) performed a retrospective review investing clinical records of cognitive behavioral therapy (CBT) in 22 patients as well as clinical observations from supervisory discussion and subjective reports from patients and their family members. The study found that 55% of the patients reported an improvement in interpersonal skills and effectiveness, 32% reported improvements in obsessive–compulsive symptoms, and 18% reported improvements in social anxiety (Abdul Salam et al., 2013). Fourteen patients received medication (antipsychotics, antidepressants, anxiolytics, or polypharmacy) during the study.

Two studies investigated the rate of transition to psychosis in patients with schizotypal disorder who received integrated treatment compared to standard treatment (Albert et al., 2017; Nordentoft et al., 2006). The integrated treatment consisted of a combination of family therapy, psychoeducation, social skill training, psychotherapy, and medication. It could also comprise help with housing and vocational functioning. Nordentoft et al. (2006) performed a randomized clinical trial and found that participants who received the integrated treatment had a reduced risk of transitioning to psychosis at the end of the two-year follow-up (RR 0.36 CI (0.16–0.85)) and a reduced level of negative symptoms at one-year follow-up (−0.71 CI (−1.21 – −0.21)), which were, however, lost at the two-year follow-up. Contrary to this finding, a randomized clinical trial by Albert et al. (2017) reported an overall decrease in negative symptoms and increased level of functioning at

3.5 years follow-up in the sample of patients with schizotypal disorder, but there was no significant effect of the prolonged integrated intervention on psychosis development or other clinical outcomes. This difference in findings could be due to the Albert et al. (2017) trial including patients with a longer duration of symptoms (1.5–5 years) than those included in the Nordentoft et al. (2006) study (0–2 years).

Pharmacological Interventions

A total of seven studies investigating pharmacological treatments for schizotypal disorder were identified. Four studies examined the effect of antipsychotic medication on patients with schizotypal disorder (Goldberg et al., 1986; Keshavan et al., 2004; Koenigsberg et al., 2003; Rabella et al., 2016). One study investigated the effect of a nonstimulant usually used for attention deficit hyperactivity disorder or high blood pressure (centrally acting alpha 2A-adrenergic receptor agonists) (McClure et al., 2019) and two studies investigated the effect of different dopamine receptor agonists (McClure et al., 2010; Rosell et al., 2015).

Antipsychotic medications One open-label study with flexible dose design found 26 weeks of low-dose olanzapine (2.5–12.5 mg/day) (average 9.32 + −2.75 mg/day) to significantly improve positive and negative symptoms ($p = 0.001$), depressive symptoms ($p = 0.035$), and overall level of functioning (p = 0.005) (Keshavan et al., 2004). Weight gain (4.9–25.9 KG) was reported in all subjects who completed the 26-week study (8 subjects). Another RCT found 9 weeks of low-dose risperidone (0.25 mg/day – 2 mg/day) to be effective in reducing positive ($p = 0.009$) and negative symptoms ($p = 0.094$) of schizotypal disorder (Koenigsberg et al., 2003). The clinical global impression was improved by 22% in the risperidone group compared to 4% in the placebo group, but this did not reach significance. Side effects were reported in 50% of subjects receiving risperidone and in 55.56% of patients in the placebo group (Koenigsberg et al., 2003). A double-blind randomized cross-over study by Rabella et al. (2016) found treatment with 1 mg risperidone to improve self-monitoring in patients with schizotypal personality disorder reported as increased performance in selective attention (spatial) and executive control (on the Eriksen Flanker task) and increased amplitude in cognitive event-related brain potentials measured via electroencephalogram (EEG). Finally, an RCT by Goldberg et al. (1986) found 12 weeks of low-dose treatment with Thiothexine (mean dose 8.7 mg/day) to have an effect on illusions, ideas of reference, psychoticism, obsessive–compulsive symptoms, and phobic anxiety in a sample of patients with schizotypal disorder (Goldberg et al., 1986).

Dopamine agonist A randomized, double-blind, placebo-controlled clinical trial by McClure et al. (2010) investigated the use of Pergolide, a long-acting dopamine agonist, in treating cognitive deficits in schizotypal disorder. They found increased performance in the domains of visual-spatial working memory, executive functioning, and verbal learning and memory after 4 weeks compared to placebo. The study did, however, raise concerns regarding the possibility for valvular heart disease as a side effect of treatment. Another RCT found a short-term intervention with a D1 receptor agonist to significantly enhance verbal working memory compared to placebo (Cohen's $d = 1.14$) (Rosell et al., 2015).

Nonstimulant Another RCT found a pro-cognitive effect of an intervention comprising the nonstimulant medication Guanfacine as an augment to a cognitive remediation intervention and social skills training (McClure et al., 2019). McClure et al. (2019) reported this combined intervention to result in improved cognition in the domain of reasoning and problem-solving along with improved functional skills when compared to cognitive remediation and social skills training alone.

Treatment Study Findings and Clinical Staging

This literature review indicated that there is a lack of evidence-based guidelines for treating schizotypal disorder due to the paucity of research in this area. Drawing firm conclusions is also complicated by the fact that schizotypal disorder is not often researched as a distinct disorder but is combined with other disorders, such as borderline personality disorder or with high risk for psychosis samples. Nevertheless, there is some evidence in favor of psychotherapies, particularly metacognitive therapy, CBT, and integrated treatments. Metacognitive therapy may reduce global severity of symptoms and improve metacognition, CBT may improve interpersonal skills, obsessive-compulsive and social anxiety symptoms, and integration treatment may reduce the risk of progression to frank psychosis in this patient population. Pharmacological research is also nascent in this group. The current state of evidence indicates that antipsychotic medication may have some effect on improving clinical symptoms and functioning in schizotypal disorder and that other pharmacotherapies may have benefit for neurocognitive functioning. There is indication, however, that there may be significant side effects associated with this treatment approach, particularly with antipsychotics.

From a clinical staging perspective, given the lack of notable side effects, the indication that they may be useful in reducing risk of progression to frank psychosis, and the possible benefit for negative symptoms and functioning, psychotherapies seem appropriate for all stages of schizotypal disorder, but particularly appropriate for early stages of the disorder. Further work needs to be done to identify the most effective psychotherapies, match therapy to individual patients, and refine which therapies might be most useful for which components of the disorder. Identification of psychological treatment mechanisms is also required. Rosell et al. (2014) suggest that antipsychotic medication should be used cautiously and not as a first line of treatment for schizotypal disorder.

Conclusions and Future Directions

It is clear that it is premature to develop an adequate clinical staging model of schizotypal disorder given the lack of empirical studies in this area. As argued above, longitudinal studies with enriched populations, probably with childhood and youth cohorts, are required to map symptom/disorder trajectory and to identify whether there are certain components of schizotypal psychopathology that follow a stage-based framework compared to others.

It is important to be reminded from psychopathological research that schizotypal disorder is characterized by a complex constellation of symptoms that varies between patients. The phenotype can include different attenuated symptoms (positive, negative, and disorganized symptoms), self-disorders and other subjective experiential anomalies, and often also co-morbid mental symptoms. These symptoms should not be approached as atomistic and isolated symptoms that are independent of the broader clinical picture (Parnas et al., 2013). We suspect that this "symptom checking" approach is currently frequently leading to under-recognition and misdiagnosis. The phenotypic complexity has implications for treatment planning. Psychotherapeutic and psychosocial treatment must be flexible and capable of addressing numerous co-occurring or shifting symptoms in a common framework rather than treating specific symptoms or comorbidities as separate siloes. Outcomes studies need to take this broad, and sometimes subtle, range of psychopathology into account, rather than overemphasize single symptom dimensions as outcomes. The range of symptomatology also increases the risk of excessive polypharmacy.

Coupling the suggestion that certain features of the disorder may follow a more stage-based framework than others is the possibility that some features may be more responsive to treatment than others. This should not lead to a therapeutic nihilism but rather to nuanced planning and goals of treatment. Heuristically, it can be argued that psychotherapeutic or psychosocial treatment naturally involves goals and strategies for *reducing* or eliminating symptoms as well as for *coping* with symptoms. In schizotypal disorder, treatment planning can include both perspectives but may often involve helping the patient to cope and function despite the fact that certain symptoms may persist. It must also be taken into account that certain phenomena, regarded as "symptoms" by the clinician, may appear natural and meaningful to the patient, e.g., withdrawal, magical or "odd" ideas, or eccentric behaviors. In addition, certain symptoms and behaviors might play a function of assisting an individual compensate for or cope with other symptoms or disturbances, e.g., certain forms of hyperreflectivity, compulsions (Rasmussen & Parnas, 2022), so-called "positive withdrawal," and rigid social interactions and daily routines (Nilsson et al., 2019). We note that the historical literature on pseudoneurotic schizophrenia emphasizes the clinical importance of long-term, stable therapeutic relationships (Hoch et al., 1962; Vanggaard, 1979). Similar points have been made about the positive impact of the relational aspect of therapy on basic self disturbances (Skodlar & Henriksen, 2019). Given both domains are relevant to the psychopathology of schizotypal disorder, this relational aspect of therapy should be given more direct attention in research studies in this area.

Mining existing data sets offers an immediate path forward. As indicated at the outset, psychosis risk research is paying increasing attention to ultra-high-risk patients who do not transition to psychosis yet who have persistent levels of attenuated psychotic symptoms at follow up ("non-remitters" or "persistent" cases) (Polari et al., 2018), often with high levels of comorbidity and subjective experiential anomalies (Rasmussen et al., 2019). Are these cases in fact early-stage schizotypal disorder whose clinical and biopsychosocial characteristics could be examined in more detail? Similarly, it may be possible to reexamine existing treating studies, including the ultra-high risk for psychosis intervention studies, and identify subgroups with schizotypal disorder in order to examine particular treatment effects for these patients. These analyses can inform the design of future observational and treatment studies needed for this under-recognized and under-researched clinical population, incorporating the considerations presented above.

References

Abdul Salam, K. P., Manjula, M., Sudhir, P. M., & Sharma, M. P. (2013). Cognitive behavior therapy for patients with schizotypal disorder in an Indian setting: A retrospective review of clinical data.

Albert, N., Glenthoj, L. B., Melau, M., Jensen, H., Hjorthoj, C., & Nordentoft, M. (2017). Course of illness in a sample of patients diagnosed with a schizotypal disorder and treated in a specialized early intervention setting. Findings from the 3.5year follow-up of the OPUS II study. *Schizophrenia Research, 182*, 24–30. https://doi.org/10.1016/j.schres.2016.10.013

Asarnow, J. R. (2005). Childhood-onset schizotypal disorder: A follow-up study and comparison with childhood-onset schizophrenia. *Journal of Child and Adolescent Psychopharmacology, 15*(3), 395–402. https://doi.org/10.1089/cap.2005.15.395

Beck, K., Andreou, C., Studerus, E., Heitz, U., Ittig, S., Leanza, L., & Riecher-Rössler, A. (2019). Clinical and functional long-term outcome of patients at clinical high risk (CHR) for psychosis without transition to psychosis: A systematic review. *Schizophrenia Research, 210*, 39–47. https://doi.org/10.1016/j.schres.2018.12.047

Blankenburg, W. (1971). Der Verlust der natürlichen Selbstverständlichkeit. Ein Beitr. Z. Psychopathologie symptomarmer Schizophrenien. Enke.

Bleuler, E. (1911/1950). *Dementia praecox or the group of schizophrenias*. International University Press.

Caspi, A., Houts, R. M., Ambler, A., Danese, A., Elliott, M. L., Hariri, A., Harrington, H., Hogan, S., Poulton, R., Ramrakha, S., Rasmussen, L. J. H., Reuben, A., Richmond-Rakerd, L., Sugden, K., Wertz, J., Williams, B. S., & Moffitt, T. E. (2020). Longitudinal assessment of mental health disorders and comorbidities across 4 decades among participants in the Dunedin birth cohort study [Article]. *JAMA Network Open, 3*(4), e203221. https://doi.org/10.1001/jamanetworkopen.2020.3221

Cheli, S. (2020). Assessment and treatment planning for schizotypal personality disorder: A metacognitively oriented point of view. *Psychiatric Rehabilitation Journal, 43*(4), 335.

Cheli, S., Lysaker, P. H., & Dimaggio, G. (2019). Metacognitively oriented psychotherapy for schizotypal personality disorder: A two-case series. *Personality and Mental Health, 13*(3), 155–167.

Cropley, V. L., Lin, A., Nelson, B., Reniers, R., Yung, A. R., Bartholomeusz, C. F., Klauser, P., Velakoulis, D., McGorry, P., Wood, S. J., & Pantelis, C. (2016). Baseline grey matter volume of non-transitioned "ultra high risk" for psychosis individuals with and without attenuated psychotic symptoms at long-term follow-up. *Schizophrenia Research, 173*(3), 152–158. https://doi.org/10.1016/j.schres.2015.05.014

DeYoung, C. G., Chmielewski, M., Clark, L. A., Condon, D. M., Kotov, R., Krueger, R. F., Lynam, D. R., Markon, K. E., Miller, J. D., Mullins-Sweatt, S. N., Samuel, D. B., Sellbom, M., South, S. C., Thomas, K. M., Watson, D., Watts, A. L., Widiger, T. A., & Wright, A. G. C. (2022). The distinction between symptoms and traits in the Hierarchical Taxonomy of Psychopathology (HiTOP). *Journal of Personality, 90*(1), 20–33. https://doi.org/10.1111/jopy.12593

Esterberg, M. L., Goulding, S. M., & Walker, E. F. (2010). Cluster a personality disorders: Schizotypal, schizoid and paranoid personality disorders in childhood and adolescence. *Journal of Psychopathology and Behavioral Assessment, 32*(4), 515–528. https://doi.org/10.1007/s10862-010-9183-8

Fusar-Poli, P., Salazar de Pablo, G., Correll, C. U., Meyer-Lindenberg, A., Millan, M. J., Borgwardt, S., Galderisi, S., Bechdolf, A., Pfennig, A., Kessing, L. V., van Amelsvoort, T., Nieman, D. H., Domschke, K., Krebs, M. O., Koutsouleris, N., McGuire, P., Do, K. Q., & Arango, C. (2020). Prevention of psychosis: Advances in detection, prognosis, and intervention. *JAMA Psychiatry, 77*(7), 755–765. https://doi.org/10.1001/jamapsychiatry.2019.4779

Goldberg, S. C., Schulz, S. C., Schulz, P. M., Resnick, R. J., Hamer, R. M., & Friedel, R. O. (1986). Borderline and schizotypal personality disorders treated with low-dose thiothixene vs placebo. *Archives of General Psychiatry, 43*(7), 680–686.

Gundersen, K. B., Rasmussen, A. R., Sandström, K. O., Albert, N., Polari, A., Ebdrup, B. H., Nelson, B., & Glenthøj, L. B. (2023a). Treatment of schizotypal disorder: A protocol for a systematic review of the evidence and recommendations for clinical practice. *In preparation.*

Gundersen, K. B., Sandström, K. O., Albert, N., Rasmussen, A. R., Ebdrup, B. H., Polari, A., Nelson, B., & Glenthøj, L. B. (2023b). Treatment of schizotypal disorder: A systematic review of the evidence and recommendations for clinical practice. *In preparation.*

Henriksen, M. G., Raballo, A., & Nordgaard, J. (2021). Self-disorders and psychopathology: A systematic review. *Lancet Psychiatry, 8*(11), 1001–1012. https://doi.org/10.1016/S2215-0366(21)00097-3

Hoch, P. H., Cattell, J. P., Strahl, M. O., & Pennes, H. H. (1962). The course and outcome of pseudoneurotic schizophrenia. *The American Journal of Psychiatry, 119*, 106–115. https://doi.org/10.1176/ajp.119.2.106

Jansson, L., & Parnas, J. (2020). 'The schizophrenic basic mood (self-disorder)' by Hans W Gruhle (1929). *History of Psychiatry, 31*(3), 364–375. https://doi.org/10.1177/0957154X20915147

Jones, H. P., Testa, R. R., Ross, N., Seal, M. L., Pantelis, C., & Tonge, B. (2015). The Melbourne assessment of Schizotypy in kids: A useful measure of childhood schizotypal personality disorder. *BioMed Research International, 2015*, 635732. https://doi.org/10.1155/2015/635732

Keshavan, M., Shad, M., Soloff, P., & Schooler, N. (2004). Efficacy and tolerability of olanzapine in the treatment of schizotypal personality disorder. *Schizophrenia Research, 71*(1), 97–101. https://doi.org/10.1016/j.schres.2003.12.008

Koenigsberg, H. W., Reynolds, D., Goodman, M., New, A. S., Mitropoulou, V., Trestman, R. L., Silverman, J., & Siever, L. J. (2003). Risperidone in the treatment of schizotypal personality disorder. *The Journal of Clinical Psychiatry, 64*(6), 628–634. https://doi.org/10.4088/jcp.v64n0602

Lingiardi, V., & Boldrini, T. (2019). The diagnostic dilemma of psychosis: Reviewing the historical case of pseudoneurotic schizophrenia. *The Journal of Nervous and Mental Disease, 207*(7), 577–584. https://doi.org/10.1097/NMD.0000000000001008

McClure, M. M., Harvey, P. D., Goodman, M., Triebwasser, J., New, A., Koenigsberg, H. W., Sprung, L. J., Flory, J. D., & Siever, L. J. (2010). Pergolide treatment of cognitive deficits associated with schizotypal personality disorder: Continued evidence of the importance of

the dopamine system in the schizophrenia spectrum. *Neuropsychopharmacology, 35*(6), 1356–1362. https://doi.org/10.1038/npp.2010.5
McClure, M. M., Graff, F., Triebwasser, J., Perez-Rodriguez, M., Rosell, D. R., Koenigsberg, H., Hazlett, E. A., Siever, L. J., Harvey, P. D., & New, A. S. (2019). Guanfacine augmentation of a combined intervention of computerized cognitive remediation therapy and social skills training for schizotypal personality disorder. *American Journal of Psychiatry, 176*(4), 307–314.
McGhie, A., & Chapman, J. (1961). Disorders of attention and perception in early schizophrenia. *The British Journal of Medical Psychology, 34*, 103–116. https://doi.org/10.1111/j.2044-8341.1961.tb00936.x
McGorry, P. D. (2007). Issues for DSM-V: Clinical staging: A heuristic pathway to valid nosology and safer, more effective treatment in psychiatry [Editorial]. *The American Journal of Psychiatry, 164*(6), 859–860. https://doi.org/10.1176/ajp.2007.164.6.859
McGorry, P. D., & Hickie, I. B. (Eds.). (2019). *Clinical staging in psychiatry: Making diagnosis work for research and treatment*. Cambridge University Press.
McGorry, P. D., & Mei, C. (2021). Clinical staging for youth mental disorders: Progress in reforming diagnosis and clinical care. *Annual Review of Developmental Psychology, 3*, 15–39. https://doi.org/10.1146/annurev-devpsych-050620-030405
McGorry, P. D., Hickie, I. B., Yung, A. R., Pantelis, C., & Jackson, H. J. (2006). Clinical staging of psychiatric disorders: A heuristic framework for choosing earlier, safer and more effective interventions [Review]. *The Australian and New Zealand Journal of Psychiatry, 40*(8), 616–622. https://doi.org/10.1111/j.1440-1614.2006.01860.x
McGorry, P. D., Nelson, B., Goldstone, S., & Yung, A. R. (2010). Clinical staging: A heuristic and practical strategy for new research and better health and social outcomes for psychotic and related mood disorders. *Canadian Journal of Psychiatry, 55*(8), 486–497. https://doi.org/10.1177/070674371005500803
McGorry, P., Keshavan, M., Goldstone, S., Amminger, P., Allott, K., Berk, M., Lavoie, S., Pantelis, C., Yung, A., Wood, S., & Hickie, I. (2014). Biomarkers and clinical staging in psychiatry. *World Psychiatry, 13*(3), 211–223. https://doi.org/10.1002/wps.20144
McGorry, P. D., Hartmann, J. A., Spooner, R., & Nelson, B. (2018). Beyond the "at risk mental state" concept: Transitioning to transdiagnostic psychiatry. *World Psychiatry, 17*, 133–142.
Meehl, P. E. (1962). Schizotaxia, schizotypy, schizophrenia. *Amrican Psychologist, 17*, 827–838. https://doi.org/10.1037/h0041029
Minkowski, E. (1927). La schizophrénie. Psychopathologie des schizoïdes et des schizophrenes.
Nagy, J., & Szatmari, P. (1986). A chart review of schizotypal personality disorders in children. *Journal of Autism and Developmental Disorders, 16*(3), 351–367. https://doi.org/10.1007/bf01531664
Nilsson, L. S., Urfer Parnas, A., & Nordgaard, J. (2019). Social life in the schizophrenia spectrum: A phenomenological study of five patients. *Psychopathology, 52*(4), 232–239. https://doi.org/10.1159/000501833
Nordentoft, M., Thorup, A., Petersen, L., Ohlenschlaeger, J., Melau, M., Christensen, T. O., Krarup, G., Jorgensen, P., & Jeppesen, P. (2006). Transition rates from schizotypal disorder to psychotic disorder for first-contact patients included in the OPUS trial. A randomized clinical trial of integrated treatment and standard treatment. *Schizophrenia Research, 83*(1), 29–40. https://doi.org/10.1016/j.schres.2006.01.002
Nordgaard, J., Nilsson, L. S., Saebye, D., & Parnas, J. (2017). Self-disorders in schizophrenia-spectrum disorders: A 5-year follow-up study. *European Archives of Psychiatry and Clinical Neuroscience*. https://doi.org/10.1007/s00406-017-0837-3
Nordgaard, J., Nilsson, L. S., Sæbye, D., & Parnas, J. (2018). Self-disorders in schizophrenia-spectrum disorders: A 5-year follow-up study. *European Archives of Psychiatry and Clinical Neuroscience, 268*(7), 713–718. https://doi.org/10.1007/s00406-017-0837-3
Olin, S. S., Raine, A., Cannon, T. D., Parnas, J., Schulsinger, F., & Mednick, S. A. (1997). Childhood behavior precursors of schizotypal personality disorder. *Schizophrenia Bulletin, 23*(1), 93–103. https://doi.org/10.1093/schbul/23.1.93

Parnas, J. (2011). A disappearing heritage: The clinical core of schizophrenia. *Schizophrenia Bulletin, 37*(6), 1121–1130. https://doi.org/10.1093/schbul/sbr081

Parnas, J., & Schulsinger, H. (1986). Continuity of formal thought disorder from childhood to adulthood in a high-risk sample. *Acta Psychiatrica Scandinavica, 74*(3), 246–251. https://doi.org/10.1111/j.1600-0447.1986.tb06240.x

Parnas, J., Licht, D., & Bovet, P. (2005). Cluster A personality disorders: A review. In M. Maj, H. S. Akiskal, J. E. Mezzich, & A. Okasha (Eds.), *Personality disorders, Volume 8*. John Wiley & Sons, Ltd.

Parnas, J., Raballo, A., Handest, P., Jansson, L., Vollmer-Larsen, A., & Saebye, D. (2011). Self-experience in the early phases of schizophrenia: 5-year follow-up of the Copenhagen Prodromal Study. *World Psychiatry, 10*(3), 200–204. https://doi.org/10.1002/j.2051-5545.2011.tb00057.x

Parnas, J., Sass, L. A., & Zahavi, D. (2013). Rediscovering psychopathology: The epistemology and phenomenology of the psychiatric object [Historical Article]. *Schizophrenia Bulletin, 39*(2), 270–277. https://doi.org/10.1093/schbul/sbs153

Plana-Ripoll, O., Pedersen, C. B., Holtz, Y., Benros, M. E., Dalsgaard, S., De Jonge, P., Fan, C. C., Degenhardt, L., Ganna, A., Greve, A. N., Gunn, J., Iburg, K. M., Kessing, L. V., Lee, B. K., Lim, C. C. W., Mors, O., Nordentoft, M., Prior, A., Roest, A. M., Saha, S., Schork, A., Scott, J. G., Scott, K. M., Stedman, T., Sørensen, H. J., Werge, T., Whiteford, H. A., Laursen, T. M., Agerbo, E., Kessler, R. C., Mortensen, P. B., & McGrath, J. J. (2019). Exploring comorbidity within mental disorders among a Danish national population [Article]. *JAMA Psychiatry, 76*(3), 259–270. https://doi.org/10.1001/jamapsychiatry.2018.3658

Polari, A., Lavoie, S., Yuen, H. P., Amminger, P., Berger, G., Chen, E., deHaan, L., Hartmann, J., Markulev, C., Melville, F., Nieman, D., Nordentoft, M., Riecher-Rossler, A., Smesny, S., Stratford, J., Verma, S., Yung, A., McGorry, P., & Nelson, B. (2018). Clinical trajectories in the ultra-high risk for psychosis population. *Schizophrenia Research, 197*, 550–556. https://doi.org/10.1016/j.schres.2018.01.022

Rabella, M., Grasa, E., Corripio, I., Romero, S., Mañanas, M. À., Antonijoan, R. M., Münte, T. F., Pérez, V., & Riba, J. (2016). Neurophysiological evidence of impaired self-monitoring in schizotypal personality disorder and its reversal by dopaminergic antagonism. *NeuroImage: Clinical, 11*, 770–779.

Rado, S. (1953). Dynamics and classification of disordered behavior. *The American Journal of Psychiatry, 110*(6), 406–416. https://doi.org/10.1176/ajp.110.6.406

Rasmussen, A. R., & Parnas, J. (2022). What is obsession? Differentiating obsessive-compulsive disorder and the schizophrenia spectrum. *Schizophrenia Research, 243*, 1–8. https://doi.org/10.1016/j.schres.2022.02.014

Rasmussen, A. R., Reich, D., Lavoie, S., Li, E., Hartmann, J. A., McHugh, M., Whitford, T. J., & Nelson, B. (2019). The relation of basic self-disturbance to self-harm, eating disorder symptomatology and other clinical features: Exploration in an early psychosis sample. *Early Intervention in Psychiatry*. https://doi.org/10.1111/eip.12850

Rasmussen, A. R., Zandersen, M., Nordgaard, J., Sandsten, K. E., & Parnas, J. (2022). Pseudoneurotic symptoms in the schizophrenia spectrum: An empirical study. *Schizophrenia Research, 250*, 164–171. https://doi.org/10.1016/j.schres.2022.11.011

Robins, L. N. (1966). *Deviant children grown up: A sociological and psychiatric study of sociopathic personality*. The Williams & Wilkins Company.

Roff, M. (1963). Childhood social interactions and young adult psychosis. *Journal of Clinical Psychology, 19*, 152–157. https://doi.org/10.1002/1097-4679(196304)19:2<152::aid-jclp2270190203>3.0.co;2-8

Rosell, D. R., Futterman, S. E., McMaster, A., & Siever, L. J. (2014). Schizotypal personality disorder: A current review. *Current Psychiatry Reports, 16*(7), 452. https://doi.org/10.1007/s11920-014-0452-1

Rosell, D. R., Zaluda, L. C., McClure, M. M., Perez-Rodriguez, M. M., Strike, K. S., Barch, D. M., Harvey, P. D., Girgis, R. R., Hazlett, E. A., Mailman, R. B., Abi-Dargham, A., Lieberman, J. A., & Siever, L. J. (2015). Effects of the D1 Dopamine Receptor Agonist

Dihydrexidine (DAR-0100A) on Working Memory in Schizotypal Personality Disorder. *Neuropsychopharmacology, 40*(2), 446–453. https://doi.org/10.1038/npp.2014.192

Schultze-Lutter, F. (2009). Subjective symptoms of schizophrenia in research and the clinic: The basic symptom concept. *Schizophrenia Bulletin, 35*(1), 5–8. https://doi.org/10.1093/schbul/sbn139

Skodlar, B., & Henriksen, M. G. (2019). Toward a phenomenological psychotherapy for schizophrenia. *Psychopathology, 52*(2), 117–125. https://doi.org/10.1159/000500163

Tienari, P., Wynne, L. C., Sorri, A., Lahti, I., Laiksy, K., Moring, J., Naarala, M., Nieminen, P., Wahlberg, K. E., & Miettunen, J. (2002). Genotype-environment interaction in the Finnish adoptive family study. Interplay between genes and environment? In H. Häfner (Ed.), *Risk and protective factors in schizophrenia. Towards a conceptual model of the disease process* (pp. 29–38). Steinkopff.

Tonge, B. J., Testa, R., Díaz-Arteche, C., Brereton, A. V., Stephanou, K., & Pantelis, C. (2020). Schizotypal disorder in children—A neglected diagnosis. *Schizophrenia Bulletin Open, 1*(1). https://doi.org/10.1093/schizbullopen/sgaa048

Vanggaard, T. (1979). *Borderlands of sanity : Neuroses, schizophrenic borderline states, atypical endogenous depression : Clinical pictures, psycho-dynamics*. Munksgaard.

Wolff, S., & Chick, J. (1980). Schizoid personality in childhood: A controlled follow-up study. *Psychological Medicine, 10*(1), 85–100. https://doi.org/10.1017/s0033291700039623

Wolff, S., Townshend, R., McGuire, R. J., & Weeks, D. J. (1991). 'Schizoid' personality in childhood and adult life. II: Adult adjustment and the continuity with schizotypal personality disorder. *The British Journal of Psychiatry, 159*(620–629), 634–625. https://doi.org/10.1192/bjp.159.5.620

Yung, A. R., Yuen, H. P., Berger, G., Francey, S., Hung, T. C., Nelson, B., Phillips, L., & McGorry, P. (2007). Declining transition rate in ultra high risk (prodromal) services: Dilution or reduction of risk? *Schizophrenia Bulletin, 33*(3), 673–681. https://doi.org/10.1093/schbul/sbm015

Zalesky, A., Pantelis, C., Cropley, V., Fornito, A., Cocchi, L., McAdams, H., Clasen, L., Greenstein, D., Rapoport, J. L., & Gogtay, N. (2015). Delayed development of brain connectivity in adolescents with schizophrenia and their unaffected siblings. *JAMA Psychiatry, 72*(9), 900–908. https://doi.org/10.1001/jamapsychiatry.2015.0226

Zandersen, M., Henriksen, M. G., & Parnas, J. (2018). A recurrent question: What is borderline? *Journal of Personality Disorders*, 1–29. https://doi.org/10.1521/pedi_2018_32_348

Chapter 21
Schizotypy and Hikikomori, A Severe Form of Social Withdrawal Syndrome

Kohei Hayakawa and Takahiro A. Kato

Introduction

It is not uncommon for patients with schizophrenia to be forced to live in a physically withdrawn state due to various positive and negative symptoms including social withdrawal. Patients with schizophrenia who have social withdrawal may become withdrawn from their homes and go out less frequently, leading to a decrease in social interactions, including the support they receive from others, which may not only result in lost opportunities for treatment, but also in a worsening of their illness. Although social withdrawal is a typical symptom of schizophrenia, it does not lead to severe agitation like positive symptoms such as hallucinations and delusions. Therefore, it is often overlooked, clinically underestimated, and not considered a primary treatment target because it does not motivate those around the patient to respond immediately to the problem, partly because pharmacotherapy is not well effective. The concept of schizotypy has been proposed as a continuum that includes schizophrenia. Social withdrawal is a symptom that can be problematic in both patients with schizophrenia and individuals with high schizotypy (Miller et al., 2002). Although there is a need to establish effective interventions to prevent individuals with high schizotypy from developing schizophrenia, social withdrawal reduces the chances of receiving interventions, and makes it difficult to continue preventive interventions, even if they are initiated. Therefore, in exploring and establishing effective interventions for individuals with high schizotypy, it is important and urgent to deepen our understanding of social withdrawal and to resolve the problem.

K. Hayakawa · T. A. Kato (✉)
Department of Neuropsychiatry, Graduate School of Medical Sciences, Kyushu University, Fukuoka, Japan
e-mail: kato.takahiro.015@m.kyushu-u.ac.jp

S. Cheli, P. H. Lysaker (eds.), *A Dimensional Approach to Schizotypy*,
https://doi.org/10.1007/978-3-031-41788-7_21

Social withdrawal is social isolation caused by illness, and here, we must be clearly aware of the difference between social isolation and loneliness. Loneliness is a negative emotion caused by social isolation, and social isolation itself does not necessarily lead to loneliness. It is known that there is no strong correlation between social isolation and loneliness (Coyle & Dugan, 2012). People sometimes regain mental peace through social isolation, which can even give them time to recover physically and mentally. Nevertheless, social isolation has many negative aspects. Recently, many people are facing social isolation due to various factors such as changes in family structure, including an increase in lifetime unmarried rates and the shift to nuclear families, diversification of sense of values and interpersonal relationships in response to social changes, and turning points in life, such as divorce and bereavement. Social isolation has become a growing problem worldwide, and it is well remembered that in 2018, the UK created the world's first-ever Minister for Loneliness as "loneliness is one of the greatest public health challenges of our time". During the COVID-19 pandemic that recently struck the world, many people experienced a situation of forced social isolation due to government restrictions on leaving home or voluntary refraining from leaving home and social contact (Kato et al., 2020b). When isolation becomes so prolonged that one begins to feel loneliness, pathological reactions may occur. For example, as physical reactions, social isolation is associated with increased mortality (Steptoe et al., 2013), and loneliness is associated with dysregulation of adrenocortical hormone secretion (Doane & Adam, 2010) and inflammatory cytokine reactivity to mental stress (Hackett et al., 2012). As mental reactions, loneliness is closely related to cognitive function in the elderly (Shankar et al., 2013), and various mental health problems such as anxiety, depression, and substance dependence (Matthews et al., 2019; Cacioppo et al., 2006). In terms of behavior, lonely youth tend to use the Internet more frequently and as an emotional support tool (Morahan-Martin & Schumacher, 2003). Also, loneliness is associated with suicide (Stravynski & Boyer, 2001). A recent meta-analysis even points to a significant interrelationship between loneliness and psychosis (Michalska da Rocha et al., 2018), suggesting the magnitude of the impact of social withdrawal in schizotypy.

To consider social withdrawal in schizophrenia or schizotypy, insight into hikikomori, a severe form of social withdrawal syndrome, may be helpful. It was around the 1990s that hikikomori attracted attention as a social problem. It was initially thought to be a social and cultural phenomenon unique to Japan, but a number of subsequent studies have revealed that hikikomori is in fact a psychosocial problem that is not unique to Japan, but is found all over the world. Hikikomori is not limited to a few countries, but may be an indicator of a pandemic of psychological problems that the global Internet-connected society will have to face in the near future (Kato et al., 2011). Although hikikomori is considered principally non-psychotic, it is actually difficult to distinguish from social withdrawal due to autistic spectrum disorders, schizophrenia, or schizotypy. Also, the Japanese Ministry of Health, Labour and Welfare's 2010 guidelines on hikikomori stated that "schizophrenia is not included in the definition of hikikomori in principle", however, it did not deny the possibility of schizophrenia being included, and the definition of hikikomori was vague without any reference to individuals with high schizotypy. Although hikikomori overlaps with social withdrawal caused by various psychiatric conditions, some common psychopathological mechanisms may exist in the act of withdrawing from society, regardless of the psychiatric diagnosis (Kato et al., 2019). Although the hikikomori concept itself was originally proposed by focusing on the behavioral trait of social withdrawal and avoidance of direct interpersonal relationships or its unique lifestyle, it may be a useful concept for the study of social withdrawal in other psychiatric disorders or mental health conditions.

Here, we focus on hikikomori, which overlaps with schizotypy in its behavior of withdrawal from society, and discuss the similarities between the two conditions for a deeper understanding of each condition and to find the seeds for new future intervention strategies for people in a state of withdrawal from society.

Hikikomori

Introduction

The existence of individuals with hikikomori was already recognized in the 1970s. It was around the 1990s that hikikomori became highlighted as one of unique social problems in Japan. In 2010, the Japanese Ministry of Health, Labour, and Welfare (MHLW) issued a guideline that defined this phenomenon as "a condition in which an individual avoids social engagement (schooling including compulsory education, employment including part-time jobs, and socializing outside the home) as a result of various factors and generally remains in the home for six months or longer in principle (even if he or she goes out without socializing with other people)" (Ministry of Health Labour and Welfare in Japan, 2010). It also states, "In principle, it is a non-psychotic phenomenon that is distinct from a withdrawn state based on positive or negative symptoms of schizophrenia, but it should be noted that it is not uncommon for schizophrenia to be included before a definite diagnosis is made". It was a milestone when it was clearly stated that hikikomori is a different concept from social withdrawal in the conventional psychopathological sense, and at the same time, it was pointed out that some hikikomori patients may have coexisting psychiatric disorders such as schizophrenia. Initially, hikikomori was thought to be a problem unique to Japanese society and culture, but subsequent international epidemiological studies have revealed that it is also found in various regions and ethnic groups outside Japan, including Hong Kong, urban China, India, Korea, Spain, and the United States (Kato et al., 2012; Malagón-Amor et al., 2015; Teo & Kato, 2015; Wong et al., 2015, 2017; Wu et al., 2019).

Epidemiology of Hikikomori

An epidemiological study of Japanese adults in the early 2000s reported a lifetime prevalence of hikikomori was 1.2%, with 54.5% of hikikomori individuals experiencing psychiatric disorders such as mood disorder, anxiety disorder, impulse control disorder, and substance use disorder during their lifetime (Koyama et al., 2010), but that study did not consider possible comorbidity of personality disorder, psychotic disorder, or neurodevelopmental disorder. In the Survey on the Lives of Young People conducted by Japan's Cabinet Office in 2016 (Cabinet Office Director General for Policies on Cohesive Society, 2016) and the Survey on the Living Conditions in 2019 (Cabinet Office Director General for Policies on Cohesive Society, 2019), the number of individuals with hikikomori in the broad sense who fulfill the conditions of "going out only for hobbies", "going to nearby convenience stores", or "leaving their own room but not leaving the house" was estimated to be 541,000 for those aged 15–39 and 613,000 for those aged 40–64, suggesting that there are at least 1.1 million individuals with hikikomori in the broad sense of the term in Japan. However, both surveys had limitations because they extracted hikikomori by asking only a few questions, such as "How long do you usually go out?". Therefore, more rigorous diagnostic criteria and evaluation methods for hikikomori were considered essential to obtain accurate information.

Diagnostic Tool for Hikikomori (Diagnostic Criteria/Assessment Method)

Therefore, we developed diagnostic criteria and an evaluation method for rigorously diagnosing hikikomori based on the results of about 10 years of research, and conducted an international survey. First, we developed an interview to assess for the presence of suspected hikikomori as an international diagnostic tool (Teo et al., 2015a). The tool focuses on four key factors: (1) spending most of the day and nearly every day at home, (2) avoiding social situations (such as attending school or going to a workplace)/social relationships (such as friendships or contact with family members), (3) duration of at least 6 months, and (4) significant distress or impairment due to social isolation. Through the international survey using this diagnostic tool, we found that there are individuals with hikikomori in Korea, the United States, and India (Teo et al., 2015a). Subsequently, we developed a questionnaire to assess hikikomori at an earlier stage in order to detect and prevent hikikomori at an early stage, and conducted a preliminary validation. First, we developed the HQ-25M, a self-report scale of hikikomori consisting of 25 items with three subscales: (1) socialization, (2) isolation, and (3) emotional support. In March 2022, we conducted an online survey of 762 unemployed males living in Japan and found that total HQ-25M scores were significantly positively correlated with duration of hikikomori and intensity of psychological distress. Each of the three factors of the HQ-25M also had a significant positive correlation with the duration of social withdrawal (Kato et al., 2022). In addition to direct assessment of patients using structured interviews and questionnaires, and gathering information from family members, supervisors, and colleagues, we are developing an early hikikomori assessment tool. In addition, we are also focusing on biological factors and practicing multi-axial assessment of hikikomori using blood biomarkers that are expected to be useful in the future. In the course of this work, we have found that there are cases in which it is difficult to appropriately assess the reality of social engagement and social interaction using the existing definition of hikikomori (e.g., "I don't go out because I have nothing to do" or "I have friends and talk every day in online games"). Therefore, we further revised the above interview to assess for the presence of suspected hikikomori and developed the following new diagnostic criteria for hikikomori in 2020 (Kato et al., 2020a).

[New Diagnostic Criteria for Hikikomori]

Hikikomori is a form of pathological social withdrawal or social isolation whose essential feature is physical isolation in one's home. The person must meet the following criteria:

(a) Marked social isolation in one's home
(b) Duration of continuous social isolation of at least 6 months
(c) Significant functional impairment or distress associated with the social isolation

Severity is defined as follows.

Mild. Occasionally leave their home (2–3 days/week)
Moderate. Rarely leave their home (1 day/week or less)
Severe. Rarely leave a single room

An exclusion criterion is defined as follows.

Exclusion criteria. Individuals who leave their home frequently (4 or more days/week)

Pre-hikikomori is defined as follows.

Pre-hikikomori. Individuals with a duration of at least 3 (but not 6) months of social isolation

Although the age of onset of hikikomori is usually in adolescence or early adulthood, later onset is not uncommon, and housewives and the elderly who meet the above criteria can also be diagnosed. The new hikikomori diagnostic criteria include four important points: first, it clarifies how frequently a person must go out to meet the criteria for hikikomori's definition of "marked social isolation in one's home"; second, it clarifies how often a person must go out to meet the criteria for hikikomori's definition of "marked social isolation in one's home"; third, it clarifies how much time is needed for the person to be able to participate in social activities.

Second, the requirement of "avoiding social situations/social relationships" was removed. When hikikomori are interviewed, they often deny avoiding social interactions, even though they affirm that they have few social relationships and little social interaction. This lack of social avoidance is one of the primary differentiating features of social anxiety disorder. Third, he pointed out that significant functional impairment or distress associated with social isolation must be carefully assessed. In-depth clinical interviews with hikikomori, especially in the early stages, have revealed that many feel satisfied with their social withdrawal and are often filled with a sense of relief at being free of their painful external life. It has been found that many people are satisfied with their social withdrawal and are filled with a sense of relief at being free from their suffering external life. However, as the duration of hikikomori increases, most individuals with hikikomori begin to complain of distress, such as loneliness. Fourth, we did not include the presence of other psychiatric disorders in the exclusion criteria for hikikomori. It is clear that hikikomori tends to co-occur with other psychiatric disorders. We hypothesize that hikikomori may coexist with various psychiatric disorders as "a contributor to psychopathology" in the same way that catatonic and melancholic features are designated as specifiers of depression in The Diagnostic and Statistical Manual of Mental Disorders, Fifth Edition (the DSM-5).

Comorbidity of Hikikomori

We also investigated the comorbidity of hikikomori with psychiatric disorders in both Japan and the United States (Teo et al., 2015b). Twenty-two patients diagnosed with hikikomori by an interview to assess for the presence of suspected hikikomori were examined for comorbid psychiatric disorders other than schizophrenia and developmental disorders. Results showed that 5 of the 22 (23%) had primary hikikomori with no comorbid psychiatric disorders, all of whom were Japanese. Sixty-eight percent of the participants met multiple psychiatric diagnostic criteria, of which 59% had three or more diagnoses and 9% had two diagnoses. The most common comorbidity was avoidant personality disorder (41%), followed by major depressive disorder (32%), paranoid personality disorder (32%), post-traumatic stress disorder (27%), and social anxiety disorder (27%). Although the frequency of each comorbidity was not high, obsessive-compulsive personality disorder was found in 18%, schizoid and dependent personality disorder were found in 9%, narcissistic personality disorder, schizotypal personality disorder, borderline personality disorder, and antisocial personality disorder were found in 5% of individuals with hikikomori. These results, in which personality disorder comorbidity was prominent, suggest the possibility that personality pathology may exist in the background of the occurrence of hikikomori. We did not evaluate schizophrenia comorbidity in our report, but Kondo et al. reported that 33.3% of people with hikikomori had been diagnosed with either schizophrenia, mood disorder, or anxiety disorder (Kondo et al., 2013). Hikikomori has also been suggested to be an important risk factor for behavioral problems such as suicide, obsessive-compulsive behaviors, and addictive behaviors (Yong & Nomura, 2019). The causal relationship between Hikikomori and psychiatric disorders currently has no definitive answer. However, social withdrawal is often observed in patients with psychosis such as schizophrenia, depression, social anxiety disorder, and autism spectrum disorder, and may be a contributing factor to hikikomori. For example, in social anxiety disorder, symptoms such as "marked fear or anxiety about social situations," "fear of embarrassment or rejection," and "avoidance of anxiety-producing social situations" may lead to hikikomori. Symptoms of depression can lead to difficulty going out for long periods of time due to "inability to enjoy or be interested in activities that used to be enjoyable", and "inability to sleep or sleeping too much", which can lead to a life in which day and night are reversed, making it difficult to go to work or school, which can lead to hikikomori. The "modern type depression" (Kato et al., 2011, 2016; Kato & Kanba, 2017, 2018) that has emerged in recent years mainly among young people has also been shown to be characterized by avoidant and narcissistic personality traits. It is possible that prolonged social avoidance due to maladjustment, anxiety, and fear of school and work may lead to hikikomori. Of course, even if not diagnosed as psychosis, the latent or prodromal state of schizophrenia may also overlap with hikikomori, suggesting that some common psychopathological mechanism may exist in the behavior of withdrawal.

A "Bio-psycho-socio-cultural Model" to Understand the Whole Picture of Hikikomori Pathology from Multiple Perspectives

We have proposed a bio-psycho-socio-cultural model of hikikomori (Kato et al., 2019). This model is designed to provide a multifaceted understanding of hikikomori's pathophysiology. The pathophysiology of hikikomori is still largely unknown. In order to further deepen the psychiatric understanding of hikikomori, we believe that it is necessary to elucidate its pathophysiology, focusing not only on its psychiatric aspects but also on its psychological aspects, including loneliness and distrust, social and cultural aspects, such as information technology and social globalization, and biological aspects, including inflammation, immunity, and oxidative stress.

The Japanese social and cultural context in which hikikomori has become known includes the traditional concepts of "Amae (culture-based dependence)" and "Haji (shame)", which may be the cultural background of not only hikikomori but also the disease called "taijin kyofusho". "Amae" describes the characteristics of the Japanese parent–child relationship. The Japanese parent–child relationship is characterized by an extremely long and close bond between the child and mother in the absence of the father, which has been considered to facilitate acceptance of hikikomori within the family, enabling the child to withdraw into the home for prolonged periods and making it difficult for the child to become independent (Kato et al., 2018). In addition, a systematic review of hikikomori suggests that family dysfunction for various reasons, the way parents communicate and teach their children, the problem of parents who overprotect and parasitize their children, an educational system that tends to exclude dropouts, the loss of a sense of direction and the failure to find a place in society, are important social and cultural factors in the development of hikikomori (Li & Wong, 2015). The shift from direct to indirect communication and the physical isolation of individuals from each other as a result of the shift to IT in society, and in particular the fact that social interactions that previously required face-to-face contact in real physical space can now occur, at least in part, in virtual worlds (Kato et al., 2018), may also be behind the situation where hikikomori is becoming a global problem that transcends the framework of cultural spheres. From a developmental perspective, the culture of "Amae" from childhood, overprotection by parents, a close relationship between mother and child, changes in the schooling environment during the school years, the harsh working environment during adolescence and young adulthood, and reduced opportunities for direct communication due to the spread of the Internet, all contribute to stress reactivity, including reduced resilience and easy traumatization. In particular, basic interpersonal skills in the early stages of life may be inadequately developed in individuals with hikikomori, leading to stress vulnerability in the school/work environment. It is then assumed that stress-induced depressive reactions, anxiety, fear, and shame are more likely to occur, leading to avoidance of social situations, which may result in the hikikomori condition (Kato et al., 2018). Of course, to deeply understand hikikomori, not only these psychological and social aspects, but also biological perspectives such as neurotransmitters, inflammation/immunity, and oxidative stress are indispensable. Therefore, in clinical settings, it is necessary to conduct a multi-axial assessment based on the bio-psycho-social-cultural model.

Biological Basis of the Pathology of Hikikomori

In previous studies, only psychological, social, and cultural aspects of hikikomori have been focused on, while the biological aspects have been completely neglected. Recently, there has been a large amount of research on the biological aspects of psychiatric disorders, and the biological basis of their pathophysiology is gradually being clarified. Not only psychiatric disorders, but also personalities and behaviors that at first glance appear to be mostly caused by psychological and social factors are now known to have a biological background. For example, suicide is usually thought to be a behavior with psychological and socio-cultural factors, caused by psychological distress or physical distress such as severe pain, but biological factors have been suggested to be involved in suicide as well (Suzuki et al., 2019). According to a postmortem study of suicide victims, microglial activation (Steiner et al., 2008), increased glial cell density (Hercher et al., 2009), and increased mRNA expression of cytokines such as interleukin (IL)-4 and IL-13 have been observed in the brains of suicide victims (Tonelli et al., 2008). Suicide is not uncommon among individuals with hikikomori, and we are examining the possibility that hikikomori, like suicide, may have a biological pathological basis (Kato et al., 2019). Actually, we conducted a study to explore the biological basis of the pathophysiology of hikikomori. Individuals diagnosed with hikikomori using a structured interview designed for the study ($n = 55$) and healthy controls ($n = 78$) were evaluated for personality traits by psychological examinations, and underwent blood biochemical tests for biomarker exploration. Results showed that hikikomori individuals had higher avoidant personality traits in both males and females. Hikikomori males had lower blood UA levels than healthy males, and hikikomori females had lower blood HDL-C levels than healthy females (Hayakawa et al., 2018). In addition, the drug-naive hikikomori group ($n = 42$) and healthy controls ($n = 41$) were evaluated for hikikomori and depression severity by psychological examinations, and underwent blood biochemical tests and plasma metabolome analysis. Results showed that blood levels of long-chain acylcarnitines were significantly higher in individuals with hikikomori. In hikikomori males, blood bilirubin and arginine levels were low, and ornithine and serum arginase levels were high (Setoyama et al., 2021). The results of these two studies suggest that hikikomori may have some biological basis for the pathophysiology. We propose to classify hikikomori biotypes by measuring biomarkers during the early stages of hikikomori support. Based on the results of the above studies, we suggest that biological approaches, such as nutritional therapy, may be effective for those with hikikomori who are presumed to be significantly affected by biological factors.

The Latest Treatment and Intervention for Hikikomori

Currently, it is completely unclear what biological approaches are effective in therapeutic intervention for hikikomori and we are in the process of exploring therapeutic approaches from various directions. In order to establish effective treatment and intervention methods for hikikomori, we have launched the "Hikikomori Clinical Research Unit" within the University Hospital and are working to develop evidence-based support programs in collaboration with hikikomori support centers in the public and private sectors. As a first step, we are attempting to establish an evidence-based educational program for families of hikikomori persons. In the case of hikikomori, only parents often come for the first visit. However, family members are not only unable to deal directly with a hikikomori individual in many cases due to prejudice and lack of knowledge about hikikomori, but also tend to turn a blind eye for many years without seeking help from others, so we believe that parental education is essential for early detection of hikikomori. Therefore, we have first developed an educational program for families of hikikomori people, based on Mental Health First Aid (MHFA) and Community Reinforcement and Family Training (CRAFT), incorporating role-play and homework. This is a 5-day family program with a total of 5 weekly sessions (2 hours per session). A 6-month follow-up was conducted after the program and its effectiveness was evaluated using various self-assessment questionnaires. The results showed improvements in cognitive skills for hikikomori cases of depression, stigma held by participants, and some of the behaviors of participants with hikikomori, as well as increased social engagement, etc. Thus, positive behavioral changes in hikikomori patients were reported (Kubo et al., 2020). The program was subsequently shortened from five days to three days and modified as a three-day family program (one session every other week, 180 minutes per session). As a result, participants' own mental health improved at the 4-month follow-up, while their confidence in hikikomori support decreased and their stigma toward mental health issues remained unchanged. However, in the short term, preliminary validity was confirmed, with improved skills in approaching individuals with hikikomori, and actual behavioral changes observed, such as social engagement and use of support by participants with hikikomori (Kubo et al., 2021b).

For individuals with hikikomori, we are also attempting a therapeutic intervention using group psychotherapy in our university hospital. Although we have not yet accumulated a sufficient number of cases, a hikikomori male with schizoaffective disorder who participated in group psychotherapy showed steady improvement in his hikikomori tendency, with a decrease in HQ-25 from 28 at the beginning of treatment to 12 and a recovery to a level where he can go out almost every day (including 5 workdays a week) (Kubo et al., 2021a). We have also observed steady improvement of other hikikomori sufferers in hikikomori tendencies.

In addition, the possibility of therapeutic intervention using robots is being explored to solve the problem that individuals with hikikomori themselves often do not come to the doctor's office, but their parents come as proxies. For example, in a case where a tele-operated robot called OriHime was used, it enabled a patient with ASD who presented with hikikomori to come to the office at his own pace without the threat of being "watched by the doctor", thereby reducing his fear of strangers and his alertness. It has also been reported that by shaking OriHime's head, the patient became able to politely say "no" to the doctor and learned that communicating "no" to others is an important skill for his own well-being, and gradually expanded his range of activities and became able to attend school (Kumazaki et al., 2021). As described above, evidence-based effective treatments and interventions for individuals with hikikomori are still being explored, but the budding of effective approaches from many directions is gradually beginning to emerge.

Schizotypy and Hikikomori

The details of the concept of schizotypy are described in another section of this book (*Part 1. Schizotypy as a Feature of Personality and Psychopathology*). The main focus of this section is to compare schizotypy and hikikomori and to discuss the differences between the two concepts.

Similarities Between Schizotypy and Hikikomori in Psychological and Social Aspects

Similarities between schizotypy and hikikomori can be noted in several aspects. Then, what are the similarities between them in terms of psychological and social aspects? There are conflicting reports on how individuals with high schizotypy are affected by socially isolated situations. One is that individuals with high schizotypy are less affected by social isolation. This is because high schizotypy correlates with decreased perceptions of social support (Blanchard et al., 2011), and schizotypy acts as a buffer to alleviate stress-related negative emotions (Blanchard et al., 2011), individuals with high schizotypy are less susceptible to social isolation (Leigh-Hunt et al., 2017; Wang et al., 2018). During the period of time following the COVID-19 pandemic in 2020, people were more prone to forced/voluntary social isolation. It has been reported that in such a particular situation, negative schizotypy acted as a buffer to reduce the effects of social dysfunction caused by the social isolation (Masucci et al., 2022). In other words, individuals with high negative schizotypy demonstrated a tolerance to the stresses of specific and extreme situations of isolation, such as the COVID-19 pandemic. It has been noted in some patients with schizophrenia that pathological traits can serve as a buffer against the negative emotions that arise in stressful situations (Cohen et al., 2003). Hikikomori is also a trait that can exhibit an affinity for socially isolated situations. This is especially true in the early stages of hikikomori, when many hikikomori often feel content and filled with a sense of relief at being socially withdrawn. Of course, even for hikikomori, prolonged social isolation can gradually increase feelings of loneliness and become an important risk factor for psychiatric disorders such as anxiety, depression, and addiction. However, it is also true that, even within the limited period of time of the beginning of hikikomori, there is an aspect of protecting oneself by withdrawing (i.e., retreating) from society for individuals with hikikomori (Kato et al., 2020b). As indicated by these findings, affinity for social isolation situations is one of the similarities between schizotypy and hikikomori. However, there are conflicting opinions about the characteristics that pathological traits exhibit in a socially isolated situation. The positive schizotypy trait "suspiciousness" and the negative schizotypy trait "no close friends" are both positively correlated with loneliness (Chau et al., 2022), suggesting that individuals with high schizotypy do in fact feel a strong sense of loneliness. On the other hand, both positive and negative schizotypy are associated with a desire for solitude when in the company of others. This is because individuals with high positive schizotypy have high social anxiety, which is reduced by social isolation, and individuals with high negative schizotypy are less likely to experience positive emotions in interpersonal interactions (Kwapil et al., 2012). This dilemma that individuals with high schizotypy often face in desiring a socially isolated life but at the same time being prone to loneliness is incompatible with the affinity of schizotypy for social isolation. Such a dilemma is also observed in hikikomori. We assessed 103 individuals with hikikomori and 221 healthy controls for social isolation using psychological tests. The results revealed that individuals with hikikomori tend to prefer isolation (i.e., higher Preference for Solitude Scale) and also feel more lonely (i.e., higher on the Revised UCLA Loneliness Scale) than healthy controls (Katsuki et al., 2020). Thus, individuals with hikikomori have the dilemma of being easily socially isolated and at the same time feeling loneliness, which is a psychological response to social isolation common to schizotypy.

Similarities in Personalities in the Background of Schizotypy and Hikikomori

We can point out the similarities found between schizotypy and hikikomori, not only in psychological and social aspects, but also in the personality traits underlying them. Various personality pathologies can be assumed to underlie schizotypy. Previous studies have reported that both positive and negative schizotypy may be associated with schizotypal and avoidant personality traits. Individuals with high positive schizotypy had low self-esteem, high social anxiety, and fear of social rejection. They were also more likely to avoid social interactions with others. In contrast, individuals with high negative schizotypy showed a tendency to avoid others due to decreased positive emotions in interpersonal relationships, such as a desire to interact with others and pleasure from interacting with others. This negative schizotypy is a characteristic of the schizoid personality. Indeed, the association between negative schizotypy and schizoid personality traits has been shown repeatedly in the past (Barrantes-Vidal et al., 2013; Kwapil et al., 2008, 2013, 2022). This is consistent with the prevalence of avoidant personality disorder and schizoid personality disorder in the premorbid personality of schizophrenia (Rodríguez Solano & González De Chávez, 2000), suggesting the existence of a continuum lying between schizotypy and schizophrenia in terms of personality pathology. Meanwhile, individuals with hikikomori are characterized by high feelings of resentment, irritability, aggression (Frankova, 2019), frequent indirect expressions of emotions, and a tendency to expect others to guess their feelings and thoughts (Katsuki et al., 2019). In some hikikomori individuals with strong autistic tendencies, this is accompanied by low self-esteem and a high tendency to complain (Katsuki et al., 2020). Behind these traits are personality traits with diverse characteristics such as avoidant, depressive, narcissistic, paranoid, passive-aggressive, schizoid, and schizotypal, which may lead individuals with hikikomori to primitive dependency and attachment to significant others, making it difficult for them to be mentally independent (Katsuki et al., 2019). It is possible to point out that individuals with hikikomori have a variety of personality traits, including characteristics of avoidant and schizoid personalities, which have certain similarities with schizotypy.

Biomarkers of Avoidant and Schizoid Personalities in the Background of Schizotypy and Hikikomori

Here, we would like to present our findings on the biological basis of the common personality pathology between schizotypy and hikikomori, the avoidant and schizoid personality traits, both of which tend to be socially isolated.

Biomarkers of Avoidant Personality Traits

We previously conducted an international survey in Japan and the United States and suggested that the most common comorbidity in hikikomori may be avoidant personality disorder (Teo et al., 2015b). Based on the findings, we hypothesized that avoidant personality traits are associated with hikikomori. Then, to investigate what biological factors are associated with hikikomori, we conducted two preliminary studies using this hypothesis in young healthy volunteers. First, the SCID-II personality questionnaire was used to investigate avoidant personality traits in healthy male participants. Next, a computer-based trust game was administered to assess behavioral characteristics in interpersonal relationships. Actual social relationships in the real world are considered to be influenced by people's unconscious behaviors and feelings, and there is a gap between actual social relationships and self-assessments of sociability. Therefore, it is difficult to assess actual social relationships by self-administered questionnaires or interviews alone. Economic games, developed in the fields of social psychology and economics, are useful for assessing actual behaviors and personalities in the real world (Watabe et al., 2015), and it is hoped that economic games may be a revolutionary method for assessing interpersonal problems that patients with psychiatric disorders face in the real world (King-Casas et al., 2008). One of such economic games is the trust game, which has been used to evaluate trust in others. We developed our own computer-based trust game between two players (Watabe et al., 2013, 2015). In this two-player game, each player initially receives an explanation of the game rules and is given 1300 yen (JPY). The first player then decides how much of the 1300 JPY to give to the second player (partner) and rates the partner's attractiveness and trustworthiness based on their photographs presented on a computer screen (both of the score ranges: 0–9). The amount of money given to the partner by the first player (i.e., Monetary Scores) is tripled. The second player then decides whether to split the money equally with the first player or take away the entire amount of money. In this PC experiment, all the participants were actually assigned to be the first player, and the second players were virtual players on a computer screen. The participants had no information about their partners except for the facial photographs including the head and shoulders with a neutral facial expression. We randomly selected 40 pictures for the trust game. The first player was not aware of the partner's decision. The first player's decision as to how much money to give to the second player is thought to reflect their level of trust in the second player. After the experiments, each participant was actually paid the amount of money corresponding to the result of a randomly selected game from all games as a reward. After the trust game was administered, non-fasting venous blood was collected and various biomarkers were measured. The items measured are those that have attracted attention in the research field of various psychiatric disorders such as schizophrenia, and all of them can be easily measured in a normal clinical setting (high-density lipoprotein cholesterol (HDL-C), serum low-density lipoprotein cholesterol (LDL-C), serum total bilirubin, serum uric acid (UA), serum high-sensitivity C-reactive protein (hsCRP), and plasma fibrin degeneration products (FDP)). In determining the measurement items, we referred to the items used in the Midlife in Japan (MIDJA), a health survey of middle-aged and older adults in Japan. All analyses of the obtained data were performed separately by sex. Various models were created and evaluated using structural equation modeling (SEM) to create models of the assumed causal relationships between avoidant personality traits, psychological traits, behavioral traits, and blood biomarkers. The results showed that in the optimal model by gender using SEM, the higher the avoidant personality trait, the greater the loneliness and the lower the social support network in both sexes. In addition, in males, lower serum HDL-C and serum UA levels were associated with higher avoidant personality traits and lower cooperativeness. In females, higher plasma FDP and serum hsCRP levels were associated with higher avoidant personality traits and a tendency toward interpersonal distrust. The blood biomarker candidates found in this study were all markers related to oxidative stress and inflammation. Oxidative stress is known to decrease serotonin in the brain (Arora & Chopra, 2013). Considering the association between dysregulation of the serotonergic nervous system and avoidant personality disorder (Blom et al., 2011), we speculated that a decrease in antioxidants such as uric acid and HDL-C could cause social anxiety and avoidant behavior in males via oxidative stress. In addition, previous studies have shown that males with high uric acid tend to have a hyperthymic temperament (Lorenzi et al., 2010), and the financial generosity found in males with high serum uric acid levels in the present study may be associated with hyperthymic and altruistic traits. Both hsCRP and FDP, which were associated with trust and avoidance of the partner in females, are biomarkers of inflammation that are widely used in clinical practice. Given that inflammation has been noted to be associated with various psychiatric disorders, including depression, it is possible that women judge whether a person is trustworthy under the direct influence of inflammation or indirectly through aversive personality traits, suggesting an impact of inflammation on the social decision-making system.

Biomarkers of Schizoid Personality Traits

This study suggested that in young healthy females, lower serum LDL-C levels were associated with higher levels of loneliness, social phobia, isolated lifestyle with little social support, and less trust in others. Considering that the personality closely linked to loneliness and social isolation is schizoid personality trait, we hypothesized that LDL-C is associated with schizoid personality trait. Based on this hypothesis, we examined the association between serum LDL-C levels and schizoid personality traits using data from the MIDJA database and data obtained from young healthy volunteers we independently recruited. We also examined the relationship between serum LDL-C levels and social decision-making in patients with schizophrenia by administering the aforementioned trust game to them. The results showed that blood LDL-C level was a predictor of schizoid personality traits in females, and there was a negative correlation between them. In female patients with schizophrenia, a tendency to distrust females was observed when blood LDL-C level was low (Hayakawa et al., 2022).

In summary, the findings regarding biomarkers of avoidant and schizoid personality traits suggested that drugs targeting the regulation of oxidative stress and inflammation may lead to future treatments for hikikomori which may also be applicable to the treatment of social withdrawal in schizotypy. Furthermore, our study results consistently showed sex differences, suggesting that cultural and social factors may have influenced the results. Therefore, the usefulness of varying the therapeutic approach according to gender in the clinical practice of hikikomori or social withdrawal in schizotypy may be a consideration. The findings of our study are just based on preliminary research, and it is important to continue to clarify the biological basis of social withdrawal or hikikomori from the aspects of oxidative stress and inflammation, and to develop effective preventive and therapeutic strategies from the biological aspects.

Conclusion

Here, we discussed the similarities between hikikomori and social withdrawal often observed in schizotypy. Both schizotypy and hikikomori are associated with a tendency to stay inside home, which does not easily lead to medical examinations or treatment opportunities. In addition, from actual clinical experience with hikikomori, it seems that there is a great deal of prejudice and shame toward hikikomori and comorbid psychiatric disorders, and in many cases, such problems have deprived people of opportunities to visit a doctor and receive treatment. It is an important issue how to connect individuals with schizotypy or hikikomori who present with social withdrawal to opportunities for medical consultation and treatment, and to overcome this issue, it will be useful to deepen our understanding of the pathophysiology of social withdrawal, focusing on the similarities between schizotypy and hikikomori. Then, it is expected to establish treatment strategies for social withdrawal/hikikomori, including non-pharmacological therapies such as psychotherapy, psychological and social support, and treatment approaches grounded in the elucidation of the biological basis of the pathophysiology.

References

Arora, V., & Chopra, K. (2013). Possible involvement of oxido-nitrosative stress induced neuro-inflammatory cascade and monoaminergic pathway: Underpinning the correlation between nociceptive and depressive behaviour in a rodent model. *Journal of Affective Disorders, 151*(3), 1041–1052. https://doi.org/10.1016/j.jad.2013.08.032

Barrantes-Vidal, N., Gross, G. M., Sheinbaum, T., Mitjavila, M., Ballespí, S., & Kwapil, T. R. (2013). Positive and negative schizotypy are associated with prodromal and schizophrenia-spectrum symptoms. *Schizophrenia Research, 145*(1–3), 50–55. https://doi.org/10.1016/j.schres.2013.01.007

Blanchard, J. J., Collins, L. M., Aghevli, M., Leung, W. W., & Cohen, A. S. (2011). Social anhedonia and schizotypy in a community sample: The Maryland longitudinal study of schizotypy. *Schizophrenia Bulletin, 37*(3), 587–602. https://doi.org/10.1093/schbul/sbp107

Blom, R. M., Samuels, J. F., Riddle, M. A., Joseph Bienvenu, O., Grados, M. A., Reti, I. M., Eaton, W. W., Liang, K.-Y., & Nestadt, G. (2011). Association between a serotonin transporter promoter polymorphism (5HTTLPR) and personality disorder traits in a community sample. *Journal of Psychiatric Research, 45*(9), 1153–1159. https://doi.org/10.1016/j.jpsychires.2011.03.003

Cabinet Office Director General for Policies on Cohesive Society. (2016). *Report of the Survey on the Lives of Young People*. https://www8.cao.go.jp/youth/kenkyu/hikikomori/h27/pdf-index.html

Cabinet Office Director General for Policies on Cohesive Society. (2019). *Report of the Survey on the Living Conditions*. https://www8.cao.go.jp/youth/kenkyu/life/h30/pdf-index.html

Cacioppo, J. T., Hughes, M. E., Waite, L. J., Hawkley, L. C., & Thisted, R. A. (2006). Loneliness as a specific risk factor for depressive symptoms: Cross-sectional and longitudinal analyses. *Psychology and Aging, 21*(1), 140–151. https://doi.org/10.1037/0882-7974.21.1.140

Chau, A. K. C., So, S. H., Sun, X., Zhu, C., Chiu, C.-D., Chan, R. C. K., & Leung, P. W.-L. (2022). A network analysis on the relationship between loneliness and schizotypy. *Journal of Affective Disorders, 311*, 148–156. https://doi.org/10.1016/j.jad.2022.05.057

Cohen, A. S., Docherty, N. M., Nienow, T., & Dinzeo, T. (2003). Self-reported stress and the deficit syndrome of schizophrenia. *Psychiatry, 66*(4), 308–316. https://doi.org/10.1521/psyc.66.4.308.25440

Coyle, C. E., & Dugan, E. (2012). Social isolation, loneliness and health among older adults. *Journal of Aging and Health, 24*(8), 1346–1363. https://doi.org/10.1177/0898264312460275

Doane, L. D., & Adam, E. K. (2010). Loneliness and cortisol: Momentary, day-to-day, and trait associations. *Psychoneuroendocrinology, 35*(3), 430–441. https://doi.org/10.1016/j.psyneuen.2009.08.005

Frankova, I. (2019). Similar but different: Psychological and psychopathological features of primary and secondary hikikomori. *Frontiers in Psychiatry, 10*, 558. https://doi.org/10.3389/fpsyt.2019.00558

Hackett, R. A., Hamer, M., Endrighi, R., Brydon, L., & Steptoe, A. (2012). Loneliness and stress-related inflammatory and neuroendocrine responses in older men and women. *Psychoneuroendocrinology, 37*(11), 1801–1809. https://doi.org/10.1016/j.psyneuen.2012.03.016

Hayakawa, K., Kato, T. A., Watabe, M., Teo, A. R., Horikawa, H., Kuwano, N., Shimokawa, N., Sato-Kasai, M., Kubo, H., Ohgidani, M., Sagata, N., Toda, H., Tateno, M., Shinfuku, N., Kishimoto, J., & Kanba, S. (2018). Blood biomarkers of hikikomori, a severe social withdrawal syndrome. *Scientific Reports, 8*(1), 2884. https://doi.org/10.1038/s41598-018-21260-w

Hayakawa, K., Watabe, M., Horikawa, H., Sato-Kasai, M., Shimokawa, N., Nakao, T., & Kato, T. A. (2022). Low-density lipoprotein cholesterol is a possible blood biomarker of schizoid personality traits among females. *Journal of Personalized Medicine, 12*(2). https://doi.org/10.3390/jpm12020131

Hercher, C., Parent, M., Flores, C., Canetti, L., Turecki, G., & Mechawar, N. (2009). Alcohol dependence-related increase of glial cell density in the anterior cingulate cortex of suicide completers. *Journal of Psychiatry & Neuroscience: JPN, 34*(4), 281–288. http://www.pubmedcentral.nih.gov/articlerender.fcgi?artid=2702445&tool=pmcentrez&rendertype=abstract

Kato, T. A., & Kanba, S. (2017). Modern-type depression as an "adjustment" disorder in Japan: The intersection of collectivistic society encountering an individualistic performance-based system. *The American Journal of Psychiatry, 174*(11), 1051–1053. https://doi.org/10.1176/appi.ajp.2017.17010059

Kato, T. A., & Kanba, S. (2018). Is a socio-cultural analysis of depressive disorders a matter of concern? Response to Kaiya. *The American Journal of Psychiatry, 175*(5), 483–484. https://doi.org/10.1176/appi.ajp.2018.17121404r

Kato, T. A., Shinfuku, N., Sartorius, N., & Kanba, S. (2011). Are Japan's hikikomori and depression in young people spreading abroad? *Lancet (London, England), 378*(9796), 1070. https://doi.org/10.1016/S0140-6736(11)61475-X

Kato, T. A., Tateno, M., Shinfuku, N., Fujisawa, D., Teo, A. R., Sartorius, N., Akiyama, T., Ishida, T., Choi, T. Y., Balhara, Y. P. S., Matsumoto, R., Umene-Nakano, W., Fujimura, Y., Wand, A., Chang, J. P.-C., Chang, R. Y.-F., Shadloo, B., Ahmed, H. U., Lerthattasilp, T., & Kanba, S. (2012). Does the "hikikomori" syndrome of social withdrawal exist outside Japan? A preliminary international investigation. *Social Psychiatry and Psychiatric Epidemiology, 47*(7), 1061–1075. https://doi.org/10.1007/s00127-011-0411-7

Kato, T. A., Hashimoto, R., Hayakawa, K., Kubo, H., Watabe, M., Teo, A. R., & Kanba, S. (2016). Multidimensional anatomy of "modern type depression" in Japan: A proposal for a different diagnostic approach to depression beyond the DSM-5. *Psychiatry and Clinical Neurosciences, 70*(1), 7–23. https://doi.org/10.1111/pcn.12360

Kato, T. A., Kanba, S., & Teo, A. R. (2018). Hikikomori: Experience in Japan and international relevance. *World Psychiatry: Official Journal of the World Psychiatric Association (WPA), 17*(1), 105–106. https://doi.org/10.1002/wps.20497

Kato, T. A., Kanba, S., & Teo, A. R. (2019). Hikikomori: Multidimensional understanding, assessment, and future international perspectives. *Psychiatry and Clinical Neurosciences, 73*(8), 427–440. https://doi.org/10.1111/pcn.12895

Kato, T. A., Kanba, S., & Teo, A. R. (2020a). Defining pathological social withdrawal: Proposed diagnostic criteria for hikikomori. *World Psychiatry: Official Journal of the World Psychiatric Association (WPA), 19*(1), 116–117. https://doi.org/10.1002/wps.20705

Kato, T. A., Sartorius, N., & Shinfuku, N. (2020b). Forced social isolation due to COVID-19 and consequent mental health problems: Lessons from hikikomori. *Psychiatry and Clinical Neurosciences, 74*(9), 506–507. https://doi.org/10.1111/pcn.13112

Kato, T. A., Suzuki, Y., Horie, K., Teo, A. R., & Sakamoto, S. (2022). One month version of Hikikomori Questionnaire-25 (HQ-25M): Development and initial validation. *Psychiatry and Clinical Neurosciences*. https://doi.org/10.1111/pcn.13499

Katsuki, R., Inoue, A., Indias, S., Kurahara, K., Kuwano, N., Funatsu, F., Kubo, H., Kanba, S., & Kato, T. A. (2019). Clarifying deeper psychological characteristics of hikikomori using the Rorschach comprehensive system: A pilot case-control study. *Frontiers in Psychiatry, 10*, 412. https://doi.org/10.3389/fpsyt.2019.00412

Katsuki, R., Tateno, M., Kubo, H., Kurahara, K., Hayakawa, K., Kuwano, N., Kanba, S., & Kato, T. A. (2020). Autism spectrum conditions in hikikomori: A pilot case-control study. *Psychiatry and Clinical Neurosciences, 74*(12), 652–658. https://doi.org/10.1111/pcn.13154

King-Casas, B., Sharp, C., Lomax-Bream, L., Lohrenz, T., Fonagy, P., & Montague, P. R. (2008). The rupture and repair of cooperation in borderline personality disorder. *Science (New York, N.Y.), 321*(5890), 806–810. https://doi.org/10.1126/science.1156902

Kondo, N., Sakai, M., Kuroda, Y., Kiyota, Y., Kitabata, Y., & Kurosawa, M. (2013). General condition of hikikomori (prolonged social withdrawal) in Japan: Psychiatric diagnosis and outcome in mental health welfare centres. *The International Journal of Social Psychiatry, 59*(1), 79–86. https://doi.org/10.1177/0020764011423611

Koyama, A., Miyake, Y., Kawakami, N., & Tsuchiya, M. (2010). Lifetime prevalence, psychiatric comorbidity and demographic correlates of "hikikomori" in a community population in Japan. *Psychiatry Research, 176*(1), 69–74. https://doi.org/10.1016/j.psychres.2008.10.019

Kubo, H., Urata, H., Sakai, M., Nonaka, S., Saito, K., Tateno, M., Kobara, K., Hashimoto, N., Fujisawa, D., Suzuki, Y., Otsuka, K., Kamimae, H., Muto, Y., Usami, T., Honda, Y., Kishimoto, J., Kuroki, T., Kanba, S., & Kato, T. A. (2020). Development of 5-day hikikomori intervention program for family members: A single-arm pilot trial. *Heliyon, 6*(1), e03011. https://doi.org/10.1016/j.heliyon.2019.e03011

Kubo, H., Aida, N., & Kato, T. A. (2021a). Psychodynamic group psychotherapy for hikikomori: The case of a socially withdrawn male with schizoaffective disorder. *Journal of Clinical Psychology, 77*(8), 1851–1864. https://doi.org/10.1002/jclp.23216

Kubo, H., Urata, H., Sakai, M., Nonaka, S., Kishimoto, J., Saito, K., Tateno, M., Kobara, K., Fujisawa, D., Hashimoto, N., Suzuki, Y., Honda, Y., Otsuka, K., Kanba, S., Kuroki, T., & Kato, T. A. (2021b). Development of a 3-day intervention program for family members of hikikomori sufferers. *Japanese Psychological Research*. https://doi.org/10.1111/jpr.12368

Kumazaki, H., Muramatsu, T., Yoshikawa, Y., Kato, T. A., Ishiguro, H., Kikuchi, M., & Mimura, M. (2021). Use of a tele-operated robot to increase sociability in individuals with autism spectrum disorder who display Hikikomori. *Asian Journal of Psychiatry, 57*, 102588. https://doi.org/10.1016/j.ajp.2021.102588

Kwapil, T. R., Barrantes-Vidal, N., & Silvia, P. J. (2008). The dimensional structure of the Wisconsin Schizotypy scales: Factor identification and construct validity. *Schizophrenia Bulletin, 34*(3), 444–457. https://doi.org/10.1093/schbul/sbm098

Kwapil, T. R., Brown, L. H., Silvia, P. J., Myin-Germeys, I., & Barrantes-Vidal, N. (2012). The expression of positive and negative schizotypy in daily life: An experience sampling study. *Psychological Medicine, 42*(12), 2555–2566. https://doi.org/10.1017/S0033291712000827

Kwapil, T. R., Gross, G. M., Silvia, P. J., & Barrantes-Vidal, N. (2013). Prediction of psychopathology and functional impairment by positive and negative schizotypy in the Chapmans' ten-year longitudinal study. *Journal of Abnormal Psychology, 122*(3), 807–815. https://doi.org/10.1037/a0033759

Kwapil, T. R., Clark, H. E., Rbeiz, K. S., Bathery, A. J., Kemp, K. C., & Barrantes-Vidal, N. (2022). Association of positive, negative, and disorganized schizotypy with cluster a, borderline, and avoidant personality disorders and traits. *Personality Disorders, 13*(2), 182–191. https://doi.org/10.1037/per0000488

Leigh-Hunt, N., Bagguley, D., Bash, K., Turner, V., Turnbull, S., Valtorta, N., & Caan, W. (2017). An overview of systematic reviews on the public health consequences of social isolation and loneliness. *Public Health, 152*, 157–171. https://doi.org/10.1016/j.puhe.2017.07.035

Li, T. M. H., & Wong, P. W. C. (2015). Youth social withdrawal behavior (hikikomori): A systematic review of qualitative and quantitative studies. *The Australian and New Zealand Journal of Psychiatry, 49*(7), 595–609. https://doi.org/10.1177/0004867415581179

Lorenzi, T. M., Borba, D. L., Dutra, G., & Lara, D. R. (2010). Association of serum uric acid levels with emotional and affective temperaments. *Journal of Affective Disorders, 121*(1–2), 161–164. https://doi.org/10.1016/j.jad.2009.05.023

Malagón-Amor, Á., Córcoles-Martínez, D., Martín-López, L. M., & Pérez-Solà, V. (2015). Hikikomori in Spain: A descriptive study. *The International Journal of Social Psychiatry, 61*(5), 475–483. https://doi.org/10.1177/0020764014553003

Masucci, M. D., Martin, V., Le, T. P., & Cohen, A. S. (2022). Negative schizotypy attenuates the effect of momentary stress on social dysfunction related to COVID-19 social distancing. *Schizophrenia Research, 243*, 24–31. https://doi.org/10.1016/j.schres.2022.02.028

Matthews, T., Danese, A., Caspi, A., Fisher, H. L., Goldman-Mellor, S., Kepa, A., Moffitt, T. E., Odgers, C. L., & Arseneault, L. (2019). Lonely young adults in modern Britain: Findings from an epidemiological cohort study. *Psychological Medicine, 49*(2), 268–277. https://doi.org/10.1017/S0033291718000788

Michalska da Rocha, B., Rhodes, S., Vasilopoulou, E., & Hutton, P. (2018). Loneliness in psychosis: A meta-analytical review. *Schizophrenia Bulletin, 44*(1), 114–125. https://doi.org/10.1093/schbul/sbx036

Miller, P., Byrne, M., Hodges, A., Lawrie, S. M., Owens, D. G. C., & Johnstone, E. C. (2002). Schizotypal components in people at high risk of developing schizophrenia: Early findings from the Edinburgh High-Risk Study. *The British Journal of Psychiatry: The Journal of Mental Science, 180*, 179–184. https://doi.org/10.1192/bjp.180.2.179

Ministry of Health Labour and Welfare in Japan. (2010). *Guidelines for the assessment and support of Hikikomori.*

Morahan-Martin, J., & Schumacher, P. (2003). Loneliness and social uses of the Internet. *Computers in Human Behavior, 19*(6), 659–671. https://doi.org/10.1016/S0747-5632(03)00040-2

Rodríguez Solano, J. J., & González De Chávez, M. (2000). Premorbid personality disorders in schizophrenia. *Schizophrenia Research, 44*(2), 137–144. https://doi.org/10.1016/S0920-9964(99)00203-0

Setoyama, D., Matsushima, T., Hayakawa, K., Nakao, T., Kanba, S., Kang, D., & Kato, T. A. (2021). Blood metabolic signatures of hikikomori, pathological social withdrawal. *Dialogues in Clinical Neuroscience, 23*(1), 14–28. https://doi.org/10.1080/19585969.2022.2046978

Shankar, A., Hamer, M., McMunn, A., & Steptoe, A. (2013). Social isolation and loneliness: Relationships with cognitive function during 4 years of follow-up in the English Longitudinal Study of Ageing. *Psychosomatic Medicine, 75*(2), 161–170. https://doi.org/10.1097/PSY.0b013e31827f09cd

Steiner, J., Bielau, H., Brisch, R., Danos, P., Ullrich, O., Mawrin, C., Bernstein, H.-G., & Bogerts, B. (2008). Immunological aspects in the neurobiology of suicide: Elevated microglial density in schizophrenia and depression is associated with suicide. *Journal of Psychiatric Research, 42*(2), 151–157. https://doi.org/10.1016/j.jpsychires.2006.10.013

Steptoe, A., Shankar, A., Demakakos, P., & Wardle, J. (2013). Social isolation, loneliness, and all-cause mortality in older men and women. *Proceedings of the National Academy of Sciences of the United States of America, 110*(15), 5797–5801. https://doi.org/10.1073/pnas.1219686110

Stravynski, A., & Boyer, R. (2001). Loneliness in relation to suicide ideation and parasuicide: A population-wide study. *Suicide and Life-threatening Behavior, 31*(1), 32–40. https://doi.org/10.1521/suli.31.1.32.21312

Suzuki, H., Ohgidani, M., Kuwano, N., Chrétien, F., Lorin de la Grandmaison, G., Onaya, M., Tominaga, I., Setoyama, D., Kang, D., Mimura, M., Kanba, S., & Kato, T. A. (2019). Suicide and microglia: Recent findings and future perspectives based on human studies. *Frontiers in Cellular Neuroscience, 13*, 31. https://doi.org/10.3389/fncel.2019.00031

Teo, A. R., & Kato, T. A. (2015). The prevalence and correlates of severe social withdrawal in Hong Kong. *The International Journal of Social Psychiatry, 61*(1), 102. https://doi.org/10.1177/0020764014554923

Teo, A. R., Fetters, M. D., Stufflebam, K., Tateno, M., Balhara, Y., Choi, T. Y., Kanba, S., Mathews, C. A., & Kato, T. A. (2015a). Identification of the hikikomori syndrome of social withdrawal: Psychosocial features and treatment preferences in four countries. *The International Journal of Social Psychiatry, 61*(1), 64–72. https://doi.org/10.1177/0020764014535758

Teo, A. R., Stufflebam, K., Saha, S., Fetters, M. D., Tateno, M., Kanba, S., & Kato, T. A. (2015b). Psychopathology associated with social withdrawal: Idiopathic and comorbid presentations. *Psychiatry research, 228*(1), 182–183. https://doi.org/10.1016/j.psychres.2015.04.033

Tonelli, L. H., Stiller, J., Rujescu, D., Giegling, I., Schneider, B., Maurer, K., Schnabel, A., Möller, H.-J., Chen, H. H., & Postolache, T. T. (2008). Elevated cytokine expression in the orbitofrontal cortex of victims of suicide. *Acta Psychiatrica Scandinavica, 117*(3), 198–206. https://doi.org/10.1111/j.1600-0447.2007.01128.x

Wang, J., Mann, F., Lloyd-Evans, B., Ma, R., & Johnson, S. (2018). Associations between loneliness and perceived social support and outcomes of mental health problems: a systematic review. *BMC Psychiatry, 18*(1), 156. https://doi.org/10.1186/s12888-018-1736-5

Watabe, M., Kato, T. A., Tsuboi, S., Ishikawa, K., Hashiya, K., Monji, A., Utsumi, H., & Kanba, S. (2013). Minocycline, a microglial inhibitor, reduces “honey trap” risk in human economic exchange. *Scientific Reports, 3*, 1685. https://doi.org/10.1038/srep01685

Watabe, M., Kato, T. A., Teo, A. R., Horikawa, H., Tateno, M., Hayakawa, K., Shimokawa, N., & Kanba, S. (2015). Relationship between trusting behaviors and psychometrics associated with social network and depression among young generation: a pilot study. *PLoS One, 10*(3), e0120183. https://doi.org/10.1371/journal.pone.0120183

Wong, P. W. C., Li, T. M. H., Chan, M., Law, Y. W., Chau, M., Cheng, C., Fu, K. W., Bacon-Shone, J., & Yip, P. S. F. (2015). The prevalence and correlates of severe social withdrawal (hikikomori) in Hong Kong: A cross-sectional telephone-based survey study. *The International Journal of Social Psychiatry, 61*(4), 330–342. https://doi.org/10.1177/0020764014543711

Wong, P. W. C., Liu, L. L., Li, T. M. H., Kato, T. A., & Teo, A. R. (2017). Does hikikomori (severe social withdrawal) exist among young people in urban areas of China? *Asian Journal of Psychiatry, 30*, 175–176. https://doi.org/10.1016/j.ajp.2017.10.026

Wu, A. F. W., Ooi, J., Wong, P. W. C., Catmur, C., & Lau, J. Y. F. (2019). Evidence of pathological social withdrawal in non-Asian countries: A global health problem? *The Lancet Psychiatry, 6*(3), 195–196. https://doi.org/10.1016/S2215-0366(18)30428-0

Yong, R., & Nomura, K. (2019). Hikikomori is most associated with interpersonal relationships, followed by suicide risks: A secondary analysis of a National Cross-Sectional Study. *Frontiers in Psychiatry, 10*, 247. https://doi.org/10.3389/fpsyt.2019.00247

A Disorder of Engaging in the World: Concluding Remarks and Future Directions

Simone Cheli and Paul H. Lysaker

In this book, a wide range of experts in the field have made an important step forward in promoting effective treatment for schizotypy. This collection can be considered a fertile attempt to extend the knowledge of this research construct toward the direction of clinical practice. One out of ten persons in the world are supposed to present with schizotypal traits along the wide and complex continuum of the possible manifestations. That said, there are no guidelines for treating, for example, schizotypal personality disorder (SPD) or early pathological onset of schizotypal traits. The more studies that were published about research on schizotypy, the less attention was seemingly paid to the clinical counterpart of this phenomenon. Little has been done, and much needs to be done.

On one hand, recent advances in dimensional and transdiagnostic approaches to personality disorders (PDs) and psychopathology may be considered still at an initial phase. Several pivotal papers and books have been published, but clinicians struggle to find reference books or guidelines for their daily practice. On the other hand, psychotherapy has paid limited attention to tailored treatments for schizotypal traits. Cluster A PDs are an understudied area of personality and the use of modern constructs such as psychoticism is limited in clinical work. As we anticipated in our Preface, the lessons learned from great forerunners such as Harry Stack Sullivan are almost forgotten. Even when we review treatments that rely on robust evidence, the target is always the severest extreme of schizotypy, that is schizophrenia or psychosis. Although it is not within the scope of this contribution to understand the reasons

S. Cheli
Department of Psychology, St. John's University, Rome, Italy

Center for Psychology and Health, Tages Charity, Florence, Italy
e-mail: chelis@stjohns.edu

P. H. Lysaker
Richard L Roudebush VA Medical Center, Department of Psychiatry, Indianapolis, IN, USA

Indiana University School of Medicine, Department of Psychiatry, Indianapolis, IN, USA

S. Cheli, P. H. Lysaker (eds.), *A Dimensional Approach to Schizotypy*,
https://doi.org/10.1007/978-3-031-41788-7

for this lack of evidence, we can acknowledge how prominent it is and hypothesize how the dominance of a reductionistic psychopathological paradigm oriented to symptoms (rather than general functioning), diagnostic categories (rather than dimensions), and ultimate organic causes (rather than biopsychosocial mechanisms) may have hindered a wider research program in psychotherapy for schizotypy. It is noteworthy how many grants and funds have been devoted to find a sort of *Saint Graal* of psychopathology, namely a single gene or locus responsible for schizophrenia. Recent advances confirm what we suspected in the past: there could be at least 120 genes, none of them uniquely related to schizophrenia. Indeed, Bleuler's intuition of considering a group of clinical manifestations rather than a clear-cut category is still valid. Furthermore, evolutionary psychopathology urges scholars to value the complexity of a life history approach rather than focusing on a single trait responsible for a specific disorder. Again, all attempts to identify a single trait or strategy related to either schizophrenia or schizotypy have failed at the test of experimental research. That said, several authors of this book have shown how these limitations must not be a ban on neuroscientific, genetic, or evolutionary studies. These very studies must be informed and stimulated by the intriguing complexity of schizotypy and human experience. Once they incorporate this stance, their contribution is pivotal in supporting clinical decisions about conceptualization and treatment.

We do not think that a polarized debate between a tightly reductionistic and loosely relativistic approach is useful here. A few centuries ago, the Italian philosopher Giambattista Vico (1668–1744) faced the same antithesis between a certain dogmatism of *cogito ergo sum* and Skepticism as the impossibility of an indisputable knowledge. Vico realized that the way out of this dilemma was in considering that *verum est ipsum factum*, to be true is the same as to be made. Since humans are the active constructors of their own knowledge, true and made are interchangeable terms. That is – from a more clinically oriented perspective – the therapist should be interested in how persons make sense of their own realities. The complexity we were referring to helps us understand the intertwined path between genetic, epigenetic, socio-cultural, psychological, and broadly speaking life history factors.

We can go a step further if we start from this practical mid-point between reductionism and relativism. The initial section of this book showed how the symptomatological heterogeneity of schizotypy and SPD is consistent with experimental research. First, when we talk about these constructs, we are referring to a wide spectrum that, due to the intersection between diathesis and stress, may lead to a variety of categorical diagnoses along the life history of a person. Psychometric and evolutionary evidence clearly supports the innumerable studies on neurophysiological data. Second, this latter data underlines a specific – even if multifaceted – risk for psychopathology. Having prominent schizotypal traits expose an individual to a heightened probability to manifest positive, negative, and disorganized symptoms. Third, evolutionary and cross-cultural research suggests that the link between schizotypy and potential psychosocial advantages may be reliable. Either schizotypy is a sustainable cost associated with enormous phylogenetic and ontogenetic benefits for our social brain, or (eventually and) schizotypy would be a sort of failure in socializing advantageous traits such as openness to experience. Fourth, a phenomenological stance seemingly supports an integrated look at all these elements in the form of schizotypy, resulting in a fragmented experience of the self. The higher the clinical manifestations associated with these traits, the more disrupted is the inner experience.

In order to overcome Vico's dilemma we previously described, we invited – for the second and third sections – authors who would support a recovery-oriented and person-centered approach to psychotherapy. We acknowledge the limits of our own subjective understanding of the phenomenon, possibly excluding perspectives that would have been inconsistent with this very understanding. At the same time, the paucity of publications about psychosocial treatments for schizotypal traits and a long-standing tradition (e.g., Sullivan, Fromm-Reichman) that we consider an inspiration for the present book may have reduced this bias. Thus, we hypothesized five main transdiagnostic mechanisms that are supported by both broader studies on conceptualization and emerging evidence on the clinical utility of treatments based on these mechanisms. We also reputed how constructs such as attachment, interpersonal situation, mentalizing, metacognition, and self-criticism are related to one another. The more the proposed treatments have an integrated approach the more they seem to work in terms of promoting recovery. Indeed, all these mechanisms are rooted in the complexity of the social brain and human experience that has been debated in the first section. The idea at the core is that subjective and intersubjective experiences are two sides of the same coin and that the suffering that may emerge from schizotypy is related to a sort of disorder of engaging in the world. Due to early and continuous relational experiences, the person's vulnerability is structured in maladaptive self-to-self and self-to-other patterns, finally manifesting a rigid and inflexible way of making sense of the world. A vicious cycle emerges where subtle schizotypal traits activate defensive responses in the forms of odd and bizarre behaviors and emotional and social withdrawal. The more these defensive strategies are used, the more a self-fulfilling prophecy of social rejection, threats, inner confusion, and disorganization is manifested.

The numerous interventions presented in the third section explicitly target this disorder of engaging in the world. They do that starting from different perspectives. The majority of the proposed treatments were originally designed as transdiagnostic forms of psychotherapy (cognitive behavioral therapy, compassion-focused therapy, mentalization-based treatment, psychoanalysis), in a few cases as therapy for specific disorders or clusters of disorders (clinical staging psychiatry, integrative treatment for hikikomori, metacognitive and interpersonal therapy, metacognitive reflection and insight therapy), and in one case to specifically target schizotypal traits (evolutionary systems therapy for schizotypy). Despite the diverse techniques and models of conceptualization, the reader can easily recognize a common attempt to share with the patient a pervasive resistance in engaging in the world, both on a subjective and intersubjective level. All the authors show how challenging, fascinating, and enriching it can be for the therapist working in this field. More importantly, they prove how even the severe manifestations of schizotypy are treatable and the experiences of patients are understandable. The inevitable impasses, difficulties, and ruptures in therapeutic work can be clearly understood by considering the role of the mechanisms we referred to (attachment, interpersonal situation, mentalizing, metacognition, and self-criticism). The challenge for the therapist is not to be distracted by the stigma of severe mental disorders but to go beyond the defensive strategies of the patient as a request for help or sense of relational safety. Once the clinician discerns the patient's oddity or detachment as their ultimate attempt to hold together a fragmented world, the therapy really starts.

We are convinced that the contributions of the authors of this book will foster a better understanding of schizotypy. At the same time, the need for evidence on which to support clinical practice is urgent and manifest. In the last twenty years, only two randomized controlled trials (RCTs) were focused on psychosocial interventions for SPD and a few single cases or cases series were published. Moreover, schizotypal traits (or psychoticism, etc.) are barely quoted when summarizing evidence for either psychotherapy or psychiatry, and we can only rely on a few robust studies on mechanisms such as attachment or mentalizing. Therefore, we identify at least three main lines of future research. First, we need evidence to confirm the pivotal and possibly intertwined role of the five mechanisms we discussed, that is attachment, interpersonal situation, mentalizing, metacognition, and self-criticism. We urge researchers to explore how they interact with one another both in large nonclinical samples (since we consider schizotypy a spectrum we need to better know how healthy traits manifest diverse forms of psychopathology) and in more fine-grained in-vivo analyses of therapeutic work (we need to better know when and how to work on which mechanism). Second, the different treatments presented in the third section have to be tested through large RCTs. We need to better know if and how effective they are individually, and if one of them may be more effective in a specific clinical stage or with specific patterns of symptoms or features. Moreover, we may consider the possibility of integrated or modular treatment plans where two or more of the proposed therapies interact with one another.

Considering that one out of ten persons in the general population may report schizotypal traits and one out of twenty may manifest SPD or psychotic experiences, these two lines of research are pivotal for public healthcare systems and may be associated with a third line of necessary research. Indeed, we suggest better exploring the viability of the schizotypy label to foster a wider research program in the field and raise public awareness. Schizotypy is a construct that arose during the fifties and is linked with an era of psychopathology that seems very different with respect to the present one. Despite studies on this spectrum that anticipated the present debate on dimensional approaches, we are not sure how schizotypy/schizotypal wording may be useful for the future research we are proposing here. An etymological and historical similarity might perpetuate the misleading overlap between the wider spectrum (i.e., schizotypy) and its severer psychopathological extreme (i.e., schizophrenia). All the actors involved might implicitly be influenced by that. Patients may be overwhelmed by the stigma associated with the diagnosis of schizophrenia and psychosis with the well-known side effects on well-being and adherence to treatment. The clinicians may similarly consider schizotypal traits far from their possibilities. Researchers and public authorities may forget that schizotypy is a wide spectrum ranging from healthy or subclinical states to severe manifestations.

We do not have the evidence to address these doubts. Thus, research in this area is needed. In our clinical experience, patients ask for a working balance between knowing what they are struggling with and feeling the viability of change and recovery. In the area of autism, for example, a large survey suggests that people prefer a direct self-definition (autistic persons), whereas in the area of personality disorders, a few scholars are suggesting to discuss PDs as interpersonal disorders.

As a concluding remark, these future research challenges should be based on the same premises we started from: Schizotypy is seemingly a disorder of engaging in the world, and persons struggling with this multifaceted organization of personality may fail in socializing their healthy traits and lively power. Thus, the therapist's stance and intervention should be aimed at restoring a missing sense of social safeness that would allow, in turn, new and more adaptive strategies in relating to oneself and others. We may turn toward Harry Stack Sullivan's advice to remind us how much the therapist may influence the patient's experience of their world, primarily by maintaining the very maladaptive patterns that were the reasons why the therapy started. This is not a karmic wheel we cannot escape from, rather it is the condition we necessarily start from to help the client. We are responsible for restoring the idea of human relationships as safe and supporting rather than the difficulty – or even impossibility – of the proposed treatment.

Afterword

Simone Cheli

Paul H. Lysaker passed away just a few days after the submission of the book. It was shocking and unexpected news. We were planning new ideas and projects to work together on. And while I am writing these sentences, I can't believe there won't be more of our Tuesday calls. Paul was a brilliant thinker and the mentor we all wish for. He was never "in the place" where you would expect him. He was cooperative with students and young colleagues, assertive when necessary, and always open to the unexpected and divergent. As a researcher, he had an enviable ability to combine clarity with creativity. His personal and scientific contribution to people struggling with severe mental disorders has been fundamental and the echo of all this will reverberate over the years.

This book would never have existed without his support. The idea came from our conversations about patients we worked with and readings of authors we loved. I owe Paul for being here today to write about schizotypy. From my early experiences when he was my supervisor to collaboration on research together, I wouldn't be where I am without his kind, amused, and inspiring guidance.

S. Cheli, P. H. Lysaker (eds.), *A Dimensional Approach to Schizotypy*,
https://doi.org/10.1007/978-3-031-41788-7

Index

S. Cheli, P. H. Lysaker (eds.), *A Dimensional Approach to Schizotypy*,
https://doi.org/10.1007/978-3-031-41788-7

MIX
Papier aus verantwortungsvollen Quellen
Paper from responsible sources
FSC® C105338

If you have any concerns about our products,
you can contact us on
ProductSafety@springernature.com

In case Publisher is established outside the EU,
the EU authorized representative is:
Springer Nature Customer Service Center GmbH
Europaplatz 3, 69115 Heidelberg, Germany

Printed by Libri Plureos GmbH
in Hamburg, Germany